A Research Agenda for DSM-V

Contents

Contributors

Renato D. Alarcón, M.D., M.P.H.
Professor and Vice-Chairman, Department of Psychiatry and Behavioral Sciences, Emory University School of Medicine; Chief, Mental Health Service Line, Atlanta Department of Veterans Affairs Medical Center, Atlanta, Georgia

Margarita Alegria, Ph.D.
Professor of Health Services Administration; Director of the Center for Evaluation and Sociomedical Research, University of Puerto Rico, San Juan, Puerto Rico

George S. Alexopoulos, M.D.
Professor, Department of Psychiatry, The New York Hospital, Cornell Medical Center, Westchester Division, White Plains, New York

Gavin Andrews, M.D.
Professor, School of Psychiatry, University of New South Wales at St. Vincent's Hospital, Anxiety Disorders Unit, Darlinghurst, New South Wales, Australia

David H. Barlow, Ph.D.
Professor, Center for Adaptive Systems, Department of Psychology, Boston University, Boston, Massachusetts

Carl C. Bell, M.D.
President/CEO, Community Mental Health Council/Foundation, Inc.; Professor of Psychiatry, Department of Psychiatry, School of Medicine, and Professor of Public Health, School of Public Health, University of Illinois at Chicago, Chicago, Illinois

Kelly Botteron, M.D.
Assistant Professor, Department of Psychiatry, Washington University School of Medicine, St. Louis, Missouri

Dennis S. Charney, M.D.
Chief, Mood and Anxiety Disorders Research Program, National Institute of Mental Health, Bethesda, Maryland

Jonathan D. Cohen, M.D.
Professor, Department of Psychology; Director, Center for Study of Brain, Mind and Behavior, Princeton University, Princeton, New Jersey; Professor, Department of Psychiatry, University of Pittsburgh, Pittsburgh, Pennsylvania

Edwin H. Cook Jr., M.D.
Professor of Psychiatry and Pediatrics, Department of Child and Adolescent Psychiatry, University of Chicago, Chicago, Illinois

E. Jane Costello, Ph.D.
Professor, Department of Psychiatry and Behavioral Sciences, Duke University Medical Center, Durham, North Carolina

Bruce Cuthbert, Ph.D.
Chief, Adult Psychopathology and Prevention Research Branch, Division of Mental Disorders, Behavioral Research and AIDS, National Institute of Mental Health, Bethesda, Maryland

Ronald E. Dahl, M.D.
Associate Professor of Psychiatry and Pediatrics, Western Psychiatric Institute and Clinic, Pittsburgh, Pennsylvania

Michael B. First, M.D.
Research Psychiatrist, New York State Psychiatric Institute; Associate Professor of Clinical Psychiatry, Columbia University College of Physicians and Surgeons, New York, New York

David Goldman, M.D.
Chief, Laboratory of Neurogenetics, National Institute on Alcohol Abuse and Alcoholism, Bethesda, Maryland

Howard Goldman, M.D., Ph.D.
Professor, Department of Psychiatry, University of Maryland, Baltimore, Maryland

Raquel E. Gur, M.D., Ph.D.
Professor, Director of Neuropsychiatry, Departments of Psychiatry, Neurology, and Radiology, University of Pennsylvania, Philadelphia, Pennsylvania

James S. Jackson, Ph.D.
Daniel Katz Distinguished University Professor of Psychology, College of Literature, Science, and the Arts; Professor of Health Behavior and Health Education, School of Public Health; and Director and Research Scientist, Research Center for Group Dynamics, Institute for Social Research, University of Michigan, Ann Arbor, Michigan

Dilip Jeste, M.D.
Professor, University of California San Diego, Department of Veterans' Affairs San Diego Healthcare System, San Diego, California

Robert E. Kendell, M.D.
Professor, University Department of Psychiatry, Royal Edinburgh Hospital, Edinburgh, Scotland

Kenneth Kendler, M.D.
Professor, Department of Psychiatry and Human Genetics, Medical College of Virginia, Virginia Commonwealth University and Virginia Institute for Psychiatric and Behavioral Genetics, Richmond, Virginia

Laurence J. Kirmayer, M.D.
Professor, Department of Psychiatry, and Director, Division of Social and Transcultural Psychiatry, McGill University, Montreal, Quebec, Canada

Doreen Koretz, Ph.D.
Associate Director for Prevention, Division of Mental Disorders, Behavioral Research and AIDS, National Institute of Mental Health, Bethesda, Maryland

John H. Krystal, M.D.
Albert E. Kent Professor and Deputy Chairman for Research, Department of Psychiatry, Yale University School of Medicine, New Haven, and Psychiatry Service, Veterans' Administration Connecticut Health System, West Haven, Connecticut

David J. Kupfer, M.D.
Thomas Detre Professor and Chair, Department of Psychiatry, Western Psychiatric Institute and Clinic, University of Pittsburgh, Pittsburgh, Pennsylvania

Anthony F. Lehman, M.D., M.S.P.H.
Professor and Chair, Department of Psychiatry, University of Maryland School of Medicine, Baltimore, Maryland

Keh-Ming Lin, M.D., M.P.H.
Professor, Department of Psychiatry, School of Medicine, University of California at Los Angeles; Director, Research Center on the Psychobiology of Ethnicity, Harbor–University of California Los Angeles Medical Center, Torrance, California

Juan F. López, M.D.
Assistant Professor, Department of Psychiatry, University of Michigan; Assistant Research Scientist, Mental Health Research Institute, Ann Arbor, Michigan

Robert Malison, M.D.
Associate Professor of Psychiatry and Associate Director, Clinical Neuroscience Research Unit, Connecticut Mental Health Center, Yale University School of Medicine, New Haven, Connecticut

James H. Meador-Woodruff, M.D.
Associate Professor, Department of Psychiatry, University of Michigan; Senior Associate Research Scientist, Mental Health Research Institute, Ann Arbor, Michigan

Kathleen R. Merikangas, Ph.D.
Chief, Section on Developmental Genetic Epidemiology, Mood and Anxiety Disorders Program, National Institute of Mental Health, Bethesda, Maryland

Steven O. Moldin, Ph.D.
Chief, Genetics Research Branch, Division of Neuroscience and Basic Behavioral Science, National Institute of Mental Health, Bethesda, Maryland

Eric J. Nestler, M.D., Ph.D.
Professor and Chairman, Department of Psychiatry, University of Texas Southwestern Medical Center, Dallas, Texas

David R. Offord, M.D.
Coordinator of Research Programs, Center for Studies of Children at Risk, McMaster University, Hamilton, Ontario, Canada

Daniel S. Pine, M.D.
Chief, Section on Development and Affective Neuroscience, National Institute of Mental Health, Bethesda, Maryland

Darrel A. Regier, M.D., M.P.H.
Executive Director, American Psychiatric Institute for Research and Education, and Director, Division of Research, American Psychiatric Association, Washington, DC

Allan L. Reiss, M.D.
Professor and Associate Chair, Department of Psychiatry and Behavioral Science, Stanford University School of Medicine, Stanford, California

David Reiss, M.D.
Vivian Gill Distinguished Research Professor of Psychiatry, Psychology, and Medicine, George Washington University Medical Center, Washington, DC

Bruce J. Rounsaville, M.D.
Professor, Yale University School of Medicine; Director, Mental Illness Research Education and Clinical Center, Department of Veterans Affairs Connecticut Healthcare, West Haven, Connecticut

M. Tracie Shea, Ph.D.
Associate Professor, Department of Psychiatry and Human Behavior, Brown University, Providence, Rhode Island

Bedirhan Üstün, M.D.
Coordinator, Classification, Assessment, Surveys and Terminology, EIP/GPE, World Health Organization, Geneva, Switzerland

Benedetto Vitiello, M.D.
Chief, Child and Adolescent Treatment and Preventive Intervention Research Branch, Division of Services and Intervention Research, National Institute of Mental Health, Bethesda, Maryland

Stanley J. Watson, M.D., Ph.D.
Professor of Psychiatry, University of Michigan; Co-Director and Senior Research Scientist, Mental Health Research Institute, Ann Arbor, Michigan

Tom Widiger, Ph.D.
Professor, Department of Psychology, University of Kentucky, Lexington, Kentucky

Katherine L. Wisner, M.D., M.S.
Gottfried and Gisella Kolb Professor of Outpatient Psychiatry and Behavioral Sciences, Obstetrics and Gynecology, and Pediatrics, and Director, Women's Health Care, Department of Psychiatry, University of Louisville School of Medicine, Louisville, Kentucky

Steven J. Zalcman, M.D.
Chief, Clinical Neuroscience Research Branch, Division of Neuroscience and Basic Behavioral Science, National Institute of Mental Health, Bethesda, Maryland

Acknowledgments

We would like to acknowledge the scientific and administrative contributions to this book made by the following staff of the American Psychiatric Association: Natalie Ivanovs, Tina Marshall, Ph.D., William Narrow, M.D., M.P.H., and Sarah Tracy.

Introduction

This volume, made up of six "white papers" in six chapters, completes the initial phase of a DSM-V planning process, which began in 1999. It is important to underscore that this work should not be construed as the initial stages of the DSM-V revision process. As far as we participants in the white-paper process are concerned, the beginning of the DSM-V revision process is still several years in the future. These chapters are an attempt to stimulate research and discussion in the field in preparation for the eventual start of the DSM-V revision process. The chapters were produced under a partnership between the American Psychiatric Association (APA) and the National Institute of Mental Health (NIMH), with the goal of providing direction and potential incentives for research that could improve the scientific basis of future classifications. Given the relatively short time frame for generating breakthrough research findings between now and the probable publication of DSM-V in 2010, it is anticipated that some of the research agendas suggested in these chapters might not bear fruit until the DSM-VI or even DSM-VII revision processes! Nonetheless, we feel that we cannot ignore this opportunity to identify and stimulate broad research fields that could fundamentally alter the limited classification paradigm now in use. Those of us who have worked for several decades to improve the reliability of our diagnostic criteria are now searching for new approaches to an understanding of etiological and pathophysiological mechanisms—an understanding that can improve the validity of our diagnoses and the consequent power of our preventive and treatment interventions.

Background

There were two primary reasons for supporting designated work groups responsible for the development of these chapters: 1) to stimulate research that would enrich the empirical database before the start of the DSM-V revision process and 2) to devise a research and analytic agenda that would facilitate the integration of findings from research and experience in animal studies, genetics, neuroscience, epidemiology, clinical research, and cross-cultural clinical services—all of which would lead to the eventual development of an etiologically based, scientifically sound classification system.

Need to Reconsider the Relationship Between the DSM Process and the Research Database

Since DSM-III (American Psychiatric Association 1980), disorders have been defined in terms of syndromes—that is, clusters of symptoms that covary together (see the section following, titled "Need to Explore the Possibility of Fundamental Changes . . ."). The most significant innovation adopted in DSM-IV (American Psychiatric Association 1994) was a revision process that 1) incorporated a comprehensive review of the available empirical research findings and 2) made new analyses of existing epidemiological and clinical research data sets to generate proposed diagnostic criteria sets. In addition, NIMH provided limited funding for a field-study grant to compare the reliability and utility of alternative criteria sets for diagnoses in clinical settings Although changes from DSM-II (American Psychiatric Association 1968) to DSM-III were based on more than a decade of clinical research using the Feighner (Feighner et al. 1972) and Research Diagnostic Criteria (RDC) (Spitzer et al. 1978), no systematic literature review or focused analysis was undertaken in the actual revision process. Instead, decisions on inclusion and exclusion criteria were made by individuals who were considered experts in their fields, a process that potentially allowed data to be either overlooked or, if they were at odds with the expert's perspective, willfully ignored. The major focus of field trials for DSM-III was establishing the reliability with which multiple clinicians could come to the same diagnostic conclusions when presented with a patient's expressed signs and symptoms. In this manner, it was possible to demonstrate that an atheoretical, descriptive approach could result in a reproducible diagnosis in multiple clinical and cultural settings.

Following the publication of DSM-III in 1980, data began to emerge by 1983 from some new studies that were not consistent with the syndromal definitions in DSM-III. Likewise, challenges were being made to hierarchical diagnostic conventions that precluded a diagnosis of some disorders when a more severe disorder was simultaneously present (e.g., a patient with symptoms meeting criteria for both schizophrenia and panic disorder would get only the diagnosis of schizophrenia) (Boyd et al. 1984). Overall, the major goal of DSM-III-R (American Psychiatric Association 1987) was to improve the consistency, clarity, and conceptual accuracy of DSM-III criteria but to avoid changes lacking substantial research evidence. No major data analyses or field trials to establish the reliability or validity of these changes were conducted. DSM-IV continued with the descriptive approach but added a meta-analytic, data-based approach to the revision process, described in the paragraphs following.

The DSM-IV revision process was formalized in a three-stage empirical review (Widiger et al. 1991). The first stage consisted of a systematic, comprehensive review of the published (and in some cases unpublished) literature, guided by literature searches using rules specified during a DSM-IV methods conference. Although many gaps were identified in the existing literature, only limited options were available to the work groups for filling in these gaps. One such mechanism was a data reanalysis project funded by the MacArthur Foundation, in which existing data sets collected for other studies were combined and reanalyzed, using meta-analytic methods, to try to answer certain diagnostic questions. These data reanalyses were useful in answering some diagnostic questions (e.g., determining the minimum number of panic attacks required in order to justify a diagnosis of panic disorder [Brown et al. 1998]); however, many of the reanalyses were seriously hampered by incompatibilities in the data sets and by the fact that the data needed for answering many diagnostic questions had not been collected. The only empirical data collected specifically for the DSM-IV revision process were those from the 15 NIMH-funded focused field trials. Because of the limited resources available and the short time available for conducting these trials, the goals of the trials were fairly modest. In most cases, goals were limited to comparing different criteria sets in terms of reliability and user acceptability. In cases in which some form of validity was measured, the gold standard used was conformity with a simultaneously assigned clinical diagnosis, as opposed to use of any of the more rigorous Robins-Guze validity criteria (Robins and Guze 1970).

One of the main reasons that the DSM-IV process was almost completely dependent on already collected data was the extremely short deadline imposed on the DSM-IV process. Because of the need to coordinate the development of DSM-IV with the parallel development of the *International Statistical Classification of Diseases and Related Health Problems*, 10th Revision (ICD-10) by the World Health Organization (World Health Organization 1992), work began on DSM-IV within a year of the publication of DSM-III-R in 1987. Publication of DSM-IV was also scheduled for 1994 in anticipation of worldwide adoption of ICD-10 in the mid-1990s. (Ironically, ICD-10 has still not been officially adopted in the United States, owing to many administrative matters related to financial and computer reprogramming concerns.) Although it became evident in 1993 that ICD-10 implementation was going to be delayed, the APA decided to proceed with the 1994 publication of DSM-IV so as not to compromise the currency of the literature review.

As mentioned previously, publication of DSM-V is expected about 2010 (or perhaps later), thus providing the opportunity to stimulate potentially informative research before the DSM-V revision process begins. Accordingly, the chapters in this volume provide a wide range of suggestions about fruitful areas to be further investigated well in advance of DSM-V.

Need to Explore the Possibility of Fundamental Changes in the Neo-Kraepelinian Diagnostic Paradigm

The DSM-III diagnostic system adopted a so-called neo-Kraepelinian approach to diagnosis. This approach avoided organizing a diagnostic system around hypothetical but unproven theories about etiology in favor of a descriptive approach, in which disorders were characterized in terms of symptoms that could be elicited by patient report, direct observation, and measurement. The major advantage of adopting a descriptive classification was its improved reliability over prior classification systems using nonoperationalized definitions of disorders based on unproved etiological assumptions. From the outset, however, it was recognized that the primary strength of a descriptive approach was its ability to improve communication among clinicians and researchers, not its established validity.

Disorders in DSM-III were identified in terms of syndromes, symptoms that are observed in clinical populations to covary together in individuals. It was presumed that, as in general medicine, the phenomenon of symptom covariation could be explained by a common underlying etiology. As described by Robins and Guze (1970), the validity of these identified syndromes could be incrementally improved through increasingly precise clinical description, laboratory studies, delimitation of disorders, follow-up studies of outcome, and family studies. Once fully validated, these syndromes would form the basis for the identification of standard, etiologically homogeneous groups that would respond to specific treatments uniformly.

In the more than 30 years since the introduction of the Feighner criteria by Robins and Guze, which eventually led to DSM-III, the goal of validating these syndromes and discovering common etiologies has remained elusive. Despite many proposed candidates, not one laboratory marker has been found to be specific in identifying any of the DSM-defined syndromes. Epidemiologic and clinical studies have shown extremely high rates of comorbidities among the disorders, undermining the hypothesis that the syndromes represent distinct etiologies. Furthermore, epidemiologic studies have shown a high degree of short-term diagnostic instability for many disorders. With regard to treatment, lack of treatment specificity is the rule rather than the exception.

The efficacy of many psychotropic medications cuts across the DSM-defined categories. For example, the selective serotonin reuptake inhibitors (SSRIs) have been demonstrated to be efficacious in a wide variety of disorders, described in many different sections of DSM, including major depressive disorder, panic disorder, obsessive-compulsive disorder, dysthymic disorder, bulimia nervosa, social anxiety disorder, posttraumatic stress disorder, generalized anxiety disorder, hypochondriasis, body dysmorphic disorder, and borderline personality disorder. Results of twin studies have also contradicted the DSM assumption that separate syndromes have a different underlying genetic basis. For example, twin studies have shown that generalized anxiety disorder and major depressive disorder may share genetic risk factors (Kendler 1996).

Concerns have also been raised that researchers' slavish adoption of DSM-IV definitions may have hindered research in the etiology of mental disorders. Few question the value of having a well-described, well-operationalized, and universally accepted diagnostic system to facilitate diagnostic comparisons across studies and to improve diagnostic reliability. However, reification of DSM-IV entities, to the point that they are considered to be equivalent to diseases, is more likely to obscure than to elucidate research findings.

All these limitations in the current diagnostic paradigm suggest that research exclusively focused on refining the DSM-defined syndromes may never be successful in uncovering their underlying etiologies. For that to happen, an as yet unknown paradigm shift may need to occur. Therefore, another important goal of this volume is to transcend the limitations of the current DSM paradigm and to encourage a research agenda that goes beyond our current ways of thinking to attempt to integrate information from a wide variety of sources and technologies.

Process of Developing This Volume

The DSM-V research planning process started with a brief discussion between Steven Hyman, M.D. (Director of NIMH), Steven M. Mirin, M.D. (Medical Director of APA), and David J. Kupfer, M.D. (Chair of the APA Committee on Psychiatric Diagnosis and Assessment), at NIMH in summer 1999. They felt that it was important for APA and NIMH to work together and focus on an agenda that would expand the scientific basis for psychiatric classification.

In September 1999, the initial DSM-V Research Planning Conference was held under the joint sponsorship of APA and NIMH. From the outset, it was established that this was not meant to be the first step of the DSM-V revision process per se but rather to set research priorities that might affect future classifications. Participants in this initial stage were selected primarily for their expertise in diverse areas such as family and twin studies, molecular genetics, basic and clinical neuroscience, cognitive and behavioral science, development, life span issues, and disability. To encourage thinking that went beyond the current DSM-IV framework, participant selection was made primarily among those who had not been closely involved in the DSM-IV development process. The participants were given the chance to consider new and emerging data, to identify knowledge gaps, and to suggest how data might be generated to fill those gaps. Participants were cautioned against thinking too narrowly with regard to how new information from emerging fields such as neuroscience and genetics might be used in a classification system.

A number of topics were identified as being particularly important and in need of further research. These included examining how disorders are manifested differently in child, adult, and geriatric age groups; identifying risk factors for disorders to facilitate prevention; and attempting to reconcile the Axis I–Axis II distinction with the concept of spectrum disorders. Broader considerations included the benefits of explicitly indicating that the disorders included in DSM have varying levels of empirical support for their reliability and validity. Given the addition of clear clinical significance criteria in DSM-IV, questions arose about how severity, distress, and disability should be accounted for in the classification—either as a part of the criteria set for threshold determinations, or as an orthogonal and separate construct. Finally, questions arose about the potential role for information gleaned from family studies, molecular genetics, neuroscience, cognitive fields, and behavioral science in constructing the diagnostic nomenclature. At the conclusion of the meeting, it was decided that this group of participants would develop a series of white papers that could promote further discussion of these topics and guide future research.

The task of developing the chapters was delegated to DSM-V Planning Work Groups assigned to cover the following five topic areas: Developmental Issues, Gaps in the Current System, Disability and Impairment, Neuroscience, and Nomenclature. The first step was to appoint chairs for each of the work groups: Daniel S. Pine, M.D., for the Developmental Work Group; Michael B. First, M.D., for the Gaps Work Group; Anthony Lehman, M.D., for the Disability and Impairment Work Group; Dennis S. Charney, M.D., for the Neuroscience Work Group; and Bruce J. Rounsaville, M.D., for the Nomenclature Work Group.

A second DSM-V Research Planning Conference was held on July 25, 2000, involving only the chairs of the work groups. The purpose was to discuss the membership of the work groups, consider the process that would guide the groups as they developed the chapters, develop a timeline, and discuss how the issues raised in the white papers might be integrated into a research agenda. Each work group was composed of 4–10 people with different areas of expertise. Some work group members included those who participated in the September 1999 meeting; others were invited because of their expertise in different fields. In the interests of developing a common international classification in the future, a number of members of the international research community were invited to participate. Liaisons from NIMH, the National Institute on Drug Abuse (NIDA), and the National Institute on Alcohol Abuse and Alcoholism (NIAAA) were assigned to each work group to facilitate the integration of the white papers into the research programs or requests for applications (RFAs) in these institutes. It was suggested that some of these white papers might lead to joint workshops sponsored by the three institutes.

A third DSM-V Research Planning Conference, held October 5–6, 2000, brought together all the work group members to allow each work group to begin its work on the white papers, to present initial outlines to the entire set of participants, and to elicit input reflecting perspectives from individuals outside the work groups. During the ensuing discussions, it was emphasized that the goals of improving future editions of DSM and defining a research agenda must be uncoupled and that all work groups must consider their objectives from both a short-term and a long-term perspective (i.e., must take into consideration that a proposed research agenda might not have any effect on classification until DSM-VI or later).

In addition to the five work groups mentioned previously, a cross-cultural work group was also formed, chaired by Renato D. Alarcón, M.D. Each of the other five work groups had at least one cross-cultural work group member assigned to it to provide expertise on how cross-cultural issues might pertain to the topic covered by the work group. Concurrently with their work in the original work group, the cross-cultural work group members also convened as a separate entity to review cross-cultural issues in psychopathology in a more comprehensive fashion and to produce a chapter integrating those issues across the whole range of research areas.

Subsequent to this meeting, the work groups met regularly through conference calls. All the work groups followed a similar model: developing an outline, assigning sections to individual members, integrating the individual sections into a single draft, and then circulating the draft to the full work group for additional input. Work groups were also encouraged to solicit comments from consultants outside the work groups. Finally, drafts of the white papers were circulated to outside reviewers for their comments and suggestions.

Future Steps

Following completion of this volume, it is anticipated that a series of diagnostic conferences will be convened to encourage more focused research investigations from the entire range of research areas covered in the chapters. For example, a conference focused on mood disorders, scheduled to take place at the World Congress of Psychiatry in August 2002, will present pertinent findings from preclinical animal models, genetics, pathophysiology, functional imaging, clinical treatment, epidemiology, prevention, the relationship with other cardiovascular medical conditions, and the global burden of disability associated with the spectrum of depressive disorders. By presenting different perspectives such as these on specific disorders, our plan is to maximize the potential for cross-fertilization of multiple research disciplines, which will stimulate new and creative approaches to integrating their findings. A more precise algorithm for weighing the contributions from these multiple research areas for the development of new diagnostic criteria is now only a future goal, well beyond our grasp.

By engaging an international group of research investigators in each of the proposed future diagnostic conferences, we hope to stimulate a cooperative research effort that can be supported by multiple national sources of research funding. Likewise, by paying greater attention to the potential contribution of diverse research disciplines to clinical disease and disorder entities, and by developing alternative research criteria for some disorders that are not constrained by the requirements of the neo-Kraepelinian categorical approach currently adopted in DSM-IV, we hope to accelerate the development of a research base that will be maximally informative for future revisions of the DSM and ICD classification systems for mental disorders.

The authors and editors hope that our readers will find this volume reflective of the great potential for improving the basic understanding of mental and addictive disorders in human populations, as well as for using this knowledge to improve the effectiveness of preventive and treatment interventions for our patients, our families, and our communities.

David J. Kupfer, M.D.
Michael B. First, M.D.
Darrel E. Regier, M.D., M.P.H.

References

American Psychiatric Association: Diagnostic and Statistical Manual of Mental Disorders, 2nd Edition. Washington, DC, American Psychiatric Association, 1968

American Psychiatric Association: Diagnostic and Statistical Manual of Mental Disorders, 3rd Edition. Washington, DC, American Psychiatric Association, 1980

American Psychiatric Association: Diagnostic and Statistical Manual of Mental Disorders, 3rd Edition, Revised. Washington, DC, American Psychiatric Association, 1987

American Psychiatric Association: Diagnostic and Statistical Manual of Mental Disorders, 4th Edition. Washington, DC, American Psychiatric Association, 1994

Boyd JH, Burke JD Jr, Gruenberg E, et al: Exclusion criteria of DSM-III: a study of co-occurrence of hierarchy-free syndromes. Arch Gen Psychiatry 41:983–989, 1984

Brown TA, Marten PA, Barlow DH: Empirical evaluation of the panic symptom ratings in DSM-III-R panic disorder, in DSM-IV Sourcebook, Vol 4. Edited by Widiger TA, Frances AJ, Pincus HA, et al. Washington, DC, American Psychiatric Association, 1998, pp 209–215

Feighner JF, Robins E, Guze SB, et al: Diagnostic criteria for use in psychiatric research. Arch Gen Psychiatry 26:57–63, 1972

Kendler KS: Major depression and generalised anxiety disorder: same genes, (partly) different environments—revisited. Br J Psychiatry 168(suppl 30):68–75, 1996

Robins E, Guze SB: Establishment of diagnostic validity in psychiatric illness: its application to schizophrenia. Am J Psychiatry 126:983–987, 1970

Spitzer RL, Endicott J, Robins E: Research diagnostic criteria: rationale and reliability. Arch Gen Psychiatry 35:773–782, 1978

Widiger TA, Frances AJ, Pincus HA, et al: Toward an empirical classification for the DSM-IV. Abnorm Psychol 100(3):280–288, 1991

World Health Organization: International Statistical Classification of Diseases and Related Health Problems, 10th Revision. Geneva, World Health Organization, 1992

CHAPTER 1

Basic Nomenclature Issues for DSM-V

Bruce J. Rounsaville, M.D., Renato D. Alarcón, M.D., M.P.H., Gavin Andrews, M.D., James S. Jackson, Ph.D., Robert E. Kendell, M.D., Kenneth Kendler, M.D.

Introduction

The criteria and format used in DSM-III, DSM-III-R, DSM-IV, and DSM-IV-TR (American Psychiatric Association 1980, 1987, 1994, 2000a) arose from psychiatric diagnostic traditions of North America and were crafted to be readily used by practicing psychiatrists. However, the effect of the DSMs has extended far beyond the boundaries of psychiatric practice in North America in a number of ways that have revealed limitations in the current system.

First, the American criteria are used in research and practice throughout the world, highlighting incompatibilities with the alternative diagnostic system of the *International Statistical Classification of Diseases and Related Health Problems,* 10th Revision (ICD-10) (World Health Organization 1992) and difficulties in applying DSM criteria across cultures.

Second, primary care medical practitioners have increasingly taken on the identification and initial treatment of patients with mental disorders. This laudable development promises to bring treatment to many patients whose conditions have been undiagnosed and untreated. However, the need to operationalize the diagnostic process in nonpsychiatric settings has posed important challenges to practitioners.

Third, criteria listed in the DSMs have been uncritically used by legal professionals and health care administrators as representing lapidary, received wisdom about the nature of mental disorders. This high-impact but uncritical use fails to recognize the variability in the level of empirical support for the reliability and validity of different diagnoses. If the text or criteria included a more explicit rating of empirical support for the different diagnoses, users unfamiliar with the field might be less likely to assume that criteria for all listed disorders are equally well established. Another factor underlying potential misinterpretation of DSM is the degree to which many, if not most, conditions and symptoms represent a somewhat arbitrarily defined pathological excess of normal behaviors and cognitive processes. This problem has led to criticisms that the system pathologizes ordinary experiences of the human condition, such as normal bereavement or the rebelliousness of adolescents. If the diagnostic system included criteria or decision rules that explicitly acknowledged the continuum nature of symptoms and disorders, this would place the pathological nature of more extreme symptomatic behavior into context. In particular, it may be helpful to find ways to denote a distinction between mild or borderline cases and clear-cut or severe cases.

Given this broad impact and the increasing importance of DSM criteria, these limitations in the system take on added significance. The purpose of this chapter is to address a series of basic topics for consideration in the DSM-V revision process and to outline a research agenda for issues that lend themselves to empirical testing. Topics include 1) defining *mental disorder*, 2) considerations in validating diagnostic criteria and categories, 3) establishing rationales for changing existing categories or criteria, 4) determining whether a dimensional approach should be substituted for the current categorical approach to diagnosis, 5) increasing compatibility between DSM-V and ICD-11, 6) addressing the applicability of criteria across different cultures, and 7) facilitating the diagnostic process in nonpsychiatric settings.

How to Define *Mental Disorder*

Medicine has never had agreed-on definitions of its most fundamental terms, disease and illness, and most physicians have always been content to assume that their meanings were self-evident. Significantly, the World Health Organization (WHO) has always avoided defining *disease*, *illness*, or *disorder* in the successive revisions of the *International Classification of Diseases, Injuries and Causes of Death* (now called the *International Statistical Classification of Diseases and Related Health Problems*). The current (ICD-10) *Classification of Mental and Behavioral Disorders* simply states that "the term *disorder* is used throughout the classification, so as to avoid even greater problems inherent in the use of terms such as *disease* and *illness. Disorder* is not an exact term, but it is used here to imply the existence of a clinically recognizable set of symptoms or behavior associated in most cases with distress and with interference with personal functions" (World Health Organization 1992, p. 5).

Like its predecessors DSM-III and DSM-III-R, the current edition of the *Diagnostic and Statistical Manual of Mental Disorders*, DSM-IV-TR, does provide a detailed definition of the term *mental disorder.* Although this definition is rather lengthy (146 words) and contains numerous subclauses and qualifications, it is not cast in a way that allows it to be used as a criterion for deciding what is and is not a mental disorder, and it has never been used for that purpose. The definition does include a clear statement that "neither deviant behavior nor conflicts that are primarily between the individual and society are mental disorders unless the deviance or conflict is a symptom of a dysfunction in the individual," but the definition fails to define or explain the crucial term *dysfunction*, except to say that it may be "behavioral, psychological, or biological" (p. xxxi).

Despite the difficulties involved, it is desirable that DSM-V should, if at all possible, include a definition of *mental disorder* that can be used as a criterion for assessing potential candidates for inclusion in the classification, and deletions from it. If for no other reason, this is important because of rising public concern about what is sometimes seen as the progressive medicalization of all problem behaviors and relationships. Even if it proves impossible to formulate a definition of mental disorder that provides an unambiguous criterion for judging all individual candidates, there should at least be no ambiguity about the reason that individual candidate diagnoses are included or excluded. The task force that produced DSM-IV assumed, or asserted, that there is no fundamental difference between so-called mental illnesses or disorders and physical illnesses or disorders, and that the distinction between them is simply a relic of Cartesian dualism (American Psychiatric Association 1994). Others have taken the same view (Kendell 2001). If this view is retained, the fundamental issue is the meanings of the terms *illness* and *disorder* in general.

Definitions of *Illness* and *Disorder*

The most contentious issue is whether *disease*, *illness*, and *disorder* are scientific biomedical terms or are sociopolitical terms that necessarily involve a value judgment. Usually, although not invariably, physicians have maintained that they are biomedical terms, whereas most philosophers and social scientists have argued that they are sociopolitical terms. The issue has attracted a good deal of attention in the past decade, mainly in response to a closely argued analysis of the concept of mental disorder by Wakefield (1992).

There are at least four fundamentally different types of definition reflecting differing assumptions about the nature of disease or disorder. These are described below.

Sociopolitical. Although it has been suggested in the past that disease is simply what doctors treat, there are no current advocates for such a simplistic view. The simplest plausible sociopolitical definition is that a condition is regarded as a disease if it is agreed to be undesirable (an explicit value judgment) and if it seems on balance that physicians (or health professionals in general) and their technologies are more likely to be able to deal with it effectively than are any of the potential alternatives, such as the criminal justice system (treating it as crime), the church (treating it as a sin), or social work (treating it as a social problem).

The attraction of this approach is that it is essentially pragmatic or utilitarian. Whether the antisocial behavior of habitual delinquents, for example, is best regarded as criminal behavior or as a manifestation of antisocial personality disorder would be determined by the relative success of the criminal justice system versus psychiatry and clinical psychology in reducing the antisocial behavior; and whether restless, overactive children with short attention spans are regarded as having attention-deficit/hyperactivity disorder or simply as being difficult children would depend on whether child psychiatrists were better at ameliorating the problem than parents and teachers. A further implication is that a given condition might be a mental disorder in one setting but not in another, depending on the relative efficacy of medical and other approaches to the problem in those different settings.

Although sociopolitical definitions of this kind have rarely been advocated by physicians, treatability is often a crucial consideration underlying their decisions to regard individual phenomena as diseases. For example, despite the advocacy of Thomas Trotter and Benjamin Rush at the beginning of the nineteenth century and a sustained campaign by Alcoholics Anonymous in the 1930s, the medical profession firmly resisted the proposal that alcoholism should be regarded as a disease until disulfiram (Antabuse) was introduced in the late 1940s. For a few years, this drug was widely hailed as a dramatically effective treatment for the condition, and it was in this climate that the American Medical Association and similar bodies throughout the world issued formal statements to the effect that alcoholism was a disease after all.

In fact, the most defensible justification of the steady increase in the number of officially recognized mental disorders that has occurred over the last 50 years is the development of an increasing range of at least partly effective therapies.

Biomedical. The most widely quoted purely biomedical criterion of disease is the "biological disadvantage" originally proposed by Scadding (1967). Scadding, a chest physician, defined a disease as "the sum of the abnormal phenomena displayed by a group of living organisms in association with a specified common characteristic or set of characteristics by which they differ from the norm for the species in such a way as to place them at a biological disadvantage" (p. 877). He never elaborated on what he meant by *biological disadvantage*, but Kendell (1975a) and Boorse (1975) both argued that it must at least encompass reduced fertility and life expectancy.

Although many mental disorders are associated with a reduced life expectancy and some, like schizophrenia, are associated with a conspicuously reduced fertility as well, Scadding's biological disadvantage criterion has perverse consequences when applied to the domain of mental disorder. Many milder conditions such as phobias as well as disorders with onset after the prime reproductive years would fail to qualify as disorders, whereas other conditions that are not regarded as mental disorders, such as homosexuality, would fall under Scadding's definition of *disorder.*

Combined biomedical and sociopolitical. Wakefield (1992, 1999) argues that mental disorders are biological dysfunctions that are also harmful, implying that the concept of mental disorder necessarily involves both a scientific or biomedical criterion (dysfunction) and an explicit value judgment or sociopolitical criterion (what he calls *harm* and the WHO refers to as *handicap*). This view is attractive because it meets the main requirement of both the sociopolitical and the biomedical camps, and also because it seems to reflect the often intuitive ways in which physicians make disease attributions and does not have any obviously unacceptable implications.

Wakefield originally proposed that *dysfunction* should imply the failure of a biological mechanism to perform a natural function for which it had been designed by evolution, but Lilienfeld and Marino (1995) and Kirmayer and Young (1999) subsequently pointed out that this evolutionary perspective raises many problems. Too little is known about the evolution of most of the higher cerebral functions whose malfunctioning probably underlies many mental disorders. Mood states such as anxiety and depression may have evolved as biologically adaptive responses to danger or loss rather than being failures of evolutionarily designed functions; and several important cognitive abilities, like reading, have been acquired too recently to be plausibly regarded as natural functions designed by evolution. It is, of course, perfectly possible in principle to define *dysfunction* without reference either to evolution or to biological disadvantage. The problem is that too little is known about the cerebral mechanisms underlying basic psychological functions, such as perception, abstract reasoning, and memory, for it to be possible in most cases to do more than infer the probable presence of a biological dysfunction. Furthermore, rejecting both the evolutionary (Wakefield 1992, 1999) and biological disadvantage (Scadding 1967) criteria may open the way to regarding a wide range of purely social disabilities (such as aggressive, uncooperative behavior or an inability to resist lighting fires or stealing) as mental disorders.

Ostensive. Lilienfeld and Marino (1995) contend that it is impossible even in principle to provide a "semantic" or "operational" definition of the global concept of mental illness or disorder, only of individual illnesses or disorders. The only criterion available, they suggest, is whether putative or candidate disorders are sufficiently similar to the prototypes of mental disorder, and both the term *similar* and the choice of prototypes (schizophrenia and major depressive disorder, perhaps) are obviously open to a range of interpretations.

There is a plausible argument that the fundamental reason why medicine has never succeeded in providing a satisfactory definition of disease is that it has always been primarily concerned with the identification and treatment of individual diseases, and these are very heterogeneous because they have been identified at various stages over the last 400 years with defining characteristics of quite varied kinds. Some, like migraine and torticollis, are still defined by their clinical syndromes; others, such as mitral stenosis, by their morbid anatomy; tumors of all kinds by their histopathology; most infections by the identity of the causative organism; porphyria by its biochemistry; Down syndrome by its chromosomal architecture; the thalassemias by abnormal molecular structures; and so on. Whether or not this is a convincing argument, it does not account for psychiatry's difficulty in defining mental disorders, because most mental disorders are still defined by their clinical syndromes.

Research Implications of Alternative Approaches to the Definition of *Mental Disorder*

Although the choice among the foregoing four disorder concepts will not be resolved on the basis of empirical data, research could clarify the implications of that choice and could also provide a broader, empirically derived perspective about how clinicians conceptualize *disorder*.

Research Agenda

- Analyze the concepts of mental disorder underlying disorders currently listed in DSM-IV, evaluating the degree to which they conform to similar or different general conceptualizations of disorder enumerated above. This process could eliminate constructs that fail to apply to a preponderance of currently recognized disorders.

- Conduct surveys, within the United States and internationally, to elucidate the concepts of disease or of mental illness or disorder used, explicitly or implicitly, by psychiatrists, other physicians, clinical psychologists, research workers, patients, health care providers, and members of different social and ethnic groups. This could be done either by exploring the meaning they attribute to such terms or by asking them to decide which of a list of contentious conditions they themselves regarded as diseases or mental disorders, an approach taken by Campbell and colleagues (1979) in an influential Canadian survey.
- Conduct studies (involving the same populations listed above) designed to elucidate views and assumptions about the relationship between people with recognized mental disorders and others who have the same symptoms intermittently or in milder form (i.e., the boundary between illness and normality).

Validity

Validity is a complex construct that has been extensively explored in the psychometric literature. The purpose here is not to attempt to review this large body of literature (which examines many subtypes of validity) but rather to focus on the uses of validity in psychiatric nosology. The logical starting point for any such discussion is the often-cited Robins and Guze paper of 1970. In this paper the authors proposed five phases for establishing diagnostic validity in psychiatric illness: clinical description, laboratory studies, delimitation from other disorders, follow-up study, and family study. The weight of the validation process fell, according to their system, on the final two steps, in which the goal was to demonstrate diagnostic homogeneity over time and familial aggregation of the putative syndrome. Kendler (1990) later expanded on this list of potential validators, differentiating between antecedent validators (e.g., family studies, premorbid personality, demographic factors, and precipitating factors), concurrent validators (e.g., psychological or biological test data), and predictive validators (e.g., diagnostic consistency, overall functioning over time, and response to treatment).

As we approach DSM-V, what might be said on the basis of more than 20 years of experience with such validating systems for psychiatric illness? First, they are not specific. Many things that are not valid psychiatric diagnoses (such as large noses) run in families. Second, there is no strong a priori rationale to suspect that the application of different diagnostic validators to a given nosologic problem would produce the same answer. For example, the evidence is now relatively compelling that if one wants to define schizophrenia as a disorder with high diagnostic stability and poor outcome, then choosing a narrow criteria set that requires prior chronicity (e.g., 6 months of illness) is very effective (Kendler et al. 1989). By contrast, if the validating criterion to be applied is familial aggregation, then the diagnosis would be *much* broader and would include a range of other psychotic disorders as well as schizophrenia-spectrum personality disorders (Baron et al. 1985; Kendler et al. 1994, 1995). This lack of congruence of results expected from various validators poses a profound problem for the nosologic process. It means that a hierarchy of validators must first be chosen for a given nosologic question. Unfortunately, this choice is fundamentally a value judgment and cannot be directly addressed by empirical inquiries (Kendler 1990). For the example above, the question boils down to "What is the core feature of schizophrenia—that it has a poor outcome or that it runs in families?" This is not a scientific question. At the second stage, once the critical validators are agreed on, only then can the process of formulating maximally valid criteria sets occur.

A third potential dilemma with the process of validation for psychiatric disorders is that it is based on a falsely optimistic assumption: that psychiatric disorders are discrete biomedical entities with clear phenotypic boundaries. Is it possible that—partially in reaction to the antidiagnostic approaches of psychoanalysis—the Washington University School (and later DSM-III and future additions) overreacted and grasped too firmly for the mantle of legitimacy provided by the diagnostic concepts of infectious disease and tumor pathology? It may be that medical syndromes such as hypertension, osteoarthritis, and tension headache are better models for psychiatric disorders than are pneumococcal pneumonia or stage IV glioblastoma. If psychiatric disorders are actually broad biobehavioral syndromes—fuzzy sets that inevitably blur into one another and into normality—what implications does this have for the validation process?

Fourth, is it possible to develop a coherent hierarchy of validators that would cut across all diagnostic categories in psychiatry? In medicine, the most definitive diagnoses are almost always etiologically based. Many of the most common validators used in psychiatry might be termed "practical," such as outcome or response to treatment. Should we argue that the value of a validator should be judged by the degree to which it reflects etiologic processes? Following this line of reasoning, we might conclude that family and genetic validators are of greater value than prognosis or course of illness, which would result in a rather radical redesign of the concept of schizophrenia. Alternatively, should it be argued that—although etiologically based diagnosis is the ultimate goal of psychiatric nosology—this is currently impractical and the time-honored practical validators—course, outcome, response to treatment, etc.—should continue to be used until the level of knowledge about the pathophysiology of psychiatric disorders improves far beyond its current state?

Although research cannot directly address the problem of the best hierarchy of validators, it can provide information about the nature of the problem. For example, it would be valuable to construct, from available data, the alternative criteria sets for several major diagnoses (e.g., schizophrenia, major depressive disorder) that would be developed on the basis of different critical validators (e.g., prognosis, response to treatment, or familial aggregation). This exercise would, at a minimum, give us a sense of the magnitude of the problem and might point toward possible solutions in that some of the criteria sets so developed might have obviously higher face validity than others.

System for Rating of Diagnoses

One of the most valid criticisms of DSM-III, DSM-III-R, and DSM-IV is that a naive reader would have no easy way of knowing that the knowledge base from which the different criteria were developed and validated differ markedly across diagnoses. It is potentially misleading for the manuals to imply that the criteria for major depressive disorder and histrionic personality disorder are of equal validity.

In part, the DSMs have already recognized this problem by the creation of an appendix that contains criteria sets provided for further study. But the existence of this appendix does not address the tremendous heterogeneity of information available on the many categories within the main part of the manual.

Should DSM-V contain a rating of the quality and quantity of information available to support the different diagnostic systems? The advantage of such an approach is straightforward—it would inform the reader about the highly variable state of knowledge with regard to various psychiatric disorders. One possibility would be that the highest of these ratings would be reserved for the small number of psychiatric disorders with a relatively clearly delineated pathophysiology (e.g., Alzheimer's disease).

Four questions that raise potential disadvantages are worth considering. First, what criteria would be used to rate the individual diagnostic categories? Would it be possible to be quite objective (e.g., the number of peer-reviewed publications with a given sample size), or would the complexity of the available information inevitably reduce the rating to a complex and only moderately reliable gestalt judgment? Second, what exactly would be rated? In particular, how much should the rating reflect what is generally known about the disorder versus what is known about the specific criteria? Third, what would be the effects on individuals with low-rated disorders and on the reimbursement for these disorders? Would patients become distraught? Would the insurance companies refuse to pay? Fourth, would the ratings become self-perpetuating in that it would be difficult to obtain funding to study disorders with low ratings, thereby maintaining the paucity of research?

Rationale for Changing Criteria

Traditionally, when changes in criteria in a diagnostic system are contemplated, the positive features of such changes (e.g., improvements in reliability or validity, greater ease of use, or superior discriminatory ability) are emphasized. To obtain a balanced view of the benefits and risks of changes of criteria requires a review of the disadvantages of changing criteria, of which seven deserve particular attention. First, any alterations in diagnostic criteria require that such changes be learned by thousands of clinicians. Inevitably, changes induce a certain amount of confusion (were those DSM-III-R criteria or DSM-IV?) in the mind of any busy clinician. Interestingly, small changes may be more difficult to commit to memory than large changes. Second, many health-related documents, including medical record forms and treatment algorithms, rely on DSM criteria. Changes in the criteria sometimes require changes in these forms. Third, changes in diagnostic criteria impair the cumulative capacity of research. A critical goal of psychiatric research is to develop a rigorous database examining the etiology, course, and treatment of the major psychiatric disorders. In the move toward evidence-based medicine, meta-analyses are more and more the standard form of data summary. Homogeneity of diagnostic classification would be an important criterion for any meta-analysis. Fourth, changes in diagnostic criteria pose special problems for longitudinal research projects—often the source of our best information about the causes and consequences of psychiatric illness. The longitudinal researcher is faced with the uncomfortable choice of either keeping to the older diagnostic system and risk being considered (by readers and review committees) as old-fashioned and behind the times, or changing to new criteria and thereby creating discontinuity in the nature of the data collected. Fifth, any change in diagnostic criteria necessitates the development of a new generation of structured psychiatric interviews to evaluate the new criteria. Sixth, inevitably questions will arise about differences between the new and old criteria. Do they define the same patient population? Do they differ in their ability to predict outcome or familial aggregation? Often, a small "cottage industry" of research is spawned to answer these questions. It is possible that our limited research resources could be better spent elsewhere. Finally, and probably most difficult to quantify, is the possibility that frequent changes in diagnostic criteria can potentially discredit the revision process and increase the chances of the DSMs becoming a subject of ridicule.

Given an appreciation of the important potential benefits and significant potential disadvantages of changes in diagnostic criteria, how are these two to be balanced? What justification should be established for the changing of diagnostic criteria? The obvious answer would be "when the advantages outweigh the disadvantages." But how can this be evaluated? How much improvement in reliability or simplification of criteria are worth the disadvantages of making changes?

Although it is impossible to suggest any compelling guidelines for this difficult issue, two general points can be made. First, small changes have nearly as many disadvantages as large changes but are less likely to have strong benefits. Second, despite protestations to the contrary, any committee-based review process for a diagnostic system may be biased toward making changes. For many on these committees, the common human urge to make a contribution or to do it better may be irresistible. For others, possible future career success may be affected by their ability to make changes in "their" diagnosis or to have "their" category formally recognized in DSM-V. Ultimately, these understandable human impulses, if not restrained, can have a highly negative cumulative impact on the nosologic system that we all use. Although the DSM-IV revision process had built-in safeguards to reduce the likelihood of such problems (e.g., a requirement that committee decisions be reached by consensus, reviews by large numbers of outside consultants, and veto power over committees by the DSM-IV task force), the potential remained for nonscientific biases to affect the nosologic system.

Dimensions Instead of Categories?

DSM-IV and ICD-10 are both categorical classifications or typologies, and so were all their predecessors. In principle, though, variation in the symptomatology of mental disorder could be represented by a set of dimensions rather than by multiple categories. Indeed, Wittenborn et al. (1953) developed a multidimensional representation of the phenomena of psychotic illness nearly 50 years ago, and since then others have developed dimensional models to portray the symptomatology of depressive and anxiety disorders, schizophrenia, and even the entire range of psychopathology.

In other branches of medicine, however, classifications of disease have invariably been typologies. This is partly because it is a fundamental characteristic of human mentation, embodied in the nouns of everyday speech, to recognize categories of objects (horses, chairs, planets, etc.), and partly because it has traditionally been assumed that most diseases were discrete entities. In the past most psychiatrists assumed that mental disorders were also discrete entities, separated from one another, and from normality, either by recognizably distinct combinations of symptoms or by demonstrably distinct etiologies; indeed, this has been shown to be so for a small number of conditions (Down syndrome, fragile X syndrome, phenylketonuria, Alzheimer's and Huntington's diseases, and Creutzfeldt-Jakob disease, for example). In the past 20 years, however, the disease entity assumption has been increasingly questioned as evidence has accumulated that prototypical mental disorders such as major depressive disorder, anxiety disorders, schizophrenia, and bipolar disorder seem to merge imperceptibly both into one another and into normality (Kendler and Gardner 1998) with no demonstrable natural boundaries or zones of rarity in between. Furthermore, both the genetic and environmental factors underlying these syndromes are often nonspecific (Brown et al. 1996; Kendler 1996).

As a result, well-informed clinicians and researchers have suggested that variation in psychiatric symptomatology may be better represented by dimensions than by a set of categories, especially in the area of personality traits (Widiger and Clark 2000) (see Chapter 4 in this volume for a more detailed discussion of a dimensional approach to personality). Indeed, Cloninger (1999) stated firmly that "there is no empirical evidence" for "natural boundaries between major syndromes" and that "the categorical approach is fundamentally flawed" (pp. 174–175). It is also worth noting that the philosopher Hempel observed 40 years ago that most sciences start with a categorical classification of their subject matter but often replace this with dimensions as more accurate measurement becomes possible (Hempel 1961).

Against this background it is important that consideration be given to advantages and disadvantages of basing part or all of DSM-V on dimensions rather than categories. There would be some obvious attractions in doing so (Kendell 1975b). The problems posed by patients who fulfill the criteria for two or more categories of disorder simultaneously, or who straddle the boundary between two adjacent categories, would disappear, as would the procrustean need to distort the symptoms of individual patients to fit a preconceived stereotype. More useful information would be conveyed, and a new realism might be introduced into clinicians' assumptions about the nature of mental disorders. The disadvantages are equally obvious. Clinicians are accustomed to thinking in terms of diagnostic categories, and most existing knowledge about the causes, presentation, treatment, and prognosis of mental disorder was obtained, and is organized, in relation to these categories. Prompt and appropriate decisions about the management of individual patients are also much easier if the patient can be confidently allocated to a category rather than to a locus in a multidimensional space. It is probably significant that most of the advocates of dimensional representation are not practicing clinicians but are primarily theoreticians.

Partly for these reasons, and also because no up-to-date, widely accepted dimensional representation exists at present in any field of psychopathology, it is probably premature to contemplate a largely dimensional DSM-V. At the same time, there is a clear need for dimensional models to be developed and for their utility to be compared with that of existing typologies in one or more limited fields, such as personality (see Chapter 4 in this volume). If a dimensional system of personality performs well and is acceptable to clinicians, it might then be appropriate to explore dimensional approaches in other domains (e.g., psychotic or mood disorders).

Reducing the Gaps Between DSM-V and ICD-11

The reconciliation process during the development of DSM-IV and ICD-10 made the systems more compatible and created crosswalks between the systems. However, many small and large differences persist at both syndrome and criterion levels. These persistent discrepancies suggest the need for a program of research to compare and reconcile the minor differences and, in the case of major differences, to explore the validity of the alternative constructs.

When DSM-III was published in 1980, one of its most important advantages was a radical improvement in the reliability of psychiatric diagnosis by virtue of its provision of operational criteria for each diagnosis. It was subsequently revised in 1987 as DSM-III-R and then again in 1994 as DSM-IV, the latter revision in particular being informed by a comprehensive review of the available research. ICD-10 followed a similar format, but the text was placed in one book of clinical descriptions, published in 1992, and the diagnostic criteria appeared in another book, published in 1993. To many people the classifications seemed parallel, and the American Psychiatric Association published an international edition that contained the ICD-10 numbering system applied to the DSM-IV descriptions and criteria. The classifications are not identical, however, and their parallel existence causes unnecessary confusion in international research and in the recording of health statistics.

The advent of precise diagnostic criteria in both systems meant that fully structured diagnostic interviews could be developed. The WHO Composite International Diagnostic Interview (CIDI; World Health Organization 1993), guided by an editorial committee balanced between DSM and ICD, was able to operationalize, for the common mental disorders, each and every diagnostic criterion set in both DSM-IV and ICD-10 to produce CIDI v. 2.1. This is available in computerized form and was used in the Australian national mental health survey. It is to be used in a forthcoming 10-country survey convened by Kessler and Üstün.

Data from the pilot for the Australian survey was used for an initial comparison between ICD-10 and DSM-IV. The results (Andrews et al. 1999) indicated numerous significant differences between the two systems. The sample was enriched by a two-stage sampling procedure, and 37% of respondents had symptoms that met criteria for one or more ICD-10 12-month diagnoses; 32% met criteria for the corresponding DSM-IV diagnoses. In general, DSM-IV disorders were diagnosed at lower rates (Andrews et al. 2001). Across the affective, anxiety, and substance-use diagnoses examined, only 68% of people whose symptoms met criteria on either classification met criteria on both, whereas 32% were discordant (i.e., meeting criteria only in one system). Agreement occurred in less than 75% of cases in social phobia, agoraphobia without panic disorder, panic disorder with and without agoraphobia, obsessive-compulsive disorder, posttraumatic stress disorder, and substance abuse or harmful use. Calculations of the burden of disease show substantial cross-system differences in years lived with disability with sedative dependence, alcohol harmful use, obsessive-compulsive disorder, and dysthymia, all of which were discordant by more than 40%. Thus, disagreements in the classifications do make differences. The reasons for the disagreement were explored in a series of papers and, with the exception of substance abuse/harmful use criteria (which describe quite different concepts), the intention of the other definitions seemed very similar. In a number of cases, clerical errors in the transfer of the ICD clinical descriptions into the diagnostic criteria accounted for the dissonance. For many diagnoses, however, what seem to be trivial differences in wording of the diagnostic criteria or threshold numbers of symptoms accounted for the dissonance. A program of research is needed to determine whether the DSM or ICD definition is closer to the research evidence.

In a review of the inclusion and exclusion criteria for the anxiety disorders in ICD-10 and DSM-IV, Andrews (2000) discovered that the inclusion criteria differ in what appears to be needless ways. The problem with the exclusion criteria is more fundamental: there is no agreement between the classifications, as though the exclusion criteria were written haphazardly. There is a real need for a review of the principles that should be used for the exclusion criteria before the actual criteria for each diagnosis are formulated.

All countries in the world are obliged to report health statistics in accordance with the ICD-10 classification. However, for reasons outlined above, the DSM system is becoming, exactly as First and Pincus (1999) suggested, the de facto world standard, certainly for research and therefore increasingly so for clinical discourse. This widens the discrepancy between research findings and administratively important health statistics and estimates of burden of disease. Given the importance of minimizing (if not eliminating) future differences between the two systems, the next revision process could include steps to achieve this goal. For example, with international input into each DSM-V committee, it might be possible to agree to delete nonessential differences and create a single definition for most disorders, with alternate classifications for the occasional disorders on which conceptual agreement could not be reached. If these conflicting descriptions were distinct enough, decisive research could be conducted internationally in the period before publication, so that dissonance could be minimal by the time of publication. Dissonance that is unresolved might well be an example of cultural factors influencing views of sickness.

Research Agenda

- Replicate the present ICD-DSM dissonance estimates and identify minor differences that could be simply reconciled.
- Identify procedural errors in either classification and recommend corrections.
- Define principles to govern the exclusion strategies and apply them.
- When differences are substantial, define a research strategy to assess the comparative validity and reliability of ICD and DSM disorders and criteria. Existing data sets on epidemiological or clinical samples characterized by both ICD and DSM criteria offer an immediate opportunity for research on the comparative reliability and validity of alternative definitions. In particular, more information is needed on the comparative validity of alternatively defined disorders, particularly pertaining to clinical course, including response to treatment.

We acknowledge the apparent contradiction between our dictum against unnecessary change and the potentially sweeping changes in DSM-V that would be required to develop a single international system reconciling the future DSM and ICD classifications. In the current planned timetable for revising the two systems, ICD-11 will not be developed until some time after the publication of DSM-V. Unless reconciliation is to come about by the WHO's wholesale adoption of DSM-V, numerous small and large changes in current DSM-IV criteria will need to be made to formulate a single system that is acceptable to both organizations. As noted above, even seemingly trivial changes in criterion wording or exclusion criteria can have a large impact in research settings and may be difficult to apply in practice because small changes are difficult to learn and remember. Given the very large number of changes required to reconcile the systems, it is unlikely that more than a handful of choices between DSM and ICD criteria can be informed by strong empirical evidence for superior reliability or validity of either system. Ultimately, the decision to create a single unified, worldwide system for diagnosing mental disorders must arise from a judgment by the leadership of the American Psychiatric Association and the WHO that the benefits derived from a single system outweigh the disadvantages of many changes required to create this system.

Cross-Cultural Use of DSM-V

Applying DSM criteria across cultures, even those within the same society, country, continent, or world region, poses a significant challenge to clinicians and researchers alike. This section addresses cultural issues related to nomenclature and the utility of diagnostic systems and procedures across cultures (a more comprehensive overview of cultural issues in diagnosis is presented in Chapter 6, in this volume). Although nomenclature per se may be acceptable, the cultural perspective would pay more specific attention to the meaning of statements reflecting diagnostic or clinical criteria in different parts of the world. The premise is that populations, groups, and communities living in different regions have different norms regarding instrumental functioning (work roles), different spiritual and religious beliefs and practices, different cultural habits and perceptions of mental health and mental illness, and different precepts regarding professional treatment (Kleinman 1980). The interpretation of diagnostic criteria is an idiosyncratic process related to the unique perceptions of the culture where they are to be applied. This, undoubtedly, is another aspect of the tension between the localistic and universalistic perspectives on the applicability of diagnosis (Kleinman 1988). Behaviors are judged differently, and different opportunities and treatment resources are available because of such perceptions. Professionals devoted to the care of patients with mental illness, emotional problems, or behavioral difficulties may use different therapeutic approaches ranging from herbs, natural folk rituals, counseling, or psychotherapy to the use of psychotropic medications or psychoactive substances.

To foster cross-cultural applicability of DSM constructs, norms, and guidelines, research aimed at determining the presence of symptoms, the delineation of syndromes, and ultimately the diagnostic criteria (along categorical or dimensional lines) will have to be adopted following two general directions: 1) clear delineation of core diagnostic criteria, desirably applicable to all societies, cultures, and countries throughout the world, and 2) recognition of cultural and cross-cultural variants in symptom definition and behavioral and symptomatic manifestations.

These two seemingly contradictory approaches may not necessarily exclude each other, because it is accepted that culture plays a pathogenic rather than an etiologic role in the causation of mental disorders, that is, being a contributing factor and not a primary, basic one in the process of becoming mentally ill. The cultural perspective accepts the notion that environmental factors act on or activate genetic or neurobiological predispositions. Culture is, in fact, the conceptual scaffolding of environmental circumstances in any human being's life (Hinton 1999).

Research Agenda

Research on cultural issues related to the nomenclature of psychiatric entities and psychiatric diagnostic areas will also follow the two directions noted above. In this context, a number of areas can be identified to further the acceptability of DSM outside the United States:

Cultural Variants in Symptom Definition and Symptom Manifestations

- Comparative research can be done on current major diagnostic categories aimed at confirming or dispelling the notion of categorical fallacies (assignment of Western-based nomenclatures or diagnostic criteria to clinical conditions observed in different cultures) in the diagnostic process, particularly among ethnic minorities within the United States (Kleinman 1988; Lewis-Fernandez and Kleinman 1995).These studies require comparisons of U.S. diagnostic practices with other developed and developing countries. A categorical fallacy, identified as such in any culture or society, thus becomes a hypothesis to be tested. One of the results of this type of research may be the indirect confirmation of core diagnostic criteria to be useful and usable across different cultures. In fact, there are some findings in the literature that confirm the eventual applicability of agreed-on Western-based diagnostic criteria in different countries; they include the International Pilot Study of Schizophrenia (IPSS) (World Health Organization 1973) and different studies on DSM-based diagnostic criteria (Sartorius et al. 1980), confirmed also by efforts at making DSM-IV and ICD-10 generally comparable. The biggest objection to this approach is that the epidemiologic methodology and instruments used for these comparisons resort to an overly simplified lowest common denominator in the spelling out of diagnostic criteria. According to the critics, this eliminates the possibility of introducing unique cultural variables in the different countries or societies where the instrument is to be used (Rogler 1999). Translation and meaning-assignment issues are extremely important, as are specification of context and the clinician's cultural background.

- Complementary roles should be assigned to the relative contributions of genotype and environment (the latter including psychological and sociocultural factors) to psychiatric conditions (Abroms 1981). Perhaps, as Littlewood (1990) and more so Leff (1990) propose, we should attempt to explain (or understand) each psychiatric condition vis-à-vis a theoretical spectrum ranging from the biological to the sociocultural, and adding an estimation of the cultural distance between examiners and populations being studied, or between patient groups being compared. The magnitude of the cultural component's impact on each diagnostic category could be estimated following the parameters of DSM-IV's cultural formulation (Mezzich and Goode 1994). At the same time, the culturally determined vulnerability to stressors, and the treatability by social, sociocultural, or psychosociocultural means could be assessed. The assignment of a cultural profile to each given condition would subsequently take into account conventional social and cultural criteria, a general assessment of the DSM operational criteria for each category, and the overall experience of the clinician. Some of the clinical features thus included may reflect characteristics of the cultural group from which the patient comes, and so it would be incumbent on the clinician to sort them out (Leff's [1990] assessment of the "cultural distance") and assign to them a diagnostic, as well as a therapeutic value. An analysis of the "symptoms" from the perspectives provided by different ethnic and cultural groups, using instruments such as Weiss's Explanatory Model Interview Catalogue (EMIC) scale (Weiss et al. 1992) might prove helpful to the clinician in differentiating true clinical conditions from nonpathological, culturally determined behavior.
- The two bulleted sections immediately preceding can form the basis of studies on the cultural implications and relevance of key diagnostic criteria as presented in current nomenclatures, particularly in relation to

the assessment of severity from a cultural perspective. This parameter has demonstrated variability across cultures, and its study requires the elaboration of new instruments or the improvement of existing instruments. Clear distinctions between etic measures (evaluations or observations made by outsiders—e.g., by clinicians or researchers) and emic measures (evaluations from inside—i.e., by the subjects or members of the cultural groups themselves) can reduce assessor bias and enhance fairness in descriptions of culturally different persons. Prejudices induced by ignorance and buttressed by fear of the unknown minority persons may result in an unrealistic appraisal of their aspirations and motivations; therefore it is important to apply moderator variables in the assessment of minority persons, a point also argued by Neligh (1988) in relation to the Native American population and by Escobar et al. (1987) regarding Hispanic patients. In assessing instrument deficiencies, the cultural fairness of individual items must be considered. Choca et al. (1990) ascertained that the expert's assessments against which inventories are validated or evaluated could also contain biases: this introduces a logical circularity that only adds to the complexity of bias investigation. These researchers advocate the use of factor analysis in bias studies. This line of research is promising in that it would ensure specific validation of clinical diagnoses and may eventually provide more clear criteria for the initial assessment.

Anthropological Approaches

The applicability and usefulness of anthropological research approaches have been underestimated in traditional clinical research in recent decades. This stance may change throughout, particularly in the diagnostic arena, due to the increasing prominence of cultural issues in clinical, therapeutic, regulatory, and policy-making circles.

- Research can be done on idioms of distress (e.g., extreme somatization) as possible symptomatic expressions of mental disorders in different cultures (Good 1994).The purpose of research in this area would be to delineate their special nature, meaning, and relevance to the culture in question, but also their potential value as diagnostic criteria in specific populations and regions of the world.
- Studies can be made of explanatory models of mental illness, which vary from culture to culture. Their study from both an anthropologico-cultural and a clinical perspective would help determine universally valid or culturally singular elements articulated within the etiopathogenesis of mental disorders (Alarcón 1995; Gaw 1993). Furthermore, the valid and

artifactual elements of these models would eventually serve as further diagnostic criteria or unique characteristics surrounding the core symptomatology of any psychiatric entity. For instance, the adscription of causality regarding catatonia to recent losses due to a natural disaster, or the report of hearing the voice of a recently deceased loved one calling the affected person's name may well point toward exploration of posttraumatic issues rather than the hasty assignment of a psychotic label and concurrent treatment decisions. The same applies to studies on the meaning of mental health and mental illness constructs across gender, ethnicity, and, particularly, religious and spiritual perspectives (Lukoff et al. 1995), where issues such as guilt, shame, identity, and social support affect diagnosis and treatment in significant ways: God's wrath used in different cultures (including Western groups) to explain clinical occurrences may open the way to otherwise hidden material relevant to the validity of any diagnosis.

- Research can be done on culture-specific syndromes—for example, *ataque de nervios* or *amok*—in different regions of the United States and in different parts of the world. The purpose of such research would be not only to assess the validity of these conditions but also to make advances in comparing them with existing clinical entities and to assess their eventual fitness (or lack of it) as components of any regular nomenclature (Littlewood 1990; Mezzich and Goode 1994). Research proposals in this area must address areas from linguistic issues (such as synonymy and grammar) to clinical context (such as level of emotionality and impact on individuals and groups). Repeated clinical assessments and interviews focusing on explanatory approaches will be useful. Models of this approach are offered by Guarnaccia and Rogler's (1999) study on *ataque de nervios* and Kleinman's (1980) exploration of neurasthenia in the Chinese population. Conversely, the expansion or applicability of the culture-specific syndrome concept to Western clinical entities such as anorexia nervosa or fibromyalgia (Gaines 1992; Guarnaccia and Rogler 1999) may help in the effort to homogenize, as much as possible, psychiatric nomenclature practices.

Well-coordinated efforts will only enrich the relevance of the obvious relationship between research on these items and core research issues in cultural psychiatry and culturally based diagnosis. Ultimately, the validity and potential use of DSM-V across different cultures may have to be examined and actually practiced in two dimensions or levels: first, the core symptoms of specific entities and their eventual or potential generalizability across the world, and second, the recognition of cultural specificities that could be considered either as associated conditions, second-layer diagnostic criteria, or specific cultural notations related to such diagnostic categories. This would involve projects on both retrospective evaluations or field trials of proposed criteria in multiple epidemiologic and clinical studies. It must be clear, however, that all research efforts should avoid reinforcing stereotyping tendencies, or narrowness of diagnostic criteria with exclusionary consequences. Rather, research on psychiatric nomenclature should move safely and deliberately away from these extremes.

Use of DSM-V in Nonpsychiatric Settings

As greater emphasis is placed on detection and early intervention for mental disorders in settings other than traditional psychiatric clinics and practices, there is a need to define or operationalize diagnostic criteria in ways that can be rated or detected using methods other than the traditional psychiatric interview, which requires considerable training and clinical judgment. Reliance on clinical judgment could be minimized in a number of ways. First, criteria for mental disorders could be culled to remove items that cannot be determined reliably through patient self-reporting or through objectively observable signs or behaviors. Second, standardized self-report questionnaires or rating scales could be incorporated into diagnostic criteria (e.g., requiring a Beck Depression Inventory [BDI] [Beck et al. 1961] score of 16 or above) or used to make the syndrome diagnosis. Third, criteria could include requirements to use biological laboratory studies to confirm a diagnosis or to distinguish between disorders. To date, these three strategies have not been diagnostically definitive because of limitations in both specificity (e.g., high BDI scores are reported in some individuals without a depressive disorder, such as those experiencing a normal grief reaction) and sensitivity (e.g., normal brain magnetic resonance imaging is seen in many patients with schizophrenia). The diagnostic precision of such automated or objective diagnostic procedures may be inherently limited by the descriptive nature of mental disorders as etiology and underlying pathophysiology remain unknown.

The use of psychological testing, standardized rating scales, or medical laboratory examinations as explicit parts of DSM criteria has been largely avoided to date in recognition of the poor specificity of most available tests and to enable clinicians to make diagnoses with a minimum of instrumentation. With the exception of diagnoses involving mental retardation and learning disorders, mention of these more technically challenging assessments in DSM-IV is limited to the descriptive text, and such examinations are seen as ancillary and not diagnostic. However, as laboratory tests and psychological assessments evolve, their validity and reliability may surpass those of the current criteria sets, which are based on clinical observation. Research on the extent to which psychometric scales and medical laboratory procedures can enhance current diagnostic criteria or can serve as a substitute for current criteria could have a particularly important impact on the detection and treatment of mental disorders in nonpsychiatric settings.

Issues related to diagnostic thresholds are particularly pertinent in nonspecialty settings. Patients treated in mental health settings represent only a more severely affected minority of those in the general community whose symptoms meet criteria for mental disorders (Regier et al. 1993). In contrast, patients in primary care settings with undiagnosed mental disorders are likely to be those with earlier or milder manifestations. Changes in diagnostic criteria could facilitate detection and treatment of mild or subthreshold cases either through reductions in severity thresholds for selected disorders or through the development of alternative, simplified, less severe criteria sets specially designated for use in primary care and other nonspecialty settings.

Laboratory Tests and Diagnosis

Use of laboratory tests may be particularly useful to facilitate detection of mental disorders in primary care medical settings, in which use of such tests for the diagnosis and management of general medical conditions is routine. As progress is made in identifying the underlying neuropathology and pathophysiology of mental disorders, incorporation of findings from blood tests or neuroimaging studies may provide a more objective and discriminating window into these pathological processes. At present, most candidate laboratory examinations, such as the dexamethasone suppression test for depression, are neither sensitive nor specific in discriminating between pathological and normal mental states or among different major classes of mental disorders (Frances et al. 1995). Although the sensitivity and specificity of many current diagnostic criteria are similarly limited, use of alternative laboratory procedures will require evidence of clear superiority to justify the added expense entailed. Development of definitive laboratory tests is a piecemeal process that will vary from disorder to disorder in relation to progress in uncovering etiology and pathological processes associated with each disorder. However, as pointed out by Widiger and Clark (2000), the current near-exclusion of laboratory findings from diagnostic criteria is both questionable and inconsistent, because definitive tests are currently available for selected disorders and are already used for others. For example, for the diagnosis of learning disorders and mental retardation, results of IQ testing are a key element of DSM-IV diagnostic criteria. By contrast, with sleep disorders, polysomnographic findings are not incorporated in DSM-IV despite their crucial role in making distinctions among subtypes of sleep disorders that cannot be ascertained from obtaining a medical history, mental status evaluation, or physical examination (American Sleep Disorders Association Polysomnography Task Force 1997). Notably, the criteria in the International Classification of Sleep Disorders (ICSD) (American Sleep Disorders Association 1990), developed by the American Sleep Disorders Association (Buysee et al. 1998), require polysomnographic testing for the diagnosis of sleep disorders. Therefore, the general exclusion of psychological assessments and laboratory findings from current diagnostic criteria should be reexamined in future revisions.

Because of the potentially widespread application and commercial potential for objective indicators of mental disorders, research in search of such indicators is likely to continue without special initiatives. However, too little attention is paid to potential improvements in diagnostic precision that can arise from research in understanding etiology and underlying neurobiological processes for mental disorders. Findings from neurobiological research can have profound and unexpected implications for the diagnostic nomenclature. For example, findings from genetics studies have suggested commonalities between the previously separate diagnoses of major depressive disorder and generalized anxiety disorder (Kendler et al. 1995), whereas findings from neuroimaging studies document a distinctly different pathophysiology underlying obsessive-compulsive disorder and other anxiety disorders that are currently grouped together. However, nosologic issues are seldom targeted in neurobiological research, for example, through the use of alternative systems for diagnosing the disorders being studied (e.g., ICD-10 vs. DSM-IV). Putting diagnostic questions into the neurobiological research agenda would add an important dimension to diagnostic validity that is absent for most mental disorders.

Psychological Testing and Diagnosis

The use of standardized, psychometrically sound self-reported and computer-scored symptom rating scales may be particularly useful in nonspecialty settings for the detection of mental disorders. In comparison with a clinician interview to diagnose according to DSM-IV criteria, these tests offer advantages in reducing requirements for staff time and clinical judgment and in improving accurate reporting through such devices as use of multiple items to cover each diagnostic criterion, use of items that disguise the face validity of questions, and use of lie scales. In addition, most such scales yield a rating of symptom severity that can be used to determine treatment needs and to assess treatment response. Such scales have been developed for all major categories of DSM-IV mental disorders (American

Psychiatric Association 2000b). At present, results of psychological testing are not included in DSM-IV diagnostic criteria, with the exception of IQ testing and tests of academic skills to diagnose learning disorders and mental retardation. This exception points the way for research that could lead to incorporation of psychological test results as diagnostic criteria for other disorders. Determination of IQ through standardized testing offers a degree of diagnostic precision and accuracy in this area that cannot be achieved through routine clinical interview and physical examination. Although IQ tests have important limitations and are associated with social and ethical controversies (Halpern et al. 1996), the literature on reliability and validity of these tests far exceeds that for most other types of psychological assessments. For additional psychological tests to warrant incorporation into DSM diagnostic criteria, research is needed demonstrating substantial gains in reliability and validity when these are substituted for criteria based on routine clinical examination.

Development of Alternative Criteria for Primary Care and Nonspecialty Settings

To facilitate diagnosis of mild or subthreshold mental disorders in primary care settings, simplified or lower-threshold diagnostic criteria could be substituted for current systems or could be devised as an alternative official nomenclature designated for use outside of specialized mental health care settings. However, numerous costs would be associated with such a wholesale change in criteria, and such revisions should be made only in accordance with the considerations described above under "Rationale for Changing Criteria."

Diagnostic criteria need not be changed to manage diagnostic challenges presented in primary care and other nonspecialty settings. For example, existing and newly developed laboratory and psychological tests can facilitate screening, treatment planning, or diagnostic confirmation in nonspecialty settings without changing DSM categories or criteria. In fact, that is the current nondiagnostic role for examinations of this type. For example, the CAGE (Ewing 1984) questionnaire is often incorporated into routine medical screening to detect potential alcohol use disorders, and the detection of substances of abuse in urine or blood is a strong indicator of potential drug abuse, especially if use of these substances is denied on interview. Although they are useful in primary care medical settings, neither type of assessment offers sufficient advantages over current diagnostic criteria to warrant their incorporation into the section on psychoactive substance use disorders. Another strategy for adapting unchanged DSM criteria to be used in medical settings entails the development of simplified criteria sets, such as the DSM-IV Primary Care Version (DSM-IV-PC) (American Psychiatric Association 1995), and questionnaires, such as the Primary Care Evaluation of Mental Disorders (PRIME-MD) (Spitzer et al. 1994). Alternatively, the challenge in improving psychiatric diagnosis in nonspecialty settings can be seen as primarily educational, and numerous training packages have been developed to enhance accurate diagnosis in primary care settings (e.g., Andrews and Hunt 1999).

Research Agenda

- Put nomenclature issues on the neurobiological research agenda. To encourage investigators to focus on the nosologic implications of research on the neurobiology of mental disorders, supplemental grant funds could be offered to support the additional assessments and analyses entailed in validating alternative definitions of disorders or symptoms being evaluated. Review criteria should place high priority on the investigation of nosologic issues in requests for applications (RFAs) for studies of the neurobiological basis of mental disorders.
- Encourage research on automated or self-report methods to reduce reliance on clinical judgment. Self-reported diagnosis could be optimized through criterion-level research identifying and removing symptoms that cannot be reliably diagnosed through self-reporting. Subsequent research could evaluate the reliability and validity of alternative or new criterion sets composed entirely of items amenable to self-reporting. Another line of investigation could evaluate the impact on diagnostic reliability and validity of incorporating laboratory or psychological tests as criteria for mental disorders or as substitutes for assessing standard diagnostic criteria.

Conclusions

Cross-cultural and cross-setting exportation of criteria developed principally in the United States by specially trained psychiatrists forces a reassessment of fundamental issues related to how mental disorders are defined and assessed. Research conducted on basic nomenclature issues can have scientific as well as political significance, because diagnostic categories and criteria that stand up across cultures and across settings are likely to represent core processes. The research agendas suggested here pertaining to ICD/DSM differences, cross-cultural applicability, and application in nonpsychiatric settings must have value independent of their pertinence to suggested revisions to be included in DSM-V. In fact, we propose a highly conservative approach to the revision process and suggest that changes be made only when the empirical evidence or the need for change is compelling. Although much of the research proposed here may not produce definitive results in time for inclusion in DSM-V, the development of definitions of syndromes and criteria with universal applicability has implications that should affect future editions of the manual.

References

Abroms GM: Psychiatric serialism. Compr Psychiatry 22:372–378, 1981

Alarcón RD: Culture and psychiatric diagnosis. Impact on DSM-IV and ICD-10. Psychiatr Clin North Am 18:449–465, 1995

American Psychiatric Association: Diagnostic and Statistical Manual of Mental Disorders, 3rd Edition. Washington, DC, American Psychiatric Association, 1980

American Psychiatric Association: Diagnostic and Statistical Manual of Mental Disorders, 3rd Edition, Revised. Washington, DC, American Psychiatric Association, 1987

American Psychiatric Association: Diagnostic and Statistical Manual of Mental Disorders, 4th Edition. Washington, DC, American Psychiatric Association, 1994

American Psychiatric Association: DSM-IV Primary Care Version (DSM-IV-PC). Washington, DC, American Psychiatric Association, 1995

American Psychiatric Association: Diagnostic and Statistical Manual of Mental Disorders, 4th Edition, Text Revision. Washington, DC, American Psychiatric Association, 2000a

American Psychiatric Association: Handbook of Psychiatric Measures. Washington, DC, American Psychiatric Press, 2000b

American Sleep Disorders Association: International Classification of Sleep Disorders: Diagnostic and Coding Manual. Rochester, MN, American Sleep Disorders Association, 1990

American Sleep Disorders Association Polysomnography Task Force: Practice parameters for the indications for polysomnography and related procedures. Sleep 20:406–422, 1997

Andrews G: The anxiety disorder inclusion and exclusion criteria in DSM-IV and ICD-10. Current Opinion in Psychiatry 13:139–141, 2000

Andrews G, Hunt C: The education of general practitioners in the management of mental disorders, in Common Mental Disorders in Primary Care. Edited by Tansella M, Thornicroft G. London, Routledge, 1999, pp 183–193

Andrews G, Henderson S, Hall W: Prevalence, comorbidity, disability and service utilization: an overview of the Australian mental health survey. Br J Psychiatry 178:145–153, 1999

Andrews G, Slade T, Peters L: Classification in psychiatry: ICD-10 versus DSM-IV. Br J Psychiatry 174:3–5, 2001

Baron M, Gruen R, Rainer JD, et al: A family study of schizophrenia and normal control probands: implications for the spectrum concept of schizophrenia. Am J Psychiatry 142:447–455, 1985

Beck AT, Ward GH, Mendelson M: An inventory for measuring depression. Arch Gen Psychiatry 4:561–571, 1961

Boorse C: On the distinction between disease and illness. Philosophy and Public Affairs 5:49–68, 1975

Brown GW, Harris TO, Eales MJ: Social factors and comorbidity of depressive and anxiety disorders. Br J Psychiatry 168 (suppl 30):50–57, 1996

Buysee DJ, Reynolds CF, Kupfer DJ: DSM-IV sleep disorders; final overview, in DSM-IV Sourcebook, Vol 4. Edited by Widiger TA, Frances AJ, Pincus HA, et al. Washington, DC, American Psychiatric Association, 1998, pp 1103–1122

Campbell ESM, Scaddins JG, Roberts RS: The concept of disease. Br Med J (6193):757–762, 1979

Choca JP, Shanley LA, Peterson CA, et al: Racial bias and the MCMI. Journal of Personality Assessment 54:479–490, 1990

Cloninger CR: A new conceptual paradigm from genetics and psychobiology for the science of mental health. Aust N Z J Psychiatry 33:174–186, 1999

Escobar JI, Karno M, Golding J: Psychosocial inferences on psychiatric symptoms: the case of somatization, in Health and Behavior Research Agenda for Hispanics. Edited by Gaviria FM, Arana JD. Chicago, IL, University of Illinois Press, 1987 pp 207–215

Ewing JA: Detecting alcoholism: the CAGE questionnaire. JAMA 252:1905–1907, 1984

First MB, Pincus HA: Classification in psychiatry: ICD-10 vs DSM-IV, a response. Br J Psychiatry 175:205–209, 1999

Frances AJ, First MB, Pincus HA: DSM-IV Guidebook. Washington, DC, American Psychiatric Press, 1995

Gaines AD: Medical/psychiatric knowledge in France and the United States: culture and sickness in history and biology, in Ethnopsychiatry: A Cultural Construction of Professional and Folk Psychiatrists. Edited by Gaines AD. Albany, NY, State University of New York, 1992, pp 125–132

Gaw A (ed): Culture, ethnicity and mental illness. Washington, DC, American Psychiatric Press, 1993

Good BJ: Medicine, Rationality, and Experience: An Anthropological Perspective. Cambridge, England, Cambridge University Press, 1994

Guarnaccia PJ, Rogler LH: Research on culture-bound syndromes: new directions. Am J Psychiatry 156:1322–1327, 1999

Halpern SJ, Loehlin, DF, Perloff R, et al: Intelligence: knowns and unknowns. Am Psychol 51:77–101, 1996

Hempel CG: Introduction to problems of taxonomy, in Field Studies in the Mental Disorders. Edited by Zubin J. New York, Grune & Stratton, 1961, pp 3–22

Hinton AL: Biocultural approaches to the emotions. Cambridge, England, Cambridge University Press, 1999

Kendell RE: The concept of disease and its implications for psychiatry. Br J Psychiatry 127:305–315, 1975a

Kendell RE: The Role of Diagnosis in Psychiatry. Oxford, Blackwell Scientific, 1975b, pp 119–136

Kendell RE: The distinction between mental and physical illness. Br J Psychiatry 178:490–493, 2001

Kendler KS: Toward a scientific psychiatric nosology: strengths and limitations. Arch Gen Psychiatry 47:969–973, 1990

Kendler KS: Major depression and generalized anxiety disorder: same genes, (partly) different environments—revisited. Br J Psychiatry 168 (suppl 30):68–75, 1996

Kendler KS, Gardner CO: Boundaries of major depression: an evaluation of DSM-IV criteria. Am J Psychiatry 155:172–177, 1998

Kendler KS, Spitzer RL, Williams JB: Psychotic disorders in DSM-III-R. Am J Psychiatry 146:953–962, 1989

Kendler KS, Gruenberg AM, Kinney DK: Independent diagnoses of adoptees and relatives as defined by DSM-III in the provincial and national samples of the Danish Adoption Study of Schizophrenia. Arch Gen Psychiatry 51:456–468, 1994

Kendler KS, Neale MC, Walsh D: Evaluating the spectrum concept of schizophrenia in the Roscommon Family Study. Am J Psychiatry 152:749–754, 1995

Kirmayer LJ, Young A: Culture and context in the evolutionary concept of mental disorder. J Abnorm Psychol 108:446–452, 1999

Kleinman A: Patients and Healers in the Context of Culture. Berkeley, CA, University of California Press, 1980

Kleinman A: Rethinking Psychiatry: From Culture Category to Personal Experience. New York, Free Press, 1988

Leff J: "The new cross cultural psychiatry." A case of the baby and the bath water. Br J Psychiatry 156:305–307, 1990

Lewis-Fernandez R, Kleinman A: Cultural psychiatry: theoretical, clinical and research issues. Psychiatr Clin North Am 18:433–448, 1995

Lilienfeld S, Marino L: Mental disorder as a Roschian concept: a critique of Wakefield's "harmful dysfunction" analysis. J Abnorm Psychol 104:411–420, 1995

Littlewood R: From categories to contexts: a decade of the new crosscultural psychiatry. Br J Psychiatry 156:308–327, 1990

Lukoff D, Lu FG, Turner R: Cultural considerations in the assessment and treatment of religious and spiritual problems. Psychiatr Clin North Am 18:467–485, 1995

Mezzich JE, Goode BJ: On culturally enhancing the DSM-IV multiaxial formulation, in Cultural Issues in DSM-IV: Support Papers. Edited by Mezzich JE, Kleinman A, Fabrega H, et al. Pittsburgh, PA, University of Pittsburgh Press, 1994, pp 983–989

Neligh G: Major mental disorders and behavior among American Indians and Alaska Natives. Am Indian Alsk Native Ment Health Res 1:116–150, 1988

Regier DA, Narrow WE, Rae DS, et al: The de facto U.S. mental health and addictive disorders service system: Epidemiological Catchment Area prospective one-year prevalance rates of disorders and services. Arch Gen Psychiatry 50:85–92, 1993

Robins E, Guze SB: Establishment of diagnostic validity in psychiatric illness: its application to schizophrenia. Am J Psychiatry 126:983–987, 1970

Rogler LH: Implementing cultural sensitivity in mental health research: convergence and new directions, part I. Psychline 3:1–12, 1999

Sartorius N, Jablensky A, Gulbinat W, et al: WHO Collaborative Study: Assessment of Depressive Disorders. Psychol Med 10:743–749, 1980

Scadding JG: Diagnosis: the clinician and the computer. Lancet 2:877–882, 1967

Spitzer RL, Williams JBW, Kroenke K, et al: Utility of a new procedure for diagnosing mental disorders in primary care: the PRIME-MD study. JAMA 272:1749–1756, 1994

Wakefield JC: The concept of mental disorder: on the boundary between biological facts and social values. Am Psychol 47:373–388, 1992

Wakefield JC: Evolutionary versus prototype analyses of the concept of disorder. J Abnorm Psychol 108:374–399, 1999

Weiss MD, Doongaji DR, Siddhartha S: The Explanatory Model Interview Catalogue (EMIC): contribution to cross cultural research methods from a study of leprosy and mental health. Br J Psychiatry 160:819–830, 1992

Widiger TA, Clark LA: Towards DSM-V and the classification of psychopathology. Psychol Bull 126:946–963, 2000

Wittenborn JR, Holzberg JD, Simon B: Symptom correlates for descriptive diagnosis. Genetic Psychology Monographs 47:237–301, 1953

World Health Organization: Report of the International Pilot Study of Schizophrenia, Vol 1 (WHO Publ No 2). Geneva, World Health Organization, 1973

World Health Organization: The ICD-10 Classification of Mental and Behavioural Disorders: clinical descriptions and diagnostic guidelines. Geneva, World Health Organization, 1992

World Health Organization: Composite International Diagnostic Interview. Geneva, World Health Organization, 1993

CHAPTER 2

Neuroscience Research Agenda to Guide Development of a Pathophysiologically Based Classification System

Dennis S. Charney, M.D., David H. Barlow, Ph.D., Kelly Botteron, M.D., Jonathan D. Cohen, M.D., David Goldman, M.D., Raquel E. Gur, M.D., Ph.D., Keh-Ming Lin, M.D., M.P.H., Juan F. López, M.D., James H. Meador-Woodruff, M.D., Steven O. Moldin, Ph.D., Eric J. Nestler, M.D., Ph.D., Stanley J. Watson, M.D., Ph.D., Steven J. Zalcman, M.D.

Psychiatric classifications have historically been organized around each era's prevailing theories about the etiology of mental disorders, reflecting the sense that classifications based on etiology are most likely to be helpful in the clinical management of patients. For example, in the sixteenth century the Swiss physician Paracelsus developed a classification system based on presumed etiology, distinguishing vesania (disorders thought to be caused by poisons), lunacy (a periodic condition believed to be influenced by phases of the moon), and insanity (diseases apparently caused by heredity factors). The obvious problem with such classifications is that their utility is strictly limited by the validity (or lack thereof) of the underlying etiological assumptions. The descriptive approach adopted by the DSM allowed for the development of a classification system that met the field's need for a common language, without being mired in ideological hypotheses about the causes of psychiatric illness. Questions have been raised by many critics (McHugh [2001]) that the DSM's descriptive approach may have outlived its usefulness and is in fact potentially misleading. Although there is a large body of research that indicates a neurobiological basis for most mental disorders, the DSM definitions are virtually devoid of biology. Instead, DSM-IV definitions are based on clusters of symptoms and characteristics of clinical course.

There has been no shortage of neurobiological theories of causation for psychiatric disorders. The original monoamine hypothesis regarding mood disorders and the dopamine hypotheses regarding schizophrenia have been of substantial heuristic value. For example, the monoamine hypothesis led to more sophisticated examination of monoamine systems, including receptor subtype analysis and the study of brain systems that interact with monoamine system functions (e.g., glutamate, γ-aminobutyric acid [GABA], and substance P). However, these hypotheses were largely derived post hoc from discoveries related to the pharmacologic actions of antidepressant and antipsychotic drug treatments. There have been replicated findings suggesting abnormalities of norepinephrine and serotonin neuronal systems in mood disorders (Garlow et al. 1999) and abnormalities of glutamate and dopamine neuronal systems (Bunney and Bunney 1999; Byne et al. 1999) in schizophrenia. However, none of these findings are sufficiently robust to be of diagnostic value. For example, there is typically a large overlap between diagnostic groups and control subjects. Disturbances in sleep architecture are commonly observed in mood disorders, especially with regard to the onset and duration of rapid eye movement (REM) sleep (Nofzinger et al. 1999). Neuroendocrine abnormalities, particularly involving the hypothalamic-pituitary-adrenal (HPA) system, have been repeatedly identified in depressed patients (Holsboer 1999). Despite initial enthusiasm for the dexamethasone suppression test and REM latency diagnostic tests for depression, neither has turned out to be a reliable and valid diagnostic marker. Test findings may vary from episode to episode in the same individual, and neither is diagnostically specific (i.e., there is substantial overlap in the range of values between depressed patients and nondepressed control subjects). Cerebrospinal fluid levels of corticotropin-releasing hormone (CRH), possibly reflecting extrahypothalamic CRH concentrations, are elevated in at least a subgroup of depressed patients, but this subgroup has not been distinguished clinically, and without the availability of CRH receptor antagonists it has not been possible to identify specific treatment response patterns (Garlow et al. 1999). The situation with anxiety disorders is not any better. There are replicated findings suggesting dysfunction in brain benzodiazepine, norepinephrine, serotonin, cholecystokinin, and CRH systems in the different anxiety disorders (Charney and Bremner 1999). Abnormalities in the regulation of respiration have been well documented, especially by studies investigating responses to inhaled CO_2. Unfortunately, none of these results have led to the identification of diagnostic markers for anxiety disorders or predictors of response. As described below, genetic investigations of schizophrenia, bipolar disorder, major depressive disorder, and anxiety disorders have failed to identify vulnerability genes that are useful in predicting current and future risk of disorder. Furthermore, very few studies of the neurobiology of major psychiatric disorders have included ethnically or culturally diverse populations in their designs. This limits the applicability of research results to clinical populations.

At the risk of making an overly broad statement of the status of neurobiological investigations of the major psychiatric disorders noted above, it can be concluded that the field of psychiatry has thus far failed to identify a single neurobiological phenotypic marker or gene that is useful in making a diagnosis of a major psychiatric disorder or for predicting response to psychopharmacologic treatment. A primary purpose of this chapter is to review why progress has been so limited and to offer strategic insights that may lead to a more etiologically based diagnostic system. Such an accomplishment would represent a highly laudable achievement for psychiatry and would help move the specialty into the mainstream of modern medicine, where etiology and pathophysiology have replaced descriptive symptomatology as the fundamental basis for making diagnostic distinctions. For example, before the elucidation of its underlying pathophysiology, diabetes mellitus was classified as a single entity in simple descriptive terms (i.e., abnormally elevated blood glucose) differentiated by typical age at onset (e.g., juvenile vs. adult) and other descriptive features (such as an association with obesity). It was only with the understanding of the underlying pathophysiology that diabetes could be divided into two distinct and clinically meaningful entities, based on insulin deficiency versus insulin receptor sensitivity. Current classification in psychiatry therefore resembles the medicine of 50–100 years ago, before the underlying pathophysiology of many disease processes was understood. Diagnostic distinctions based on etiology (as opposed to descriptive symptomatology) are more likely to lead to rational treatment selection and more valid prognostications.

Despite the importance of this objective, it must be strongly stated at the outset of this discussion that it will be years—and possibly decades—before a fully explicated etiologically and pathophysiologically based classification system for psychiatry exists. Today there is only rudimentary knowledge of the genetic and nongenetic factors that cause the common psychotic, affective, anxiety, and substance use disorders that constitute the large majority of serious psychiatric disturbances. Similarly, very little is known about the molecular and cellular abnormalities that underlie the pathophysiology of psychotic, affective, anxiety, and substance use disorders, and very little specific prognostic information can be given to patients about their disorders. Some very good treatments are available for most psychotic, affective, and anxiety disorders, and the efficacy of these treatments rivals that seen in many other medical specialties in the treatment of chronic disease. However, virtually all of these treatments were discovered by serendipity a half-century ago, with newer treatments representing refinements of the original mechanism of action of these agents. Thus, the last half-century has seen the development of very few truly new treatments for psychotic, affective, and anxiety disorders, and treatment of most addictions remains highly inadequate for most individuals.

There are many reasons for this relative lack of progress in psychiatry compared with other medical specialties. The brain is far more complex than most other organ systems, and it remains relatively inaccessible, which makes the challenge in psychiatry considerably greater. In the past two decades, more psychiatric research has focused on refining descriptive symptomatology (as embodied in DSM-III, DSM-III-R, and DSM-IV) than on neurobiology and genetics. Furthermore, there has been too strong a reliance on the DSM-defined symptom clusters and too little on biologically based symptoms that may cut across the DSM-IV–defined disorders. This over-reification of the DSM categories has led to a form of closed-mindedness on the part of researchers and funding sources. For example, researchers involved in new drug development tend to focus their efforts on treatment of DSM-IV–defined categories, despite widespread evidence that pharmacologic treatments tend to be effective in treating a relatively wide range of DSM disorders. Furthermore, the erroneous notion that the DSM categories can double as phenotypes may be partly responsibility for the lack of success in discovering robust genetic markers. Although a move to an etiologically and pathophysiologically based diagnostic system for psychiatry will be extraordinarily difficult, it is nevertheless essential, based on the increasing belief that many, and perhaps most, of the current symptom clusters of DSM will ultimately not map onto distinct disease states.

Given the current predicament, then, how can the field develop a pathophysiologically based classification system? Clearly, genetic studies in humans will provide uniquely powerful information. Despite several decades of effort, no bona fide psychiatric disease gene has yet been identified with certainty, although the field is getting closer, and new advances in genetics (including the availability of the human genome sequence) portend rapid progress. Brain imaging studies in humans promise, for the first time, to provide detailed information about molecular and cellular substrates in the brain involved in a psychiatric disorder. Although currently available imaging techniques have thus far failed to provide diagnostic tests for psychotic, affective, or anxiety disorders, it is only a matter of time before such techniques have the spatial and temporal resolution and the chemical specificity to study relevant pathophysiological mechanisms. Finally, studies of brain samples obtained at autopsy should permit more detailed molecular analysis of the pathophysiology of psychiatric disorders. Over the last decade, the field has greatly increased the sophistication with which it uses postmortem tissue.

There is no question that animal research has vastly expanded the knowledge of normal brain function. It has also been invaluable in identifying the initial protein targets through which most currently used pharmacotherapeutic agents (e.g., antipsychotic, antidepressant, and antianxiety drugs) produce their beneficial clinical effects, as well as the protein targets through which most drugs of abuse cause addiction. It has also been possible to develop several animal models that have outstanding predictive value in developing new medications with the same mechanism of action as, but fewer side effects than, the older agents. The introduction of second-generation antipsychotic agents, the selective serotonin and selective norepinephrine reuptake inhibitor antidepressants, and benzodiazepine-like agents that act on selected subunits of the $GABA_A$ receptor have all derived directly from rational drug-design efforts based on animal models.

In the following sections of this chapter we review the current status of genetic, brain imaging, postmortem, and animal model research relevant to elucidating the pathophysiology of mental disorders. This is followed by a set of recommendations for a research agenda that will allow for the eventual adoption of a etiologically and pathophysiologically based diagnostic system.

Current Status of the Genetics of Psychiatric Disorders

During the past 100 years, there has been considerable interest in examining whether genes play a role in the etiology of mental disorders. If genes play such a role, their identification is expected to have a dramatic effect on improving differential diagnosis, shedding insight into pathophysiology, and developing new treatments. The first step in characterizing the genetic bases of mental disorders has been to demonstrate familial co-aggregation. Family studies of a number of mental disorders—including schizophrenia, bipolar disorder, autism, major depressive disorder, anxiety disorders (including panic disorder and obsessive-compulsive disorder [OCD]), and attention-deficit/hyperactivity disorder (ADHD)—have consistently shown that these disorders are familial and that transmission in families is, at least in part, mediated by genes.

Familial transmission may also occur as a result of environmental factors transmitted from parent to child. Consequently, twin and adoption studies have been used to disentangle genetic from shared environmental influences. When the monozygotic concordance rate is higher than the dizygotic concordance rate, a genetic basis is the most likely explanation. A measure of the degree of genetic control over a phenotype calculated from twin studies is heritability, the ratio of genetic variance to the total variance in the population.

Adoption study designs also tease apart the effects of genes and environment by studying individuals who have been raised by biologically unrelated adoptive parents and by comparing their adoptive and biological relatives. Adoption studies of schizophrenia, bipolar disorder, alcoholism, and depression support a significant role for genetic factors in their etiologies (Kelsoe 1999; Malhi et al. 2000; Riley and McGuffin 2000; Schuckit 2000; Sullivan et al. 2000).

Starting in the early 1980s, DNA polymorphisms provided a sufficiently numerous set of markers that are spaced throughout the entire genome. Such markers permit the mapping of diseases to specific genomic regions, and their widespread availability ushered in the molecular era of psychiatric genetics. By the late 1980s, promising linkages of schizophrenia to chromosome 5q and bipolar disorder to Xq and 11p were reported, but they were subsequently neither replicated nor confirmed in the original data sets (Moldin 1997b; Risch and Botstein 1996).

Linkages of schizophrenia to numerous chromosomal regions have recently been reported (Baron 2001; Riley and McGuffin 2000). Several have been implicated in multiple data sets and have become the focus of considerable interest: 1q, 5q, 6p, 6q, 8p, 10p, 13q, and 15q. Large genomic regions have been typically implicated, and failures to replicate have been reported for each region. It is difficult to distinguish which of these results (if any) are true guideposts on the path to gene discovery and which are false positives (Moldin 1997b). Weak associations of schizophrenia to several gene loci, including *NOTCH4*, hKCa3/KCNN3 potassium channel, CHRNA7, *NURR1*, SCA1, DRD_3, catechol-*O*-methyltransferase (COMT), and the serotonin (5-hydroxytryptamine) type 2A ($5\text{-}HT_{2A}$) receptor have been reported in candidate gene studies but have not been convincingly replicated (Moldin 1999; Riley and McGuffin 2000).

Linkages of bipolar disorder to numerous chromosomal regions have also been reported (Kelsoe 1999; Moldin 1999). Several have been implicated in multiple data sets: 4p, 12q, 13q, 18p, 18q, 21q, 22q, and Xq. None of the linkage statistics reported in these studies were corrected for the testing of multiple diagnostic and transmission models; other complexities concern the implication of large chromosomal regions and failures to replicate. As in the case of schizophrenia, sufficient ambiguities exist to give pause in considering any of these linkage results as unambiguously replicated. Weak associations of bipolar disorder to several loci involved in the GABAergic, serotoninergic, and dopaminergic systems (e.g., GABRA5, serotonin transporter [5-HTT], tyrosine hydroxylase), genes mediating signal transduction (e.g., phospholipase A2A), and other loci (e.g., CRH, adenosine A, receptor) have been reported, but subsequent studies produced divergent results (V. Nimgaonkar, unpublished data, December 2000).

Researchers have searched for clinical criteria to identify subtypes of depressed patients with familial unipolar illness. Recurrent major depression appears to be the subtype of major depression that most consistently identifies increased familial risk (Sullivan et al. 2000). Childhood or adolescent onset may also be associated with significantly greater risk for recurrence in adulthood (Wickramaratne et al. 2000). Molecular studies have focused on candidate genes. Weak associations have been reported between depression and 5-HTT, but not all studies agree (Malhi et al. 2000). Other candidate loci implicated include dopamine receptor genes, 5-HT receptor genes, tyrosine hydroxylase, and genes in the GABAergic system. Convincing replications of these candidates in multiple data sets have not been forthcoming.

In a genome-wide survey of panic disorder, families with a variety of kidney or bladder problems and other medical conditions were subdivided, and significant 13q linkage evidence was reported (Weissman et al. 2000) (see further discussion below). Most molecular genetic studies of anxiety disorders have focused on candidate genes chosen based on the receptor binding profile of anxiolytic compounds, or in consideration of the molecules in neurotransmitter pathways involved in therapeutic action. Association analyses of OCD patients have implicated several genes—5-HTT, serotoninergic receptors (5-HT_{2A}, 5-HT_{2C}, 5-HT_1), DRD_4, and both COMT and MAO (monoamine oxidase) A in males only—but findings typically have not been unambiguously replicated (Moldin 2000; Wolff et al. 2000). Likewise, associations between panic disorder and several genes—5-HTT, α_{2A} adrenergic receptor, A_{2a} adenosine receptor, CCK, CCK-B, DRD_4, COMT, and MAO A—have been reported but not confirmed (Moldin 2000).

Molecular genetic studies of ADHD also have focused on candidate gene studies. A meta-analysis of case-control and family-based association studies of ADHD and the 7-repeat allele of DRD_4 found evidence of a weak association (Faraone et al. 2001). Another meta-analysis of nine studies of a 480–base-pair allele of the dopamine transporter gene found very modest evidence for an association (Curran et al. 2001). Associations to other genes in the dopaminergic system (i.e., DRD1, COMT) have been reported but not confirmed.

There have been numerous reports of aberrations (e.g., deletions, translocations, and inversions) on nearly every chromosome in autism (Gillberg 1998); however, the rates of these abnormalities vary widely across studies. Most commonly reported are those on the X chromosome, followed by those on chromosome 15. One candidate gene study of 15q identified an association between autism and the $GABA_A$ β_3 receptor subunit gene (Cook et al. 1998), but this result has not been replicated. Studies of other genes in the 15q region (e.g., *UBE3A*), several serotoninergic system genes, neurofibromatosis type 1 gene, and the c-Harvey-Ras gene have failed to consistently reveal an association. A recent report of a substitution variant at HOXA1 on chromosome 7p in a subset of autistic subjects (Ingram et al. 2000) has not been replicated. Although one region—7q—has been identified in five recent genomewide scans (Lamb et al. 2000; Maestrini et al. 2000), no genomic region identified yielded significant or suggestive (Lander and Kruglyak 1995) linkage evidence. All samples comprised fewer than 200 pedigrees; thus, analyses conducted to date likely have had low statistical power to detect true linkages.

In many of the studies described above, diagnostic definitions were broadened to include related, or "spectrum," conditions. Unfortunately, such disorders (e.g., schizotypal personality, bipolar II disorder, broader autism phenotype) are diagnosed less reliably than core phenotypes, and their familial aggregation is less specific to any one disorder (Moldin 1997a). Broadening of the core phenotype has not consistently increased linkage evidence.

Individuals are differentially vulnerable to alcoholism and other substance abuse or dependence, even in societies where disease prevalences are highest and the effects most pernicious. Differential vulnerability could indicate the existence of innate differences, environmental differences, or a combination of both. However, it has been established in twins that about half of the variance in vulnerability to alcoholism is attributable to genes, and other forms of substance dependency are also substantially heritable; for example, opioid addiction is almost 50% heritable. Identification of the alleles responsible for differential vulnerability will lead to new molecular diagnostic markers to improve diagnostic precision and individualize treatment. Better understanding of mechanisms of vulnerability and gene-environment interactions will redefine these disorders in etiologic terms and lead to new molecular targets for intervention.

ADH2 and ALDH2, the two known genes for alcohol vulnerability, are substance-specific vulnerability factors. Because various drugs of addiction elicit common neurochemical responses and behaviors (intoxication, anesthetization) across individuals, it is also likely that general vulnerability factors are present in human populations. Based on evidence from twin and family studies, there are both general and substance-specific inherited factors for vulnerability to the addictive drugs (Goldman and Bergen 1998). The prediction is that vulnerability genes act in both drug-specific fashion (e.g., the alcohol metabolic gene, ALDH2) and on general vulnerability (e.g., a gene such as 5-HTT, which has been proposed to affect anxiety). Substance-specific genetic factors were particularly important for alcohol and opioids. The conclusion that drug dependence in probands is nonpredictive of alcoholism in relatives is a provocative finding that strongly implies that specific genetic factors are involved in alcoholism. Again, in a study of drug abuse and alcoholism in parents and offspring, parental history of drug abuse was found to be nonpredictive of alcoholism in offspring, and vice versa (Kendler et al. 1997). All of these findings in large and carefully characterized data sets are consistent with previous studies on the familial transmission of alcoholism and other substance abuse (Bierut et al. 1998; Kendler et al. 1997; Merikangas et al. 1998). Only nicotine dependence (True et al. 1999) has shown significant coinheritance with alcoholism. Whole genome scans for loci influencing alcohol dependence have been conducted in a population isolate (Long et al. 1998) and in families from the cosmopolitan population of the United States, with the result that linkages to several regions were detected, including plausible candidate genes such as the dopamine D_4 receptor (chromosome 11p) and a $GABA_A$ receptor complex (chromosome 4p). However, these linkages did not reach significance by the criteria of Lander and Kruglyak (1995), and the only definitive criterion—isolation of the responsible allele—has not been met.

As discussed above, descriptive classifications define diagnostic entities that are undoubtedly heterogeneous from both an etiologic and a genetic perspective. Alternative strategies for increasing diagnostic homogeneity, and thereby increasing the power of genetic analyses, include the identification of genetically distinct diagnostic subtypes. One research team analyzed a periodic catatonia subtype of schizophrenia and found significant evidence of linkage to 15q (Stober et al. 2000). Although the reliability of this phenotype across laboratories has yet to be demonstrated and its theoretical basis has yet to be established, this interesting result demonstrates the potential utility of subdividing and redefining existing diagnostic categories. In a panic disorder study, families were subdivided on the basis of kidney or bladder problems and other medical conditions, and significant evidence of 13q linkage was reported (Weissman et al. 2000). Although replication is essential, this is an intriguing result that may help define a subtype of panic disorder on the basis of pathophysiology, that is, the involvement of CRH and identifiable neural substrates of fear and anxiety in micturition.

All of the genetic studies discussed herein have involved analysis of a binary phenotype, that is, affected or unaffected status. Brzustowicz and colleagues (1997) performed linkage analysis on quantitative dimensions of psychopathology in schizophrenia and found significant evidence linking positive symptom-scale scores to 6p. Although this result has not been replicated, such an approach represents a potentially fruitful direction for significantly increasing the power of genetic studies.

Another promising approach is the detailed ongoing exploration of behavioral phenotypes and valid and robust dimensional markers that go beyond binary phenotypes. For example, the criteria sets in DSM-IV were often developed and refined by studying disorders in isolation from one another (e.g., the DSM-IV field trials) and without consideration of possible higher-order symptom structures and differential relationships to constructs of temperament or vulnerability. Cross-sectional and longitudinal studies are currently ongoing in which a wide range of clinical indicators cutting across DSM categories are subjected to sophisticated latent variable analyses to determine the first and higher-order structure of these features. Identification of the validity and stability of these behavioral phenotypes would lead to important insights on their clinical validity and would enable more sophisticated genetic and neurobiological studies (e.g., explication of a temporally stable latent dimension that does not co-vary with other dimensions of psychopathology but influences their course). Once these broader models are established, important fine-grained analyses could proceed. For instance, multiple groups latent variable solutions could make possible the evaluation of the degree of invariance of these phenotypes across salient demographic groups (e.g., races, sexes). These analyses could uncover reliable model-based differences in the expressions of psychopathology that would have considerable heuristic value for genetic or neurobiological research (e.g., evidence of ethnic variations in linkage studies). In addition to their superior validity, the use of latent model–based dimensional phenotypes would greatly enhance the statistical power of neurobiological and genetic studies and would foster the ability to detect more complex relationships that would otherwise be masked by use of diagnostic categories alone (e.g., a nonlinear relationship between a neurobiological marker and a dimensional phenotype).

Although it has been grossly underused to date, the latent variable analysis of psychopathology phenotypes could be extended to a set of analytical procedures referred to as latent class modeling (e.g., dimensional or categorical indices of psychopathological features), except that each latent class possesses a different set of parameter values (Muthen 2000). In addition to determining whether various psychopathological phenomena operate in a continuous or a taxonomic manner, these analytical procedures hold substantial promise for establishing empirically derived symptom thresholds between “disordered” and “nondisordered” classes (e.g., identify symptoms that indicate classes well; determine the number of criteria needed to be fulfilled to meet a diagnostic class) and for determining whether the heterogeneity observed (or unobserved) within a disorder is due to the existence of latent classes (i.e., natural subtypes of disorders) (Nestadt et al. 1994). These modeling possibilities have profound implications for neurobiological and genetic research endeavors, where there is a growing belief that the power to identify markers has often been mitigated (or enhanced) by the failure (or success) to adequately account for or recognize diagnostic heterogeneity. Latent class modeling holds the unrealized potential for explicating classes that represent natural cut points in the expression of psychopathology within and across disorders that would strongly guide the pursuit of the identification of genetic and neurobiological markers.

Researchers have attempted to increase power for genetic analyses by directly incorporating into linkage analyses quantitative information provided by related biological traits presumed to be correlated with underlying disease liability. It is assumed that pleiotropy is present, that is, a gene exerts an effect on both affection status and the ancillary biological trait. Researchers over the last 30 years have searched intensively for such traits, with limited success (Moldin and Erlenmeyer-Kimling 1994). Reported linkages include impaired P50 auditory sensory gating to within 500 kb of CHRNA7 on 15q (Freedman et al. 1997), and a composite biological phenotype of P50 auditory sensory gating and antisaccade ocular motor performance to 22q (Myles-Worsley et al. 1999). Linkage of eye tracking dysfunction was reported to 6p in eight schizophrenia pedigrees (Arolt et al. 1996). Other biological traits posited as vulnerability markers of mental disorders include deficits in sustained attention (Chen and Faraone 2000), eye tracking dysfunction and deficits in the auditory P300 event-related potential (Blackwood et al. 1996), reactivity to a 35% CO_2 challenge (van Beek and Griez 2000), disturbances in sleep architecture (Giles et al. 1998), N4 and P3 components of event-related brain potentials (Almasy et al. 2001), trait anxiety (Mazzanti et al. 1998), response to alcohol (Schuckit et al. 2000) and benzodiazepine drugs (Iwata et al. 1999), and therapeutic response to antipsychotic medication (Arranz et al. 2000a).

Ethnic variations are substantial in the distribution of the genotypes and haplotypes of the majority of the proposed "candidate genes" for psychiatric disorders (Burmeister 1999; Gelernter et al. 1997; McLeod et al. 1998; Palmatier et al. 1999), as well as those of interest in relation to other common medical problems with complex genetics, such as diabetes, asthma, and hypertension (Barroso et al. 1999; Drysdale et al. 2000; Pritchard et al. 2000; Roses 2000). For example, the rate of the short variant of the serotonin transporter promoter region polymorphism may be associated with risks for mood disorders as well as poor antidepressant response in Caucasians (Pollock et al. 2000; Smeraldi et al. 1998), but the reverse in Koreans (D.K. Kim et al. 2000). However, the frequency of this allele ranges from more than 70% in East Asians to approximately 50% in Caucasians and less than 30% in African Americans (Gelernter et al. 1997). The prevalence of the low-activity COMT, which has been reported to be a risk factor for a number of psychiatric disorders, ranges from 18% in Asians to 50% in Caucasians (McLeod et al. 1998; Palmatier et al. 1999). These emerging data have led to an increased awareness of the importance of "population (ethnic) stratification" and the need to always take ethnicity into consideration in genetic research (Baron 1993; Hamer 2000; Roses 2000).

In summary, considerable evidence from genetic epidemiological studies exists to support the role that genes play in producing vulnerability to mental disorders. These results are among the most robust and replicated in psychiatry. The genetic complexity of these diseases, that is, the involvement of multiple genes in interaction with each other and the environment, has resulted in circuitous pathways from the underlying genotype to the clinical phenotype. Such biological complexities present considerable analytical challenges, and genomic localization and identification of such genes has not yet occurred. These challenges are as daunting in the study of other complex diseases such as multiple sclerosis, hypertension, and diabetes. Powerful new genomic tools and technologies (e.g., high-throughput genotyping via mass spectrometry, draft sequence of the human genome, a comprehensive catalogue of human genetic variation, new statistical genetic methods), in combination with large data sets and innovative study designs in which biological traits and subtypes of existing diagnostic categories are identified, are expected to greatly accelerate gene discovery for mental disorders. Such advances have the potential for revolutionizing psychiatric nosology in subsequent editions of the DSM by providing clinicians with a biological basis for making differential diagnostic decisions.

Current Status of Neuroimaging Studies of Psychiatric Disorders

Structural Neuroimaging

Studies examining potential structural differences associated with psychiatric disorders have been reported for about 25 years. Initial studies used computed tomography (CT), with magnetic resonance imaging (MRI) following about a decade later. Early results were inconsistently replicated, although this may have been related to significant technical and study design limitations. However, differences in brain structure associated with specific disorders such as schizophrenia and bipolar disorder were eventually demonstrated in a replicable fashion. Early demonstrations of relatively global anatomical differences such as increased lateral ventricle volume, third ventricle volume, or basal ganglia changes were often nonspecific and were noted in multiple disorders such as schizophrenia, bipolar disorder, and dementia. However, significant advances in image acquisition technology and image analysis tools have enabled the closer investigation of anatomically relevant regions. Concurrent with these advances, an increasing number of recent studies have reported specific regional differences between patients and control subjects, some of which demonstrate increased diagnostic specificity. For example, decreased superior temporal gyrus volume and decreased thalamus volume are evident in schizophrenia (Shenton et al. 2001). Depression is reported to be associated with changes in amygdala volume and reduction in ventromedial prefrontal cortical regions (Drevets 2000).

Early studies limited their quantification of structural differences to estimates of regional area or volume. However, this only partially characterizes the potential neuromorphometric parameters of specific regions and ignores information such as surface area, thickness, or shape. Shape analysis for imaging has been difficult to realize. However, some newly developed, sophisticated shape analysis methods (M. Miller et al. 1997) have demonstrated increased sensitivity over volume measures in detecting anatomical differences between disorders. For example, in schizophrenia and early dementia, shape changes demonstrated in the hippocampus have had significant power to discriminate affected individuals from healthy control subjects (Csernansky et al. 1998, 2000).

Characterization of regional structure by anatomical MRI methods only is also limiting, and other functional (functional MRI [fMRI] or positron emission tomography [PET]) or chemical (magnetic resonance spectroscopy [MRS]) techniques serve complementary roles in defining pathophysiology associated with specific disorders. A number of studies have demonstrated that structural imaging data are an important adjunct to functional or metabolic imaging. Use of functional or chemical imaging techniques applied without structural data results in the erroneous underlying assumption that there are no differences in tissue composition between patients of interest and healthy control subjects. An example is illustrated in the recent demonstration of decreased gray matter volume in regions of the ventral medial prefrontal cortex in recurrent major depression and bipolar disorder (Drevets et al. 1997; Hirayasu et al. 1998). Early functional studies had reported consistent decreases in blood flow and metabolism in this region, which had been interpreted as decreased activity in the regional neuronal tissue. However, models to estimate the per-unit volume neuronal activity in the context of decreased gray matter volume in this specific region have suggested that the neuronal activity may in fact be increased on a per-unit basis (Drevets 2000). It is likely that the integration of cross-modality imaging data will result in clearer specification of distinct neuropathophysiologies associated with psychiatric disorders. Structural changes that are secondary to effects of illness via neurodegenerative mechanisms (or via changes in neurodevelopment) not only could have important treatment implications but also would be integral to clarifying current diagnostic heterogeneity. It has been demonstrated that children with ADHD have a reduction in caudate nucleus volume, and they also show a difference in the developmental pattern of change in caudate nucleus volume with increasing age. In comparison to healthy children, who have decreasing caudate nucleus volumes with advancing age, boys with ADHD show no change in volume with age (Castellanos et al. 1996). Another example is the finding that adolescents with prepubertal-onset schizophrenia are noted to have structural differences early in the course of illness, and these changes become accentuated with age as these adolescents demonstrate a clear deviation from normal developmental trends in several regions in comparison to unaffected control subjects (Giedd et al. 1999). Thus these two examples illustrate how the onset of a disorder may affect normal developmental or aging-related brain changes. An increased emphasis on longitudinal neuroimaging studies is important not only for treatment planning but also to further specify diagnostic categorization. For example, two divergent pathophysiologic mechanisms may underlie two different cases, each currently classified as major depressive disorder (MDD). In one case, an adolescent with early-onset depression with high familial loading, and with associated specific prefrontal volumetric differences, has an illness that most likely results from an altered neurodevelopmental process potentially related to specific serotonin-related polymorphisms (Todd and Botteron 2001). In the other case, late-onset MDD that may appear very similar phenotypically and symptomatically may instead be related to subtle cerebrovascular changes that disrupt connections between structures that are essential in affective regulation (Steffens and Krishnan 1998). Although these are extreme examples of divergent mechanisms, they clearly illustrate the types of pathophysiologic heterogeneity that are not well characterized by the current DSM nosology.

Functional Neuroimaging

Functional neuroimaging methods examine brain activity through measures related to energy metabolism, such as rates of glucose and oxygen utilization and cerebral blood flow (CBF). Methods include PET for glucose metabolism and CBF, single photon emission computed tomography

(SPECT) for CBF, and fMRI for changes in signal intensity attributable to CBF.

Imaging studies have examined a wide variety of psychiatric diagnoses, including schizophrenia and other psychotic disorders (Bertolino et al. 2000; Buchsbaum et al. 1996; Farde 1997; Gur et al. 1995; Kapur et al. 2000; J.J. Kim et al. 2000; Laruelle 2000; D.D. Miller et al. 2001; Mitchell et al. 2001; Perlstein et al. 2001; Ragland et al. 2001; J.A. Stanley et al. 2000), mood (Brody et al. 1999; Drevets 1999, 2000; Kennedy et al. 2001; Nobler et al. 1999; Staley et al. 1998; Stoll et al. 2000; Strakowski et al. 2000; Yildiz et al. 2001a, 2001b), anxiety (Liberzon et al. 1999; Osuch et al. 2000; Saxena et al. 1999; Tillfors et al. 2001), substance-related disorders (Childress et al. 1999; Kilts et al. 2001; London et al. 1999; Volkow et al. 1999, 2001), developmental disorders (Filipek 1999; Hashimoto et al. 2000; Hendren et al. 2000; Ohnishi et al. 2000; Rastam et al. 2001; Rumsey and Ernst 2000; Schweitzer et al. 2000; Tuama et al. 1999; Zilbovicius et al. 2000), and dementia (Arnaiz et al. 2001; Bonte et al. 2001; Reiman et al. 2001; Schroder et al. 2001). Early paradigms evaluated resting baseline topography of glucose metabolism and CBF in patients relative to healthy participants. Researchers who conducted studies across clinical populations reported abnormalities in patient groups. Most observed hypometabolism or hypoperfusion in patients with focal areas of relatively increased activity (Buchsbaum et al. 1996; Gur et al. 1995; J.J. Kim et al. 2000). It is difficult to compare findings across studies because regions of interest (ROIs) varied according to the hypothesized pathophysiology of specific disorders. However, the cortico-striato-thalamic-cortical circuitry has been implicated in most disorders, which suggests aberrations in modulation of critical pathways that regulate a wide range of behaviors related to cognition, emotion, and motivation.

Clinical features, including symptoms and treatment status, have been examined to assess relation to underlying neural dysfunction. For example, patients with schizophrenia were subclassified by DSM-IV subtypes, by positive and negative symptoms, and by neuroleptic status (Buchsbaum et al. 1996; Gur et al. 1995; J.J. Kim et al. 2000; D.D. Miller et al. 2001; Mitchell et al. 2001; Perlstein et al. 2001; Ragland et al. 2001). Similarly, resting metabolism and its change in response to pharmacologic and psychotherapeutic intervention has been related to treatment response in depression (Brody et al. 1999, 2001; Kennedy et al. 2001; Yildiz et al. 2001a) and OCD (Baxter et al. 1992; Schwartz et al. 1996).

Nonetheless, heterogeneity within DSM-IV diagnostic groups and individual differences within healthy participants yield appreciable overlap in the distribution of physiologic activity between those with the disorder and unaffected control subjects. Furthermore, the issue of specificity has received limited attention, and direct comparison among disorders that share clinical features have been rare.

The field has shifted to activation paradigms with application of specific neurobehavioral probes designed to examine recruitment of circuitry hypothesized to underlie observed abnormalities (Childress et al. 1999; Kilts et al. 2001; J.J. Kim et al. 2000; Liberzon et al. 1999; Mitchell et al. 2001; Ragland et al. 2001; Schweitzer et al. 2000; Tillfors et al. 2001). These probe paradigms rely on multiple measures of physiologic activity obtained during differing conditions such as task performance or sensory stimulation. The activation paradigms are aimed at identifying brain circuits recruited during specific processes and conditions in healthy people and relate abnormalities in patients to the behavioral manifestations of disorders. This approach requires multiple measurements, the number of which has been constrained in isotopic studies because of exposure to ionizing radiation. Because of its temporal and spatial resolution, lack of radiation, and availability, fMRI has become the major tool for this research methodology (Mitchell et al. 2001; Perlstein et al. 2001). The ability to couple CBF changes to specific stimuli using event-related approaches, analogous to event-related potentials (ERPs) used in electrophysiology, afford additional means of tracing the cascade of neural events associated with information processing (Mitchell et al. 2001; Perlstein et al. 2001). Thus, fMRI has helped push neuroscience frontiers to critical examination of fundamental processes underlying memory, emotion, reward, and executive monitoring. Understanding these processes in healthy people is a prerequisite for advancing research in psychiatric disorders where these capacities are affected.

In vivo proton and phosphorus MRS is a noninvasive method for measuring biochemical parameters in ROIs. Qualitative and quantitative spectral analyses provide information on cellular metabolism and molecular structure, such as membrane phospholipids and *N*-acetylaspartate (NAA), a measure of neuronal integrity. Whereas most MRS studies in psychiatry have been conducted in schizophrenia (Bertolino et al. 2000; J.A. Stanley et al. 2000), there is a growing literature on mood (Yildiz et al. 2001b) and developmental disorders. Although there is converging evidence of changes in membrane phospholipid metabolites and reduction in NAA in the dorsolateral prefrontal cortex and temporal lobe in schizophrenia, reports are still inconclusive (Bertolino et al. 2000; J.A. Stanley et al. 2000). Diverse methods have been applied in cross-sectional studies, which have yielded preliminary data that can advance the understanding of the pathophysiology of disorders but do not provide diagnostic specificity or reliability.

Another window for assessing brain function is the understanding of neurotransmitter systems through the application of PET and SPECT.

These efforts are guided by pharmacologic studies and advances in neuroreceptor subtyping. Human neuroreceptor studies have built on progress with in vitro binding measurements of receptor affinity and neuroreceptor autoradiography. Initial investigations have examined antipsychotic agents in patients with schizophrenia. PET studies have suggested that, across antipsychotic agents, the degree of dopamine type 2 receptor (D_2) occupancy relates to clinical response and extrapyramidal signs (Farde 1997; Kapur et al. 2000; Laruelle 2000). The introduction of atypical antipsychotics has been accompanied by PET studies of typical and atypical receptor profiles (D.D. Miller et al. 2001; Soares and Innis 1999). The role of 5-HT_{2A} receptor blockage in the therapeutic effects of atypical antipsychotic drugs is currently scrutinized, as is the role of the D_4 receptor subtype. The role of serotonin in mood regulation has prompted the development of 5-HT_{2A} and 5-HT_{1A} ligands (i.e., radioactively tagged receptors) for PET and SPECT imaging that have been applied in the study of depression (Nobler et al. 1999; Staley et al. 1998). Although reduced binding has been reported for regions implicated in depression, such as the hippocampus and orbitofrontal areas, the field is evolving and correlations with clinical measures are lacking. These efforts are important for advancing the understanding of the pathophysiology of psychiatric disorders and have therapeutic implications. However, the literature on receptor systems is developing, and specificity is yet to be addressed.

Current Status of Postmortem Studies of Psychiatric Disorders

Postmortem studies have been undertaken in psychiatric illnesses for many years. Despite numerous attempts, many of these investigations have resulted in conflicting, often unreplicable findings. These studies have often been important starting points for new lines of investigation and the generation of novel hypotheses. Most postmortem studies have targeted schizophrenia, depression and suicide, and the dementias, although more recently the postmortem brain has been studied in other conditions, including alcoholism and substance abuse. Postmortem studies in alcoholism and substance abuse are difficult to interpret, however, because at present it is not possible to differentiate between neurobiological changes that represent a vulnerability to these illnesses and the effects of the ingested substance on the brain.

Postmortem Studies in Mood Disorders

Historically, the dominant hypotheses regarding the pathophysiology and pathogenesis of mood disorders have centered on the monoamines. Therefore, the majority of postmortem studies in depression have reflected this bias by concentrating on monoamine receptors. Many of the postmortem studies on monoamines have focused on suicide victims without a clear psychiatric diagnosis, and as a consequence these findings do not necessarily apply to mood disorders. The 5-HT_{1A} and 5-HT_2 serotonin receptors and the serotonin transporter (5-HTT) have been the most studied serotonin-related molecules in suicide victims with or without a history of depression, and in depressed patients who died of natural causes. Most, but not all, postmortem studies have reported increased 5-HT_2 receptor binding in frontal cortex in suicide victims irrespective of diagnosis, compared with control subjects (Arango et al. 1990; Arora and Meltzer 1989; Gross-Isseroff et al. 1990; Mann et al. 1986; Owen et al. 1986; M. Stanley and Mann 1983). These findings, however, are less consistent in studies in which a diagnosis of depression has been ascertained (Cheetham et al. 1988; Crow et al. 1984; Hrdina et al. 1993; Lowther et al. 1994; McKeith et al. 1987; Stockmeier et al. 1997; Yates et al. 1990). Postmortem studies of 5-HT_{1A} receptor in subjects with a history of depression have also been inconsistent. Decreased 5-HT_{1A} binding in the temporal pole and lateral orbital cortex (Bowen et al. 1989) and decreases in 5-HT_{1A} mRNA levels in the hippocampus of suicide victims with a history of depression (López et al. 1998) have been reported, but these findings are not universal (Stockmeier et al. 1997). Decreased 5-HT_{1A} binding has also been reported in superficial layers of dorsolateral prefrontal cortex tissue removed neurosurgically from patients with intractable depression (Francis et al. 1993). The decreases in 5-HT_{1A} receptor found in these studies are consistent with findings from PET studies using 5-HT_{1A} ligands (Drevets et al. 1999; Sargent et al. 2000). There also seems to be strong postmortem evidence of presynaptic 5-HT dysregulation, as measured by decreases in 5-HTT binding, in the cortex of depressed subjects (Mann et al. 2000; Perry et al. 1983). Whether these reductions are a trait marker for MDD or represent a compensatory event secondary to impairment in serotoninergic functions remains to be determined.

The noradrenergic system has also been investigated in postmortem studies of MDD, and again the findings are inconsistent. For example, the presynaptic α_2 adrenoreceptor has been reported as increased in the temporal cortex (De Paermentier et al. 1997), hypothalamus (Meana et al. 1992), and frontal cortex (Callado et al. 1998; Gonzalez et al. 1994) of suicide victims with a history of depression, compared with control subjects.

However, these observations have not been replicated in other studies in which diagnoses of depression were made (De Paermentier et al. 1991; Klimek et al. 1999; Little et al. 1993). A carefully executed anatomical study found evidence of reduced norepinephrine transporter binding in the locus coeruleus of depressed subjects who died by suicide (Klimek et al. 1997), a provocative finding that needs replication.

It is not clear if the differences found in postmortem studies of monoamine receptors are due to cause of death, the presence of depressive subtypes, history of medication use before death, postmortem delay in brain tissue processing, or the type of ligand used in some of the studies. The technical difficulties intrinsic in postmortem studies require a large number of subjects as well as a consensus of anatomical regions and standardization of biochemical protocols before clear patterns emerge.

In addition to the monoaminergic systems, the hypothalamic-pituitary-adrenal (HPA) axis has also been implicated in the pathophysiology of MDD. Hypercortisolemia and increased activity of the HPA axis are well-documented phenomena in clinical studies of subjects with depression. Postmortem studies have found evidence of chronic HPA activation in suicide victims, such as adrenal hyperplasia (Dorovini-Zis and Zis 1987), downregulation of CRH receptors, the molecule responsible for adrenocorticotropic hormone (ACTH) release, in frontal cortex (Nemeroff et al. 1988), and increases in proopiomelanocortin mRNA, the precursor for ACTH, in the pituitary (López et al. 1992). It is difficult to determine whether these changes are due to the fact that a significant subset of suicide victims are patients with depressive disorders, are due to the stress surrounding the suicide itself, or are due to a neurobiological abnormality common to all suicides irrespective of diagnosis. The limited information available from studies in which an antemortem diagnosis of depression was made does suggest that evidence of HPA hyperactivity is present in the brains of depressed subjects. Increased CRH immunoreactivity and increased CRH mRNA levels have been reported in the paraventricular nucleus of the hypothalamus of depressed subjects (Raadsheer et al. 1994, 1995). Downregulation of mineralocorticoid receptors has been found in the hippocampus of medication-free suicide victims with a history of MDD (López et al. 1998). This latter observation is consistent with a history of exposure to chronic stress and/or to high peripheral glucocorticoid levels (Herman and Watson 1994; López et al. 1998).

In animal studies, the presence of chronically elevated glucocorticoids has been implicated in neuronal atrophy (Sapolsky 2000), and indeed, recent morphometric studies (Ongur et al. 1998; Rajkowska 2000; Rajkowska et al. 1999) have demonstrated that histopathological changes in neurons and glial cells are present in mood disorder. Significant reductions in glial cell number and packing density have been reported in postmortem brains of subjects with a history of major depressive disorder and bipolar disorder (Cotter et al. 2001; Ongur et al. 1998; Rajkowska 2000; Rajkowska et al. 1999). These reductions in glia have been described in the anterior cingulate cortex (Cotter et al. 2001), subgenual prefrontal region (Drevets et al. 1997), dorsolateral prefrontal cortex, and orbitofrontal region (Rajkowska 2000; Rajkowska et al. 1999). In addition to glial abnormalities, there is a decrease in neuronal cell body size and a decrease in neuronal packing density in the lateral orbitofrontal cortex and dorsolateral prefrontal cortex in major depressive disorder and bipolar disorder (Rajkowska 2000; Rajkowska et al. 1999). This reduction in cell number may be responsible for the significant reduction in gray matter volume observed in the subgenual region (Cotter et al. 2001) and the reported decrease in cortical thickness in the lateral orbitofrontal cortex (Rajkowska et al. 1999).

It is not clear if depressed patients are genetically predisposed to the cellular histopathological changes observed in these studies, whether these changes are present since birth, or whether these changes are secondary to the pathophysiological process that may occur in mood disorders. It has been proposed that, in individuals with a predisposition to depression, cellular and morphometric changes may be related to stress-induced alterations in neurotrophins, such as brain-derived neurotrophic factor (BDNF) (Duman et al. 1997). Consistent with this view, rodent studies have shown that antidepressants can increase the levels of neurotrophic factors and therefore increase neurogenesis (Duman et al. 1997). Interestingly, glucocorticoids are also capable of modulating many of the monoamine receptors that have been reported to change in suicide and in MDD (López et al. 1999), indicating that there may be a link between the monoamine and HPA alterations seen in mood disorders and the histopathological and volumetric changes observed in this population. It is important to point out, however, that changes in neurotrophic factors have yet to be reported in postmortem studies of mood disorder, although changes in cyclic adenosine monophosphate–responsive DNA-binding protein, a modulator of BDNF, have been reported in the temporal cortex of subjects with MDD (Dowlatshahi et al. 1998). This new avenue of research in postmortem studies may serve as an impetus to forge stronger links between basic and clinical studies and, it is hoped, will increase our understanding of the pathophysiology of mood disorders.

Postmortem Studies in Schizophrenia

The direct study of the brain in schizophrenia has one of the longest histories in postmortem research in psychiatry. Originally these studies took the form of examination of the brain for gross structural abnormalities, followed by microscopic studies searching for more subtle changes, including alteration of cell density, neuron number, and orientation of cells in structures in which cells are found in patterns of alignment. Numerous attempts were made to find gliosis in the brain, which would be suggestive of an active degenerative process. For the most part, gliosis was never conclusively detected in the brains of individuals with schizophrenia. More recently, well-designed systematic studies of this sort have been undertaken and have yielded more promising results. These studies have tended to find abnormalities in cell number, including reports of decreased neuronal number in the dorsomedial nucleus of the thalamus (Pakkenberg 1990).

In a second type of these studies, instead of changes in cell number, changes in cellular density were found: one of the first of these studies found decreased neurophil in the prefrontal cortex in the face of normal cell numbers, resulting in increased packing density of cells (Selemon et al. 1995). Other studies have focused on cellular morphology: there are reports of abnormal cell size, such as diminished neuron size in the hippocampus (Benes et al. 1991), as well as abnormalities of cytoarchitecture in other medial temporal lobe structures (Krimer et al. 1997). Finally, there have been a few reports of cells being found in abnormal distributions, presumably reflecting altered neuronal migration during development (Akbarian et al. 1993).

Because of pharmacologic evidence implicating D_2 and related dopamine receptors in schizophrenia, there have been a number of postmortem studies focused on the dopaminergic system in the brains of individuals with schizophrenia (Joyce and Meador-Woodruff 1997). The most robust finding in all postmortem studies in schizophrenia is increased striatal D_2 receptor expression in schizophrenia, although this may be secondary to prior neuroleptic treatment. The novel D_2-like receptors (i.e., D_3 and D_4) have recently been the subject of intense study. After some initial excitement around the role of the D_4 receptor in schizophrenia, this receptor is no longer as intensively studied, after clinical trials using D_4 analogs had negative results. On the other hand, several recent studies have found abnormalities in D_3 expression in both cortex (Schmauss et al. 1993) and striatal regions (Gurevich et al. 1997), with abnormalities found both at the level of D_3 transcript expression and at D_3 binding sites.

More recently, abnormalities of glutamatergic transmission have been implicated in schizophrenia. Like the dopamine receptors, the expression of the glutamate receptors has been determined at multiple levels of gene expression in postmortem brain samples from schizophrenic persons; although results have not been entirely consistent from study to study, several generalizations have emerged from this literature (Meador-Woodruff and Healy 2000). The α-amino-3-hydroxy-5-methyl-4-isoxazolepropionic acid (AMPA) and kainate subtypes of glutamate receptor are both abnormal, particularly in the hippocampus of the brains of individuals with schizophrenia. These findings are consistent across transcript, protein, and binding studies. In addition, the *N*-methyl-D-aspartate (NMDA) receptor may be abnormally expressed in some cortical regions in schizophrenia. A current effort for all receptor families is to examine the expression of signal transduction molecules associated with individual receptors in the brains of persons with schizophrenia.

A particularly elegant class of study in postmortem brain involves the use of immunocytochemistry to determine patterns of innervation in specific neurotransmitter systems. The most well-studied examples are abnormal GABAergic innervation (Benes 2000) of limbic cortex, as well as diminished dopaminergic innervation to frontal and temporal cortical areas (Akil et al. 1999). Currently, these types of studies target multiple markers in the service of defining intrinsic cortical circuits that are defective in schizophrenia (Lewis 2000). Finally, recent data suggest that there may be abnormalities in developmentally expressed molecules associated with neuronal migration and cell adhesion (Vawter et al. 1998, 1999), synapse-specific proteins (Vawter et al. 1999), and genes associated with neurotransmitter release (Mirnics et al. 2000).

Blueprint for the Future

How Preclinical Research Can Enhance Knowledge of the Etiology and Pathophysiology of Psychiatric Disorders

Despite the advances in understanding normal brain function and drug mechanisms of action, animal research has not yet yielded clear information about the pathophysiology of human psychotic, affective, or anxiety disorders. The development of better animal models is therefore crucial for laying the groundwork for future discoveries into the pathophysiology of these disorders. More information is available for substance use disorders, probably due to the fact that in this case the drug is a critical etiological agent. It also is not at all clear whether available animal models of psychiatric disorders have predictive value in developing treatments with novel mechanisms of action (e.g., an antidepressant with a non-monoamine-based mechanism). Given these concerns, some have argued that there are inherent limitations in the ability to model psychiatric disease in animals, particularly in rodents, given that many of the features of these diseases involve core human functions (higher cognition, complex emotions, interpretation of reality). Although such limitations must be kept in mind, there remains a general consensus that animal research will be a vital part of any combined effort to understand psychiatric disorders. Thus, although it may not be possible to generate a "schizophrenic" mouse, it certainly has been possible to generate a mouse that replicates certain key symptoms of schizophrenia, including abnormalities in cognition and motivational state.

We can identify four major areas where animal research will contribute to the formulation of an etiologically and pathophysiologically based DSM-V. The first is the development of better animal models of psychiatric disease. As alluded to above, many extant models are based on currently available medications and lack face validity in replicating the symptoms of specific human disorders. The forced swim test serves as a useful example. In this test, a rodent is placed in a water bath and the amount of time it struggles, before floating without struggle, is quantified. Short-term administration of antidepressant drugs increases the amount of time the animal struggles, and this test has been highly effective at identifying new antidepressants with the same mechanism of action as existing agents. However, there is no reason to believe that placing a normal rodent in a water bath induces a state of depression.

Better animal models of psychiatric disease will come from several sources (Table 2–1). As disease-causing variations in specific genes are identified in humans, these mutations can be placed in rodents with the goal of recreating aspects of the human disease. This approach has proved highly fruitful for many neuropsychiatric disorders, including Alzheimer's disease, Parkinson's disease, and Huntington's disease, to name a few. Such "humanized" rodents are invaluable in understanding how the genetic mutations actually lead to the abnormalities that characterize the disease and in providing in vivo systems for drug discovery efforts. Generation of such mice with psychiatric disease genes will be a major boon for the field.

TABLE 2–1. Blueprint for the future: development of better animal models

Identify disease-specific genes in humans; once this is done, mutations can be placed in rodents, which can facilitate understanding of how the disease process unfolds and can be used in drug discovery efforts
Conduct studies using genetically modified animals (induced targeted, cell-specific genetic mutations in the brain)
Conduct studies in nonmammalian organisms
Identify genes that determine abnormal behavior in animal models (quantitative trait locus, chemical mutagenesis, enhancer trapping)
Functional genomics (microarrays, proteomics, effects of stress, antidepressants, animal models)

An increasingly useful technique is to overexpress or delete a gene of interest from a mouse. Many such genetic mutant mice show interesting behavioral abnormalities that replicate certain symptoms of human psychiatric disorders. Mutations in various genes have led to mice with symptoms of schizophrenia (e.g., abnormalities of working memory), depression, anxiety, or inattention and hyperactivity. Tools for the generation of mutant mice are becoming increasingly sophisticated. It is now possible to target genetic mutations to the brain and even to overexpress or delete a gene of interest in a selected subpopulation of neurons in the brain and to induce such a mutation in the adult animal. Such inducible, cell type–specific mutations avoid the developmental complications of constitutive mutations and will greatly increase the utility of these animals in studies of neural and behavioral plasticity in adults.

Studies in nonmammalian organisms, from yeast to worm to fruit fly to zebra fish, have their place in this endeavor. The more primitive the animal, the less referable any behavioral symptoms will be for a human condition. Nevertheless, the power of genetics in these organisms makes it possible to use them to identify families of genes and biochemical pathways implicated in a particular phenomenon. For example, a mammalian protein involved in cellular adaptations to stress has been studied in model organisms, where it has been possible to identify numerous additional proteins involved in stress responses.

More ethologically based approaches promise improvements in animal models of psychiatric disorders. Abnormal behaviors can be identified in outbred populations of rodents, or abnormal social behavior of rodents can be elicited by a variety of "psychosocial" stimuli. Combinations of such psychosocial stimuli with particular genetic strains or mutants of rodents may be particularly fruitful in identifying the relevant abnormal behaviors. Greater attention should also be given to the study of nonhuman primates, although use of these animals must be confined to carefully defined circumstances, given the cost and ethical concerns involved.

A second major domain for animal research in building a better diagnostic system is to identify genes that help determine abnormal behavior in animal models. Major efforts are now under way, utilizing quantitative trait locus (QTL) analysis, to reveal the precise genetic variations that underlie naturally occurring differences in behavior exhibited among rodent strains, for example, in models of antidepressant action, stress responses, anxiety-like behavior, and addiction. In parallel efforts, investigators are inducing random mutations in mice (as well as in nonmammalian organisms) to identify genes that contribute to normal and abnormal behavior. Chemical mutagenesis and enhancer-trapping approaches are examples of the tools in current use. Finding genes that control behavior in animals will provide candidate genes to study in human populations and, more importantly, indicate whole biochemical pathways that underlie a particular behavior.

The third area for which animal studies are important is brain imaging. Imaging studies in animals are needed to better understand the nature of imaging signals in humans. For example, fMRI provides a measure of deoxygenation of hemoglobin and thereby reflects oxygen use in the tissue. Yet a majority of oxidative phosphorylation in the brain is thought to be localized to nerve terminals. As a result, brain regions that show an increase in oxygen use as deduced from the fMRI signal presumably contain more active nerve terminals, not necessarily more active neuronal cell bodies, as is often the interpretation. Obtaining fMRI signals in rodents and nonhuman primates, followed by direct histologic and molecular analysis of the brain tissue, will vastly improve the ability to derive neurobiological information from imaging studies in humans. Similarly, PET studies in animals are a necessary concomitant for the development of novel ligands for receptors and other proteins.

Finally, the newly developed tools of functional genomics and proteomics have vastly expanded the ability to study genetic and molecular factors involved in psychiatric disorders. Functional genomics, in the context of psychiatry, generally refers to the identification of genes that are regulated in particular brain regions by a given drug or behavioral state. DNA microarrays are becoming the most widely used tools in functional genomics. Here, literally thousands of DNA samples (derived from mRNAs expressed in tissue) are spotted onto a silicon chip or glass slide. Such microarrays can then be used to simultaneously study the ability of a particular stimulus to regulate the thousands of gene products represented on the arrays. DNA microarrays are being used, for example, to identify genes that are regulated in common by many classes of antidepressant or antipsychotic treatments, or after exposure to various psychosocial stresses. DNA microarrays are also being used in studies of postmortem human brain samples to identify gene products that are present at abnormal levels in specific brain regions of individuals with a particular psychiatric disorder. In addition, different types of DNA microarrays, where sequences of human genes (as opposed to mRNAs) are spotted, are now being used to identify genetic polymorphisms in human populations.

Genes and mRNAs ultimately function through the proteins they encode, hence the power of proteomics, which simultaneously evaluates hundreds or thousands of proteins present in a tissue sample. Proteomic tools are not as well developed as are DNA microarrays, but there is intense research in this area. It is now possible, through mass spectrometry and other protein separation techniques, to identify the thousands of proteins present in a tissue extract or their state of phosphorylation, to name two examples.

Scientists are just now beginning to apply proteomic tools to the study of psychotropic drugs, animal models of psychiatric disorders, and postmortem samples from humans with these disorders.

Ultimately, advances in animal research will contribute critical information toward a new diagnostic system only through an improved integration of preclinical and clinical investigations. Discoveries in animals will define and direct clinical research into the etiology and pathophysiology of human disease, whereas findings in humans will feed back and inform animal studies aimed at identifying the underlying mechanisms involved.

Identification of Disease-Related Genes

The availability of new genetic resources in the domains of information and technology are setting the stage for an exciting new era of molecular psychiatry (Table 2–2). The rough draft of the human genome includes some 3 billion nucleotides of sequence (Venter et al. 2001), a catalog of several million polymorphisms in the genetic code (primarily single-nucleotide polymorphisms, or SNPs) (Chakravarti 2001), and more than 26,000 human genes, most of which were previously unknown and 42% of which remain unknown in function. Comparative sequencing of the fruit fly (Adams et al. 2000) and nematode worm has already defined a list of more than 2,000 genes that are orthologs of human genes, potentially enabling these other species to be used as models for the functions of the orthologous genes. The forthcoming publication of the mouse sequence is likely to have an even greater impact because of the roles of the mouse and rat as model species in neurobiology and because of the very substantial level of structural and functional conservation between the brains and genomes of rodent and human. Advances in technology include faster and cheaper sequencing methods (Tang et al. 1999), high-throughput technologies (including array methods) for genotyping and analysis of gene expression, and full-length cDNA clones containing entire protein coding sequences (Strausberg et al. 1999).

The elucidation of genetic differences among patients with the same clinical diagnosis may lead to identification of new diagnostic subtypes. As noted previously, one research team has identified a subtype of schizophrenia (periodic catatonia) for which there was significant evidence of linkage to 15q (Stober et al. 2000). In a panic disorder study, families were subdivided on the basis of kidney or bladder problems and other medical conditions, and significant 13q linkage evidence was reported (Weissman et al. 2000). Although these results require replication in other samples, this methodology represents a potentially useful strategy for future research by which biologically (and clinically) meaningful subtypes may be delineated.

TABLE 2–2. Blueprint for the future: new tools and technologies in genetics

High-throughout genotyping via mass spectrometry
Draft sequence of the human genome (fruit fly, worm, mouse)
Comprehensive catalog of human genetic variation
New statistical methods
Large data sets
Intermediate phenotypes
Biological traits, disease subtypes, symptom clusters

This in turn may form the basis for a nosology in which fundamental differences in etiology, pathophysiology, course, outcome, symptomatology, and therapeutic response—all of which are of high relevance to clinical psychiatry—are identified and ultimately validated.

Pharmacogenetic factors determine both pharmacokinetics (drug absorption, distribution, biotransformation, and excretion) and pharmacodynamics (tissue response), which in turn determine the clinical effects (both therapeutic and untoward) of medications and are likely to become an important focus in clinical psychiatry. The pharmacodynamic differences may help define new disease subtypes. Across existing diagnostic categories, pharmacogenetic tools could enable psychiatrists to predict which patients would be likely to exhibit a positive therapeutic response, as well as those who would be likely to experience an increase in adverse events (Roses 2000). In a recent study, combinations of multiple SNPs were predictive of bronchodilator response to a β agonist in asthmatics (Drysdale et al. 2000). Association studies in multiple candidate genes have been used to identify the combination of polymorphisms that give the best predictive value of response to clozapine in schizophrenic patients (Arranz et al. 2000b). Such results will not only accelerate the development of a biologically based nosology and subtypes of high relevance for clinical medicine but will also facilitate development of individualized treatment regimens.

A large body of literature demonstrates the existence of substantial cross-ethnic variations in the pharmacokinetics and pharmacodynamics of most pharmaceutical agents. Correspondingly, substantial variations in the genes controlling these processes have also been reported. Research in this area also will serve to further clarify these issues and will render pharmacotherapy increasingly more individually tailored and sensitive to group differences.

Genetic research may be useful in refining clinical phenotypes through the identification and analysis of intermediate (mediating) phenotypes (i.e., biological traits that index genetic liability to mental disorders). Many complex illnesses (e.g., hypertension, cancer, coronary heart disease, epilepsy, and cutaneous melanoma) can be characterized by multiple intermediate biological traits or risk factors that play a role in producing disease vulnerability. In general, genes will not show a one-to-one relationship to diagnosis because the intermediate phenotypes themselves will be involved in more than one psychopathology. Examples in mental disorders include impaired cognitive executive function, which could be an intermediate phenotype in both substance dependence and schizophrenia. Fear and anxiety as found in several mental disorders may predispose to certain forms of substance abuse. On the other hand, the flushing reaction secondary to deficiency of aldehyde dehydrogenase (ALDH) and/or the "overproduction" of alcohol dehydrogenase (ADH) is an intermediate protective phenotype specific to alcoholism.

The potential benefits of identifying intermediate phenotypes are manifold. Such quantitative correlates of disease liability may be more amenable to genetic analysis than disease status itself (e.g., Almasy et al. 2001). The power to initially map a disease vulnerability locus of small relative effect and to then replicate the result may be enhanced through consideration of the effects of such loci on biological traits correlated with disease, and such complex multivariate phenotypes may be used to judiciously sample families for replicating genetic findings (Moldin 1997a). Genetic research on intermediate phenotypes may directly facilitate identification of new diagnostic categories or disease subtypes of high clinical relevance. Ultimately, incorporation of biological trait data into psychiatric nosology can accelerate research on underlying pathophysiologic mechanisms, increase the accuracy for identifying individuals who fall within a spectrum of illnesses related to a core disease, resolve clinical heterogeneity, and enhance prediction of therapeutic response.

Another challenge for future nosologies will be the integration of both genetic and biological trait information into diagnostic classification. For example, the observation that there is substantial overlap in the information from gene markers (e.g., ALDH2 and ADH2) with information accessible from studies of biological traits (e.g., alcohol-induced flushing, alcohol sensitivity, personality, and electroencephalographic differences) suggests a strong need for continued integrative approaches for clarifying the underlying etiology and pathophysiology of alcohol dependence.

It is very likely that most mental disorders are complex genetic diseases involving structural alterations in the genes in question, and postmortem studies may be very useful in studying many facets of gene function and expression (see below). Anatomical studies can help by indicating which cells express these genes (in the form of mRNA and by using in situ hybridization). Such studies will allow comparison of the normal and illness levels of expression of these genes. They can also be greatly informative as to which cells and circuits are directly involved. For example, analyses of postmortem tissue from the prefrontal cortex have identified differences in the expression of genes involved in the mechanics of synaptic transmission, which may form the basis for identifying schizophrenia subtypes (Mirnics et al. 2000).

Even in simple genetic diseases caused by single genes, biological defects can and do express themselves in confusing tissue-related fashion. For example, aberrations in the hemoglobin gene are the cause of sickle cell anemia, with many organs being adversely affected. The gene's primary pathological actions are exerted in red blood cells; the pathology in other organs actually reflects red blood cell dysfunction. Hence, the causative gene may have a direct impact in one or a few locations yet indirectly affect many related organs, systems, or circuits. A knowledge of the function of the physiology of such circuits and indications of how these function are altered, perhaps in genetically altered animals using the "same" alteration or mutation, could point to core dysfunctions lying at the heart of a disorder (Tarantino and Bucan 2000). To make matters more complex, the subtle impact of the several variant genes as they affect and interact within core brain circuits and systems must also be considered. The use of these gene variants as a set in animal models can allow studies ranging from pure genetics through human brain anatomy to genetically altered animals in which these gene changes can be directly evaluated.

In summary, future genetic research will yield information highly relevant for an evolving psychiatric nosology. Gene discovery and the resulting molecular characterization of mental disorders will most likely lead to the delineation of new diagnostic subtypes and to the identification of biological traits (intermediate phenotypes) that correlate with disease liability. Postmortem studies and gene expression profiling will provide enormous depth and insight into establishing new diagnostic boundaries. This in turn will accelerate efforts to localize the molecular bases of mental disorders within the brain, and thereby provide starting points for designing new treatments for mental illness. As may be the case throughout clinical medicine of the future, genetic information in psychiatry offers tremendous potential for classifying patients who have a positive therapeutic response and those who experience adverse events. Ultimately, development of a rich multivariate psychiatric nosology may be accelerated, in which complex information on clinical symptomatology, course, outcome, biological traits (intermediate phenotypes), genetic information, and therapeutic response are directly incorporated into the differential diagnostic process and into the development of individualized therapeutic regimens.

Increased Role for Postmortem Research of Psychiatric Disorders in the Future

The direct postmortem study of human brain of individuals with mental illness is likely to have important impacts in several critical areas (Table 2–3). One of these is a follow-up on gene variation studies carried out in families or populations. As noted, it is very likely that most mental illnesses are complex genetic diseases involving structural alterations in the genes in question. Postmortem studies may be very useful in studying many facets of the gene or genes in question. For example, anatomical studies can help by indicating which cells express these genes (in the form of mRNA and by using in situ hybridization). Such studies will allow comparison of the normal and illness levels of expression of these genes. They can also be greatly informative as to which cells and circuits are directly involved.

TABLE 2–3. Blueprint for the future: postmortem investigation

Is the only method to directly study structure and function of brain and gene expression (mRNA)
Can be used to validate gene variant findings from population studies
Can be used to validate neuroimaging findings specifying the impact of disease on neural circuits
Can be used to identify disease subtypes and drug targets
Can provide data for animal models that can be used to assess the impact of gene variants on development of brain circuits and systems

Another type of information obtainable from postmortem studies is in the much broader context of mRNA expression studies. The studies, in many cases, may well cover much of the entire human genome and the expression patterns of this very large set of mRNAs across many critical brain regions. Although this may sound similar to the analysis of altered genes discussed above, it is actually a much larger problem in all respects: the numbers of molecules, regions, and functions studied. In effect, these expression studies actually look at the impact of the illness in all its aspects (genes, behavior, basic brain wiring, experience, etc.). They also detect the impact of the illness on all related co-regulated downstream responsive circuits and genes. Hence, an overall set of relationships is detected. The challenge is to learn how to use this mass of information. In some cases, it might be possible to refine diagnostic systems as a function of the neural systems activated, inhibited, or modified, or even to move to a correlation between these changes and a behavior or illness of interest. Another value found in these mRNA expression studies can be seen in the nature of altered or affected neurons and circuits. It is likely that medications can be constructed that are not only targeted to repair the effort of key defective genes but are as likely to have an impact on normal genes or pathways affected by the illness. It is probable that most of the medications currently used in psychiatry act on genetically normal neural systems that are only indirectly related to the gene or genes actually involved in the genesis of the illness.

Future of Neuroimaging

Neuroimaging is a burgeoning field, with rapid developments in the methods of acquisition and analysis of data and their application to clinical research. As noted in the previous section, significant strides have already been made, such as the move from simple baseline measures of CBF to activation paradigms that can assess the highly specific regions of brain function. As yet, however, these methods have not produced specific markers for disease states. This may be because of time on task—such studies are laborious and time consuming. It may also be a result of the lack of specificity in the current generation of techniques. However, this is changing. Outlined below are advances that are occurring in the major modalities, as well as some of the new modalities that are appearing.

Positron Emission Tomography

As noted above, new ligands are being developed that have specificity for receptors relevant to psychiatric disorders. To date, these have been used primarily to assess baseline levels of receptor occupancy. However, newer methods have begun to examine displacement, in response to both pharmacologic and sensory and behavioral challenges. Administration of amphetamine has been shown to selectively displace ligand binding at striatal D_2 receptors. Similar approaches are being explored for behaviorally induced displacement. One recent study demonstrated reduced ligand binding, presumably marking increased dopamine release, in the striatum during performance of a goal-directed task that correlated with performance in the task. Such methods should permit receptor-specific assessments of neurotransmitter function in relation to cognitive performance. This has obvious relevance for the understanding, and ultimately for the diagnosis, of psychiatric disorders. When receptor activity is monitored, evaluation of neurobehavioral performance implicated in specific circuitry recruitment will enable direct examination of how neuropharmacologic agents modulate these behaviors. Thus, in addition to elucidating how neurotransmitters modulate behavior, desired effects will have therapeutic implications.

Magnetic Resonance Imaging

Currently, the most rapid advances in noninvasive neuroimaging are occurring in the development of MRI-based methods. MRI can be used for imaging structure as well as function, and dramatic progress is occurring in each area.

One important advance in structural imaging is the development of tensor diffusion imaging (TDI). This method is sensitive to the direction and degree of proton diffusion, and thus can be used to map the structure of different fluid compartments in the brain. This method is currently being developed to diagnose and track structural changes associated with stroke and neoplasm. However, because diffusion is greatest along the axonal axis, this method can also be used to trace neuronal fiber tracts. At present, this can be done at a resolution of 100 μm, providing tract tracing well into regions of gray matter. As these methods are refined and validated against standard anatomical techniques, they promise to offer a quantum level of improvement in the ability to conduct neuroanatomical studies. They will allow us to move from simple volumetric analyses of structure to studies of connectivity. At present, studies of connectivity require elaborate dye tracing methods, which are laborious and cannot be conducted in vivo. The ability to noninvasively image whole brain patterns of structural connectivity is likely to have an impact on anatomical research akin to that of "gene chips" in genomics. This promises to advance not only the basic understanding of neuroanatomy, but also the ability to identify subtle abnormalities of connectivity that may be present in psychiatric disease.

Functional MRI

The fMRI technique currently in widest use is the blood oxygen level determination (BOLD) technique. This technique provides information very similar to PET measurements of CBF. However, because it is noninvasive and nontoxic, measurements can be repeated literally thousands of times in a single scanning session. Thus, even though single measurements are less sensitive than those obtained by PET, extensive signal averaging yields greater overall sensitivity. This provides greater spatial resolution (as high as 1 mm accuracy) and, perhaps more importantly, a temporal resolution that is higher by an order of magnitude or more. Currently it is possible to acquire whole-brain images once per second, and as rapidly as four per second when focusing on particular regions of interest. This approach, like PET, is limited by the fact that it indexes a hemodynamic response rather than neural activity directly. This is problematic for several reasons: 1) the hemodynamic response is significantly slower than the neural response (appearing after about 2 seconds and peaking between 4 and 6 seconds), 2) it is not yet known, with assurance, that the characteristics of this response are uniform throughout the brain, and 3) it is not yet known whether or how neuropsychiatric disorders and/or psychopharmacologic manipulations influence the coupling between the neural and hemodynamic responses. The evidence to date indicates that the hemodynamic response is "well behaved" (that it is stable across brain regions, pharmacologic manipulations, and neuropsychiatric disease processes). However, a deeper understanding of these factors will be important to (and will presumably help improve) the reliability of fMRI applications in psychiatric research and diagnosis.

Several approaches have begun to appear for improving the temporal resolution of fMRI, by modeling the hemodynamic response and removing ("deconvolving") it from the analysis. So-called event-related designs, coupled with such techniques, have permitted detailed studies of relatively transient cognitive events (e.g., activation of hippocampus during memory encoding). The appearance of higher-field (e.g., 3 and 4 tesla) systems has also helped. By providing greater sensitivity, these systems permit the use of measurement techniques that are sensitized to more local hemodynamic processes, ensuring that the signal is closer to the parenchymal origins of neural activity. The faster scanning that is possible with higher-field systems is also being exploited to overcome signal loss that is characteristic of certain anatomical regions of particular relevance to neuropsychiatric disease, such as the orbital frontal cortex and medial temporal areas (including the amygdala and hippocampus). Finally, ultra-high-field (7 tesla) systems are currently being developed that may permit measurements of the hemodynamic response that are more closely related to neural activity, such as the initial phase of oxygen depletion thought to occur within 500 milliseconds of and more local to the site of neural activity.

Because of the limitations of the BOLD technique discussed above, considerable effort is being devoted to the development of magnetic resonance–based methods that provide more direct measures of neurophysiological function. These include methods for directly quantitating perfusion (e.g., spin tagging); imaging nuclei other than hydrogen (e.g., Na^{2+}, Ca^{2+}, or Mg^{2+}, any of which could be used to directly measure fluxes in ion concentrations associated with neural activity); and using contrast agents that selectively bind to neurotransmitter receptors, akin to the use of radioligands with radiographic techniques. Although current progress on these methods has been slow, a breakthrough along any of these dimensions could provide yet another quantum jump in the level of detail and specificity possible with magnetic resonance–based neuroimaging techniques (Table 2–4).

Another important area of progress is in the combined use of pharma-

TABLE 2–4. Blueprint for the future: neuroimaging

Positron emission tomography
New ligand development
Assessment of neurotransmitter release (drugs, behavior)
Magnetic resonance imaging
Structural tensor diffusion imaging (connectivity)
Functional "event-related" MRI (greater temporal resolution), higher magnetic fields (greater sensitivity)
New contrast agents

cologic manipulations and fMRI. A critical first step in this direction, when used with the BOLD technique, has been to establish that pharmacologic agents do not alter the nature of the coupling of neural activity and the hemodynamic response. Insofar as this can be shown, then the use of fMRI to measure changes in brain activity in response to drug administration holds great promise both as a research tool and, eventually, as a method for assessment of clinical efficacy.

Finally, a critical area of rapid development is in the methods used for statistical analysis of MRI data sets. Increasingly sophisticated methods are permitting precise localization of changes in brain activity associated with individual mental functions, ranging from basic sensory and motor processes to higher-level cognitive and emotional processes such as memory encoding and retrieval, maintenance of information in working memory, reasoning and decision making, and emotional evaluation. Identification of the normal patterns and time course of brain activity associated with such mental functions provide an important reference point for studies that seek to identify abnormalities in these functions associated with psychiatric disorders. However, most studies to date have focused on discrete patterns of activity associated with individual mental functions. In fact, normal brain function involves complex, dynamic, and highly integrated interactions among multiple brain systems and functions. Analysis of such dynamics represents a formidable technical challenge. It would be ideal to correlate the activity of every brain region with every other one and with ongoing measures of behavioral performance throughout the course of a cognitive or emotional task. However, at present this is computationally intractable. Hypothesis-driven methods (such as structural equation modeling) have seen some use, but their validity and reliability have yet to be established. Another approach currently being explored is the use of invertible data compression methods. Sufficient compression, coupled with ongoing improvements in computing power, may soon make it practical to conduct full-scale correlational analyses. The ability to do so, and to fully characterize the normal dynamics of brain function, will be particularly important for psychiatric applications, because it is likely that interactions between multiple brain systems, rather than isolated abnormalities in the function of any one system, are what are most relevant to psychiatric disorders. The ability to characterize the dynamics of brain function may be as important an advance over measurements of specific regions of brain activity as activation studies were over simple baseline measurements.

Event-Related Potentials and Magnetoencephalography

Although current MRI-based methods of neuroimaging already provide excellent spatial resolution, temporal resolution (on the order of seconds) still falls well below the time scale of many, if not most, mental operations (on the order of tenths of seconds). These methods are complemented by scalp recording of electrical potentials (event-related potentials; ERPs) and associated magnetic fields (magnetoencephalography; MEG). The primary benefit of these techniques is their high temporal resolution (on the order of milliseconds). This has great value in assessing the dynamics of brain function, as discussed above. Recording of ERPs is the most practical and widely used method and has led to several discoveries, such as the presence of attentional effects at the earliest stages of visual processing, and signals associated with violations of expectation in language and errors in task performance. Several of these signals have been found to be disturbed in psychiatric disorders, such as schizophrenia (e.g., the P300); however, none of these has yet proved to be pathognomic of any disease. The primary problem with these methods is their low spatial resolution. Because the brain is not electrically homogeneous, localizing the source of an electrical potential is problematic (it is like observing a flashbulb in a house of mirrors—the timing can be precisely determined, but it is much harder to know where it came from). One approach has been to develop high-density electrode caps (having as many as 128 electrodes) and quantitative methods to construct current source density maps. Such methods are still somewhat controversial and, at best, provide spatial resolution that remains relatively crude (on the order of centimeters). Because the brain is magnetically homogeneous, MEG permits more precise and reliable source localization. However, the apparatus is relatively expensive (approximately the same cost as an MRI scanner) and the method is primarily limited to cortical structures, where highly structured columns of cells produce magnetic fields that are suitably aligned and sufficiently proximal to be detected by sensors at the scalp. Perhaps the greatest promise of ERPs and MEG are their use in combination with fMRI, as is discussed under the section "Multimodal Approaches" below.

Optical Techniques

Another approach to improving temporal resolution has been the development of optical methods for measuring brain activity. Direct measurements at the cortical surface of animals have established that changes in blood flow (and, some have claimed, in neural activity) produce absorption changes in the visible and near-infrared ranges of the spectrum. Scalp measurements of activity-related changes in blood flow using near-infrared spectroscopy (NIRS) have also been reported. Like MEG, such measurements are limited in depth (a few centimeters) and thus are probably only useful for tracking cortical activity. Because they provide information similar to hemodynamically based methods of fMRI and PET, they are also subject to similar limitations. Nevertheless, they may have some advantages. First, the apparatus is significantly less costly than those for either MRI or PET (about one-tenth the cost) and is also much less expensive to maintain. Perhaps more importantly, like ERP, it involves a mobile head cap and thus can be used in settings (e.g., homes or remote clinics) and with subjects (e.g., infants, very young children, and patients with motor abnormalities) for whom PET or fMRI are not feasible. Furthermore, continued improvements in optical methods offer hope that they will be able to track the oxygen depletion phase of the hemodynamic response, or physiologic changes related more directly to neural activity, that would provide significantly improved temporal resolution.

Other Measures

A variety of other measures of neurophysiologic function have long been in active use, such as eye tracking, pupillometry, and measurements of galvanic skin resistance (GSR). Each of these has already produced some interesting findings (e.g., the abnormalities of smooth pursuit eye movements associated with schizophrenia). The utility of these methods will no doubt be greatly enhanced as they are integrated with more direct measurements of brain activity (see the section "Multimodal Approaches" below).

Transcranial magnetic stimulation. All of the methods discussed above provide passive measures of brain activity. Transcranial magnetic stimulation (TMS) uses focal pulses of magnetic field induction to either stimulate or interfere with brain activity. Thus, this is an interventional rather than an imaging method per se. However, it has potential to be a tremendously important tool, both in research and in clinical intervention. In research, this technique has several potentially valuable applications. First, although imaging can provide information about patterns of brain activity that are correlated with mental functions, it is difficult to use such information to establish causal relationships (e.g., that a particular brain area is responsible for a particular function). TMS can provide such information: by inducing transient disruptions of function, or exogenously generating activity in a particular brain region, TMS can be used to test whether that region is required for, or is sufficient to produce, a given function. Studies are already being undertaken to examine the effects of pulses in prefrontal cortex on working memory function and the effects of pulses in temporal and parietal areas on attentional performance. Furthermore, used in combination with PET or fMRI, TMS-induced patterns of activity can be used to trace the functional connectivity of different brain regions. Finally, TMS holds the promise of providing a focal means of therapeutic intervention, targeting specific brain areas associated with neuropsychiatric disturbances. For example, recent reports have begun to indicate that TMS in frontal cortical regions may be effective in relieving depression, providing an adjunctive treatment, and perhaps eventually an alternative, to ECT. Similarly, the utility of TMS in temporal areas is being explored for its effectiveness in interfering with auditory hallucinations in schizophrenia. Finally, it is possible to imagine that TMS could be used in conjunction with pharmacologic therapies to increase uptake and/or activity in targeted brain areas to help induce greater selectivity in the sites of drug action.

Multimodal approaches. Although the foregoing list of recent and ongoing techniques illustrates how much progress is being made, perhaps the greatest promise for the field lies in the combined use of the various methods. There are a variety of benefits that can be gained by the integrated use of different modalities, many of which are beginning to be explored. First, methods can be used to complement one another. For example, numerous efforts are under way to combine fMRI with ERP and/or MEG, using fMRI (sometimes together with MEG) to provide spatial information that can constrain efforts to conduct source localization of ERP measurement. Tensor diffusion imaging is also being used to generate better models of the resistance properties of the brain, which can further augment efforts at ERP source localization. Initial successes in these efforts have begun to produce "movies" of brain activity that have millisecond temporal precision and millimeter spatial resolution, and demonstrate the complex dynamic interactions that take place among diverse brain areas in even the simplest conditions (such as observing a flashing light). The use of independent methods can also be important in providing convergent support for a particular finding or in validating a new method. For example, validation of initial β-adrenergic receptor type I (BARI) findings against PET was an important step in validating fMRI (and establishing confidence in the results of each). Similarly, comparing findings of new methods such as optical imaging against fMRI or PET will be an important step in validating these new methods. Finally, the availability of diverse types of measurements, such as CBF, scalp electrical signals, eye movements, pupillometry, and GSR provide a rich set of constraints on the development of theories of integrated brain function. Ultimately, more comprehensive theories will have to be able to simultaneously account for changes in all of these variables. Although this sets a high benchmark for theory development, success should bring with it the rich rewards of a greater understanding of both normal brain function and the complexities of function associated with damage to any one component.

Neuroinformatics. As the use of neuroimaging techniques proliferates, both in basic and in clinical research, there is an increasing need to manage and make sense of the large amounts of data that are being generated. For example, a single fMRI scanning session can generate as much as 1 gigabyte of data, a typical study can involve as many as 20–30 subjects, and there are an estimated 1,500 new studies conducted per year. Thus, on the order of 30–50 terabytes of new fMRI data are generated each year. ERP recording generates equally large data sets. Unfortunately, most of the actual data generated never see the light of day, as findings are usually published in highly processed and summarized form (tables of brain areas activated, or two-dimensional figures). Electronic data sharing has become an important tool in most other scientific disciplines, especially for those that work with large and complex data sets, such as astrophysics, proteonomics, and, most recently, genomics. The benefits of such efforts are clear-cut: they can facilitate the comparison of findings across laboratories (to better assess the reliability of methods and reproducibility of results), encourage meta-analyses that explore phenomena not apparent in individual data sets, and provide investigators without access to neuroimaging facilities the opportunity to conduct research using existing data. All of these scenarios represent more efficient use of data that are often very expensive to collect. The public sharing of neuroimaging data faces unique technical and ethical challenges. However, the strong potential benefits have begun to attract increasing attention, and this is rapidly becoming a high priority for the field, with major efforts beginning to form. It is important that these efforts take into consideration both the technical and the ethical needs of clinical researchers if neuropsychiatric research is to participate in and benefit from such efforts. The heart of any data sharing effort is the definition of the information that will be stored and exchanged. Clinical research brings to the table a set of needs that overlap with, but go beyond, basic research. The data must contain additional descriptors (technically referred to as *meta-*

data) that define clinical evaluations, medication status, and other biological parameters that may not be of central relevance to basic research. The sharing of such clinical information on a subject-by-subject basis also significantly raises the stakes with regard to issues of confidentiality. All things considered, the clinical research community stands to benefit enormously from the sharing of neuroimaging data.

Summary

Over the past several decades, tremendous strides have been made in imaging the intact human brain, and the pace of these developments continues to accelerate. These methods promise to have a dramatic impact on psychiatry. Already they are providing a deeper understanding of the organization and function of the normal brain and of the relationship of brain disturbances to psychiatric disorders. Furthermore, an important new direction is the use of these methods in conjunction with modern genetic methods, with the goal of identifying *endophenotypes*—patterns of brain function that can be linked to a particular genotype—in an effort to further refine the understanding of the taxonomy and mechanisms associated with individual variability and psychiatric disorders.

Role of Ethnicity and Culture in Future Clinical Neuroscience Research

Ethnicity and culture represent important factors that should always be considered in clinical neuroscience research. As discussed above, a large body of recent literature now clearly indicates that ethnicity (population stratification) is crucial in the interpretation of most genetic studies. At the same time, it has long been known that factors associated with ethnicity and culture strongly influence individuals' vulnerability and resilience; determine their coping styles, cognitive response to stress, and the nature of social support; shape their psychopathology, their experiencing of distress, and their clustering of symptoms; and influence the course and outcome of psychiatric conditions. Any future research examining the relationship between genotypes and clinical (behavioral) phenotypes will thus need to carefully consider ethnic and cultural factors.

Although reports suggesting strong ethnic and cultural influences on endophenotypic manifestations of psychiatric conditions are not as robust as those related to genotype and clinical phenotype, there are theoretical reasons to believe that such associations also may be substantial. In addition to specific genetic characteristics, which may vary significantly across ethnicities (for example, the existence of *ALDH2*2* and *ADH2*2* alleles and the sensitivity to alcohol), culture also significantly determine individuals' childhood experiences and influences their social and physical milieu, which interact with genetic factors to determine neurobiological activities. For example, significant ethnic differences have been reported in sleep electroencephalographic patterns (in both nondepressed volunteers and depressed patients), response to dexamethasone suppression test (DST), patterns of HPA axis activity, cardiovascular reactivity to stress, and a number of other proposed biological markers. Together, this literature indicates that ethnicity also is an important factor in research at the endophenotypic level. This may be especially true when such data are examined in conjunction with clinical and genetic characteristics.

In addition to methodological and practical reasons (for the control of potential confounds and for ensuring the applicability of findings across ethnic groups), the inclusion of ethnic and cultural factors in neuroscience research also may be important for theory building and hypothesis generation. Cross-ethnic and cross-cultural replication of findings strengthens the validity of results, whereas discrepancies may serve as the stimuli for searching for refined or alternative hypotheses that might lead to findings with greater generalizability and more universal applicability.

Concluding Comments: A Diagnostic System for the Future?

It is our goal to translate basic and clinical neuroscience research relating brain structure, brain function, and behavior into a classification of psychiatric disorders based on etiology and pathophysiology. It is possible, even likely, that such a classification will be radically different from the current DSM-IV approach. Prognostication is a risky business. However, we speculate that single genes will be discovered that map onto specific cognitive, emotional, and behavioral disturbances but will not correspond neatly to currently defined diagnostic entities. Rather, it will be discovered that specific combinations of genes will relate to constellations of abnormalities in many brain-based functions—including but not limited to the regulation of mood, anxiety, perception, learning, memory, aggression, eating, sleeping, and sexual function—that will coalesce to form disease states heretofore unrecognized. On the other hand, genes that confer resilience and protection will also be identified, and their interaction with disease-related genes will be clarified. The impact of environmental factors on gene expression and phenotype expression will be defined. The ability to discover intermediate phenotypes will be improved with advances in techniques such as neuroimaging. This will all lead to novel therapeutic targets of greater efficacy and specificity to disease states. Prediction of therapeutic response will be possible through genetic analysis and phenotype analysis. Disease prevention will become a realistic goal. Ethnicity and culture represent important factors that should be included in all of these research endeavors.

We conclude the chapter with a speculative outline for a possible future implementation of a multiaxial system that highlights how various facets of information about the patient, each conceptualized at a different level of abstraction, need to be recorded, synthesized, and integrated in order to fully understand and manage the patient clinically (Table 2–5). In this system, Axis I would be set aside for recording the patient's *genotype*, identifying symptom- or disease-related genes, resiliency genes, and genes related to therapeutic responses and side effects to specific psychotropic drugs. Axis II could be used for recording the patient's *neurobiological phenotype*, identifying intermediate phenotypes related to the patient's genotype and behavioral phenotype. The neurobiological phenotype may be discerned by neuroimaging, cognitive evaluation, and neurophysiological testing. The neurobiological phenotype could aid in selecting targeted pharmacotherapies and psychotherapies and monitoring the neurobiological response to treatment. Axis III would be the *behavioral phenotype*, which could detail the severity and frequency of specific cognitive, emotional, and behavioral disturbances. The behavioral phenotype would be related to genotype (Axis I), neurobiological phenotype (Axis II), and environmental modifiers or precipitants (Axis IV). Furthermore, the behavioral phenotype would also be related to specific medication approaches and psychotherapies (Axis V). Axis IV would be *environmental modifiers or precipitants* and would call for the recording of environmental factors that may alter the neurobiological and behavioral phenotypes. These effects would be evaluated in the context of the patient's genotype. Finally, Axis V would be devoted to *therapeutics*. This axis would examine the range of therapeutic options, both pharmacologic and psychotherapeutic, available to the patient based on the data revealed in Axes I through IV. It is possible that certain axis patterns will be logically grouped under broad disease states resembling those that are currently classified in DSM-IV. It is also probable that new broad disease entities will be discovered.

It is our hope and expectation that through advances in animal models, genetics, neuroimaging, and postmortem investigations psychiatry will ultimately have a diagnostic system based on etiology and pathophysiology. Such a system should result in reliable and valid diagnosis, more specific and effective treatments, and therapeutic strategies to delay and even prevent the development of psychiatric disorders.

TABLE 2–5. Outline for a possible future multiaxial system

Axis I: genotype
Identification of disease- /symptom-related genes
Identification of resiliency/protective genes
Identification of genes related to therapeutic responses to and side effects of specific psychotropic drugs
Axis II: neurobiological phenotype
Identification of intermediate phenotypes (neuroimaging, cognitive function, emotional regulation) related to genotype
Relates to targeted pharmacotherapy
Axis III: behavioral phenotype
Range and frequency of expressed behaviors associated with genotype, neurobiological phenotype, and environment
Relates to targeted therapies
Axis IV: environmental modifiers or precipitants
Environmental factors that alter the behavioral and neurobiological phenotype
Axis V: therapeutic targets and response

References

Adams MD, Celniker SE, Holt RA, et al: The genome sequence of *Drosophila melanogaster.* Science 287:2185–2195, 2000

Akbarian S, Bunney WE Jr, Potkin SC, et al: Altered distribution of nicotinamide-adenine dinucleotide phosphate-diaphorase cells in frontal lobe of schizophrenics implies disturbances of cortical development. Arch Gen Psychiatry 50:169–177, 1993

Akil M, Pierri JN, Whitehead RE, et al: Lamina-specific alteration in the dopamine innervation of the prefrontal cortex in schizophrenic subjects. Am J Psychiatry 156:1580–1589, 1999

Almasy L, Porjesz B, Blangero J, et al: Genetics of event-related brain potentials in response to a semantic priming paradigm in families with a history of alcoholism. Am J Hum Genet 68:128–135, 2001

Arango V, Ernserger P, Marzuk PM, et al: Autoradiographic demonstration of increased serotonin 5-HT2 and [beta]-adrenergic receptor binding sites in the brain of suicide victims. Arch Gen Psychiatry 47:1038–1047, 1990

Arnaiz E, Jelic V, Almkvist O, et al: Impaired cerebral glucose metabolism and cognitive functioning predict deterioration in mild cognitive impairment. Neuroreport 12:851–855, 2001

Arolt V, Lencer R, Nolte A, et al: Eye tracking dysfunction is a putative phenotypic susceptibility marker of schizophrenia and maps to a locus on chromosome 6p in families with multiple occurrence of the disease. Am J Med Genet 67:564–579, 1996

Arora RC, Meltzer HY: Increased serotonin2 (5-HT2) receptor binding as measured by [3H]lysergic acid diethylamide ([3H]-LSD) in the blood platelets of depressed patients. Life Sci 44:725–734, 1989

Arranz MJ, Bolonna AA, Munro J, et al: The serotonin transporter and clozapine response. Mol Psychiatry 5:124–125, 2000a

Arranz MJ, Munro J, Birkett J, et al: Pharmacogenetic prediction of clozapine response. Lancet 355:1615–1616, 2000b

Baron M: The D2 dopamine receptor gene and alcoholism: a tempest in a wine cup. Society of Biological Psychiatry 34:821–823, 1993

Baron M: Genetics of schizophrenia and the new millennium: progress and pitfalls. Am J Hum Genet 68:299–312, 2001

Barroso I, Gurnell M, Crowley VE, et al: Dominant negative mutations in human PPARgamma associated with severe insulin resistance, diabetes mellitus and hypertension. Nature 402:880–883, 1999

Baxter LR, Schwartz JM, Bergman KS, et al: Caudate glucose metabolic rate changes with both drug and behavior therapy for obsessive-compulsive disorder. Arch Gen Psychiatry 49:681–689, 1992

Benes FM: Emerging principles of altered neural circuitry in schizophrenia. Brain Res Brain Res Rev 11:97–101, 2000

Benes FM, Sorensen I, Bird ED: Reduced neuronal size in posterior hippocampus of schizophrenic patients. Schizophr Bull 17:597–608, 1991

Bertolino A, Breier A, Callicott JH, et al: The relationship between dorsolateral prefrontal neuronal N-acetylaspartate and evoked release of striatal dopamine in schizophrenia. Neuropsychopharmacology 22:125–132, 2000

Bierut LJ, Dinwiddie SH, Begleiter H, et al: Familial transmission of substance dependence: alcohol, marijuana, cocaine, and habitual smoking: a report from the Collaborative Study on the Genetics of Alcoholism. Arch Gen Psychiatry 55:982–988, 1998

Blackwood DH, Sharp CW, Walker MT, et al: Implications of comorbidity for genetic studies of bipolar disorder: P300 and eye tracking as biological markers for illness. Br J Psychiatry 168 (suppl Jun 30):85–92, 1996

Bonte FJ, Weiner MF, Bigio EH, et al: SPECT imaging in dementias. J Nucl Med 42:1131–1133, 2001

Bowen DM, Najlerahim A, Proctor AW, et al: Circumscribed changes of the cerebral cortex in neuropsychiatric disorders of later life. Proc Natl Acad Sci U S A 86:9504–9508, 1989

Brody AL, Saxena S, Silverman DH, et al: Brain metabolic changes in major depressive disorder from pre- to post-treatment with paroxetine. Psychiatry Res 91:127–139, 1999

Brody AL, Saxena S, Stoessel P, et al: Regional brain metabolic changes in patients with major depression treated with either paroxetine or interpersonal therapy. Arch Gen Psychiatry 58:631–640, 2001

Brzustowicz LM, Honer WG, Chow EW, et al: Use of a quantitative trait to map a locus associated with severity of positive symptoms in familial schizophrenia to chromosome 6p. Am J Hum Genet 61:1388–1396, 1997

Buchsbaum MS, Someya T, Teng CY, et al: PET and MRI of the thalamus in never-medicated patients with schizophrenia. Am J Psychiatry 153:191–199, 1996

Burmeister M: Basic concepts in the study of diseases with complex genetics. Biol Psychiatry 45:522–532, 1999

Bunney WE, Bunney BG: Neurodevelopmental hypothesis of schizophrenia, in Neurobiology of Mental Illness. Edited by Charney DS, Nestler EJ, Bunney BS. New York, Oxford University Press, 1999, pp 225–235

Byne W, Kemether E, Jones L, et al: The neurochemistry of schizophrenia, in Neurobiology of Mental Illness. Edited by Charney DS, Nestler EJ, Bunney BS. New York, Oxford University Press, 1999, pp 236–245

Callado LF, Meana JJ, Grijalba B, et al: Selective increase of alpha2A-adrenoceptor agonist binding sites in brains of depressed suicide victims. J Neurochem 70:1114–1123, 1998

Castellanos FX, Giedd JN, Marsh WL, et al: Quantitative brain magnetic resonance imaging in attention-deficit hyperactivity disorder. Arch Gen Psychiatry 53(7):607–616, 1996

Chakravarti A: To a future of genetic medicine. Nature 409:822–823, 2001

Charney DS, Bremner JD: The neurobiology of anxiety disorders, in Neurobiology of Mental Illness. Edited by Charney DS, Nestler EJ, Bunney BS. New York, Oxford University Press, 1999, pp 494–517

Cheetham SC, Crompton MR, Katona CLE, et al: Brain 5HT2 receptor binding sites in depressed suicide victims. Brain Res 443:272–280, 1988

Chen WJ, Faraone SV: Sustained attention deficits as markers of genetic susceptibility to schizophrenia. Am J Med Genet 97:52–57, 2000

Childress AR, Mozley PD, McElgin W, et al: Limbic activation during cue-induced cocaine craving. Am J Psychiatry 156:11–18, 1999

Cook EH, Courchesne RY, Cox NJ, et al: Linkage-disequilibrium mapping of autistic disorder, with 15q11-13 markers. Am J Hum Genet 62:1077–1083, 1998

Cotter DR, Pariante CM, Everall IP: Glial cell abnormalities in maor psychiatric disorders: the evidence and implications. Brain Res Bul 55(5):585–595, 2001

Crow TJ, Cross AJ, Cooper SJ, et al: Neurotransmitter receptors and monoamine metabolites in the brains of patients with Alzheimer-type dementia and depression, and suicides. Neuropharmacology 23:1561–1569, 1984

Csernansky JG, Joshi SC, Wang L, et al: Hippocampal morphometry in schizophrenia by high dimensional brain mapping. Proc Natl Acad Sci U S A 95:11406–11411, 1998

Csernansky JG, Wang L, Joshi S, et al: Early DAT is distinguished from aging by high-dimensional mapping of the hippocampus. Dementia of the Alzheimer type. Neurology 55(11):1636–1643, 2000

Curran S, Mill J, Tahir E, et al: Association study of a dopamine transporter polymorphism and attention deficit hyperactivity disorder in UK and Turkish samples. Mol Psychiatry 6(4):425–428, 2001

De Paermentier F, Cheetham SC, Crompton MR, et al: Brain beta-adrenoceptor binding sites in depressed suicide victims: effects of antidepressant treatment. Psychopharmacology (Berl) 105:283–288, 1991

De Paermentier F, Mauger JM, Lowther S, et al: Brain alpha-adrenoceptors in depressed suicides. Brain Res 757:60–68, 1997

Dorovini-Zis K, Zis AP: Increased adrenal weight in victims of violent suicide. Am J Psychiatry 144:1214–1215, 1987

Dowlatshahi D, MacQueen GM, Wang JF, et al: Increased temporal cortex CREB concentrations and antidepressant treatment in major depression. Lancet 352:1754–1755, 1998

Drevets WC: Prefrontal cortical-amygdalar metabolism in major depression. Ann N Y Acad Sci 877:614–637, 1999

Drevets WC: Neuroimaging studies of mood disorders. Biol Psychiatry 48:813–829, 2000

Drevets WC, Price JL, Simpson JR Jr, et al: Subgenual prefrontal cortex abnormalities in mood disorders. Nature 386:824–827, 1997

Drevets WC, Frank E, Price JC, et al: PET imaging of serotonin 1A receptor binding in depression. Biol Psychiatry 46:1375–1387, 1999

Drysdale CM, McGraw DW, Stack CB, et al: Complex promoter and coding region beta 2-adrenergic receptor haplotypes alter receptor expression and predict in vivo responsiveness. Proc Natl Acad Sci U S A 97:10483–10488, 2000

Duman RS, Heninger GR, Nestler EJ: A molecular and cellular theory of depression. Arch Gen Psychiatry 54:597–606, 1997

Faraone SV, Doyle AE, Mick E, et al: Meta-analysis of the association between the 7-repeat allele of the dopamine D(4) receptor gene and attention deficit hyperactivity disorder. Am J Psychiatry 158(7):1052–1057, 2001

Farde L: Brain imaging of schizophrenia—the dopamine hypothesis. Schizophr Res 28:157–162, 1997

Filipek PA: Neuroimaging in the developmental disorders: the state of the science. J Child Psychol Psychiatry 40:113–128, 1999

Francis PT, Pangalos MN, Stephens PH, et al: Antemortem measurements of neurotransmission: possible implications for pharmacotherapy of Alzheimer's disease and depression. J Neurol Neurosurg Psychiatry 56:80–84, 1993

Freedman R, Coon H, Myles-Worsley M, et al: Linkage of a neurophysiological deficit in schizophrenia to a chromosome 15 locus. Proc Natl Acad Sci U S A 94:587–592, 1997

Garlow SJ, Musselman DL, Nemeroff CB: The neurochemistry of mood disorders: clinical studies, in Neurobiology of Mental Illness. Edited by Charney DS, Nestler EJ, Bunney BS. New York, Oxford University Press, 1999, pp 348–364

Gelernter J, Kranzler H, Cubells JF: Serotonin transporter protein (SLC6A4) allele and haplotype frequencies and linkage disequilibria in African- and European-American and Japanese populations and in alcohol-dependent subjects. Hum Genet 101:243–246, 1997

Giedd JN, Jeffries NO, Blumenthal J, et al: Childhood-onset schizophrenia: progressive brain changes during adolescence. Biol Psychiatry 46(7):869–870, 1999

Giles DE, Perlis ML, Reynolds CF III, et al: EEG sleep in African-American patients with major depression: a historical case control study. Depress Anxiety 8:58–64, 1998

Gillberg C: Chromosomal disorders and autism. J Autism Dev Disord 28:415–425, 1998

Goldman D, Bergen A: General and specific inheritance of substance abuse and alcoholism. Arch Gen Psychiatry 55:964–965, 1998

Gonzalez AM, Pascual J, Meana JJ, et al: Autoradiographic demonstration of increased alpha 2-adrenoceptor agonist binding sites in the hippocampus and frontal cortex of depressed suicide victims. J Neurochem 63:256–265, 1994

Gross-Isseroff R, Salama D, Israeli M: Autoradiographic analysis of [3H]ketaserin binding in the human brain postmortem: effect of suicide. Brain Res 507:208–215, 1990

Gur RE, Mozley PD, Resnick SM, et al: Resting cerebral glucose metabolism and clinical features of schizophrenia. Arch Gen Psychiatry 52:657–667, 1995

Gurevich EV, Bordelon Y, Shapiro RM, et al: Mesolimbic dopamine D3 receptors and use of antipsychotics in patients with schizophrenia. Arch Gen Psychiatry 54(3):225–232, 1997

Hamer D, Sirota L: Beware the chopsticks gene. Mol Psychiatry 5:11–13, 2000

Hashimoto T, Sasaki M, Fukumizu M, et al: Single-photon emission computed tomography of the brain in autism: effect of the developmental level. Pediatr Neurol 23:416–420, 2000

Hendren RL, De Backer I, Pandina GJ: Review of neuroimaging studies of child and adolescent psychiatric disorders from the past 10 years. J Am Acad Child Adolesc Psychiatry 39:815–828, 2000

Herman JP, Watson SJ: Glucocorticoid regulation of stress-induced mineralocorticoid receptor gene transcription in vivo. Ann N Y Acad Sci 746:485–488, 1994

Hirayasu Y, Shenton ME, Salisbury DF, et al: Subgenual prefrontal cortex reduction in first episode affective psychosis. Biol Psychiatry 43:97–103, 1998

Holsboer F: Animal models of mood disorders, in Neurobiology of Mental Illness. Edited by Charney DS, Nestler EJ, Bunney BS. New York, Oxford University Press, 1999, pp 317–332

Hrdina PD, Demeter E, Vu TB, et al: 5-HT uptake sites and 5-HT2 receptors in brain of antidepressant-free suicide victims/depressives: increase in 5-HT2 sites in cortex and amygdala. Brain Res 614:37–44, 1993

Ingram JL, Stodgell CJ, Hyman SL, et al: Discovery of allelic variants of HOXA1 and HOXB1: genetic susceptibility to autism spectrum disorders. Teratology 62:393–405, 2000

Iwata N, Cowley DS, Radel M, et al: Relationship between a GABAA alpha 6 Pro385Ser substitution and benzodiazepine sensitivity. Am J Psychiatry 156:1447–1449, 1999

Joyce JN, Meador-Woodruff JH: Linking the family of D2 receptors to neuronal circuits in human brain; insights into schizophrenia. Neuropsychopharmacology 16:375–384, 1997

Kapur S, Zipursky R, Jones C, et al: Relationship between dopamine D(2) occupancy, clinical response, and side effects: a double-blind PET study of first-episode schizophrenia. Am J Psychiatry 157:514–520, 2000

Kelsoe JR: Recent progress in the search for genes for bipolar disorder. Current Psychiatry Reports 1:135–140, 1999

Kendler KS, Davis CG, Kessler RC: The familial aggregation of common psychiatric and substance use disorders in the National Comorbidity Survey: a family history study. Br J Psychiatry 170:541–548, 1997

Kennedy SH, Evans KR, Kruger S, et al: Changes in regional brain glucose metabolism measured with positron emission tomography after paroxetine treatment of major depression. Am J Psychiatry 158:899–905, 2001

Kilts CD, Schweitzer JB, Quinn CK, et al: Neural activity related to drug craving in cocaine addiction. Arch Gen Psychiatry 58:334–341, 2001

Kim DK, Lim SW, Lee S, et al: Serotonin transporter gene polymorphism and antidepressant response. Neuroreport 11:215–219, 2000

Kim JJ, Mohamed S, Andreasen NC, et al: Regional neural dysfunctions in chronic schizophrenia studied with positron emission tomography. Am J Psychiatry 157:542–548, 2000

Klimek V, Stockmeier C, Overholser J, et al: Reduced levels of norepinephrine transporters in the locus coeruleus in major depression. J Neurosci 17:8451–8458, 1997

Klimek V, Rajkowska G, Luker SN, et al: Brain noradrenergic receptors in major depression and schizophrenia. Neuropsychopharmacology 21:69–81, 1999

Krimer LS, Herman MM, Saunders RC, et al: A qualitative and quantitative analysis of the entorhinal cortex in schizophrenia. Cereb Cortex 7:732–739, 1997

Lamb JA, Moore J, Bailey A, et al: Autism: recent molecular genetic advances. Hum Mol Genet 9:861–868, 2000

Lander ES, Kruglyak L: Genetic dissection of complex traits: guidelines for interpreting and reporting linkage results. Nat Genet 11:241–247, 1995

Laruelle M: The role of endogenous sensitization in the pathophysiology of schizophrenia: implications from recent brain imaging studies. Brain Res Brain Res Rev 31:371–384, 2000

Lewis DA: Is there a neuropathology of schizophrenia? Neuroscientist 6:208–218, 2000

Liberzon I, Taylor SF, Amdur R, et al: Brain activation in PTSD in response to trauma-related stimuli. Biol Psychiatry 45:817–826, 1999

Little KY, Clark TB, Ranc J, et al: Beta-adrenergic receptor binding in frontal cortex from suicide victims. Biol Psychiatry 34:596–605, 1993

London ED, Bonson KR, Ernst M, et al: Brain imaging studies of cocaine abuse: implications for medication development. Crit Rev Neurobiol 13(3):227–242, 1999

Long JC, Knowler WC, Hanson RL, et al: Evidence for genetic linkage to alcohol dependence on chromosomes 4 and 11 from an autosome-wide scan in an American Indian population. Am J Med Genet 81:216–221, 1998

López JF, Palkovits M, Arato M, et al: Localization and quantification of pro-opiomelanocortin mRNA and glucocorticoid receptor mRNA in pituitaries of suicide victims. Neuroendocrinology 56:491–501, 1992

López JF, Chalmers DT, Little KY, et al: Regulation of serotonin1A, glucocorticoid, and mineralocorticoid receptor in rat and human hippocampus: implications for the neurobiology of depression. Biol Psychiatry 43:547–573, 1998

López JF, Akil H, Watson SJ: Neural circuits mediating stress. Biol Psychiatry 46:1461–1471, 1999

Lowther S, De Paermentier F, Crompton MR, et al: Brain 5HT2 receptors in suicide victims: violence of death, depression and effects of antidepressant treatment. Brain Res 642:281–289, 1994

Maestrini E, Paul A, Monaco AP, et al: Identifying autism susceptibility genes. Neuron 28:19–24, 2000

Malhi GS, Moore J, McGuffin P: The genetics of major depressive disorder. Current Psychiatry Reports 2:165–169, 2000

Mann JJ, Stanley M, McBride A, et al: Increased serotonin2 and [beta]-adrenergic receptor binding in the frontal cortices of suicide victims. Arch Gen Psychiatry 43:954–959, 1986

Mann JJ, Huang YY, Underwood MD, et al: A serotonin transporter gene promoter polymorphism (5-HTTLPR) and prefrontal cortical binding in major depression and suicide. Arch Gen Psychiatry 57:729–738, 2000

Mazzanti CM, Lappalainen J, Long JC, et al: Role of the serotonin transporter promoter polymorphism in anxiety-related traits. Arch Gen Psychiatry 55:936–940, 1998

McKeith IG, Marshall EF, Ferrier IN, et al: 5-HT receptor binding in post-mortem brain from patients with affective disorder. J Affect Disord 13:67–74, 1987

McHugh P: Beyond DSM-IV: from appearances to essences. Psychiatr Res Rep Am Psychiatr Assoc 17(2):2–3, 14–15, 2001

McLeod HL, Syvanen AC, Githang'a J, et al: Ethnic differences in catechol O-methyltransferase pharmacogenetics: frequency of the codon 108/158 low activity allele is lower in Kenyan than Caucasian or South-west Asian individuals. Pharmacogenetics 8:195–199, 1998

Meador-Woodruff JH, Healy DJ: Glutamate receptor expression in schizophrenic brain. Brain Res Brain Res Rev 31:288–294, 2000

Meana JJ, Barturen F, Garcia-Sevilla JA: Alpha 2-adrenoceptors in the brain of suicide victims: increased receptor density associated with major depression. Biol Psychiatry 31:471–490, 1992

Merikangas KR, Stolar M, Stevens DE, et al: Familial transmission of substance use disorders. Arch Gen Psychiatry 55:973–979, 1998

Miller DD, Andreasen NC, O'Leary DS, et al: Comparison of the effects of risperidone and haloperidol on regional cerebral blood flow in schizophrenia. Biol Psychiatry 49:704–715, 2001

Miller M, Banerjee A, Christensen G, et al: Statistical methods in computational anatomy. Stat Methods Med Res 6:267–299, 1997

Mirnics K, Middleton FA, Marquez A, et al: Molecular characterization of schizophrenia viewed by microarray analysis of gene expression in prefrontal cortex. Neuron 28:53–67, 2000

Mitchell RL, Elliott R, Woodruff PW: fMRI and cognitive dysfunction in schizophrenia. Trends in Cognitive Science 5:71–81, 2001

Moldin SO: Detection and replication of linkage to a complex human disease. Genet Epidemiol 14:1023–1028, 1997a

Moldin SO: The maddening hunt for madness genes. Nat Genet 17:127–129, 1997b

Moldin SO: Summary of research—appendix to the report of the NIMH's Genetics Workgroup. Biol Psychiatry 45:573–602, 1999

Moldin SO: Neurobiology of anxiety and fear: challenges for genomic science of the new millennium. Biol Psychiatry 48:1144–1146, 2000

Moldin SO, Erlenmeyer-Kimling L: Measuring liability to schizophrenia, progress report 1994: editors' introduction. Schizophr Bull 20:25–29, 1994

Muthen BO: Latent variable mixture modeling, in New Developments and Techniques in Structural Equation Modeling. Edited by Marcoulides GA, Schumacker RE. Mahwah, NJ, Erlbaum, 2000, pp. 167–189

Myles-Worsley M, Coon H, McDowell J, et al: Linkage of a composite inhibitory phenotype to a chromosome 22q locus in eight Utah families. Am J Med Genet 88:544–550, 1999

Nemeroff CB, Owens MJ, Bissette G, et al: Reduced corticotropin releasing factor binding sites in the frontal cortex of suicide victims. Arch Gen Psychiatry 45:577–579, 1988

Nestadt G, Hanfeld J, Liang KY, et al: An evaluation of the structure of schizophrenia spectrum personality disorders. J Personal Disord 8:288–298, 1994

Nobler MS, Mann JJ, Sackeim HA: Serotonin, cerebral blood flow, and cerebral metabolic rate in geriatric major depression and normal aging. Brain Res Rev 30:250–263, 1999

Nofzinger EA, Keshavan M, Buysse DJ, et al: The neurobiology of sleep in relation to mental illness, in Neurobiology of Mental Illness. Edited by Charney DS, Nestler EJ, Bunney BS. New York, Oxford University Press, 1999, pp 915–929

Ohnishi T, Matsuda H, Hashimoto T, et al: Abnormal regional cerebral blood flow in childhood autism. Brain 123:1838–1844, 2000

Ongur D, Drevets WC, Price JL: Glial reduction in the subgenual prefrontal cortex in mood disorders. Proc Natl Acad Sci U S A 95:13290–13295, 1998

Osuch EA, Ketter TA, Kimbrell TA, et al: Regional cerebral metabolism associated with anxiety symptoms in affective disorder patients. Biol Psychiatry 48:1020–1023, 2000

Owen F, Chambers DR, Cooper SJ, et al: Serotonergic mechanisms in brains of suicide victims. Brain Res 362:185–188, 1986

Pakkenberg B: Pronounced reduction of total neuron number in mediodorsal thalamic nucleus and nucleus accumbens in schizophrenics. Arch Gen Psychiatry 47:1023–1028, 1990

Palmatier MA, Kang AM, Kidd KK: Global variation in the frequencies of functionally different catechol-O-methyltransferase alleles. Biol Psychiatry 46:557–567, 1999

Perlstein WM, Carter CS, Noll DC, et al: Relation of prefrontal cortex dysfunction to working memory and symptoms in schizophrenia. Am J Psychiatry 158:1105–1113, 2001

Perry EK, Marshall EF, Blessed G, et al: Decreased imipramine binding in the brains of patients with depressive illness. Br J Psychiatry 142:188–192, 1983

Pollock BG, Ferrell RE, Mulsant BH, et al: Allelic variation in the serotonin transporter promoter affects onset of paroxetine treatment response in late-life depression. Neuropsychopharmacology 23:587–590, 2000

Pritchard JK, Stephens M, Rosenberg NA, et al: Association mapping in structured populations. Am J Hum Genet 67:170–181, 2000

Raadsheer FC, Hoogendijk WJ, Stam FC, et al: Increased numbers of corticotropin-releasing hormone expressing neurons in the hypothalamic paraventricular nucleus of depressed patients. Neuroendocrinology 60:436–444, 1994

Raadsheer FC, van Heerikhuize JJ, Lucassen P J, et al: Corticotropin-releasing hormone mRNA levels in the paraventricular nucleus of patients with Alzheimer's disease and depression. Am J Psychiatry 152:1372–1376, 1995

Ragland JD, Gur RC, Raz J, et al: Effect of schizophrenia on frontotemporal activity during word encoding and recognition: a PET cerebral blood flow study. Am J Psychiatry 158:1114–1125, 2001

Rajkowska G: Postmortem studies in mood disorders indicate altered numbers of neurons and glial cells. Biol Psychiatry 48:766–777, 2000

Rajkowska G, Miguel-Hidalgo JJ, Wei J, et al: Morphometric evidence for neuronal and glial prefrontal cell pathology in major depression. Biol Psychiatry 45:1085–1098, 1999

Rastam M, Bjure J, Vestergren E, et al: Regional cerebral blood flow in weight-restored anorexia nervosa: a preliminary study. Dev Med Child Neurol 43:239–242, 2001

Reiman EM, Caselli RJ, Chen K, et al: Declining brain activity in cognitively normal apolipoprotein E varepsilon 4 heterozygotes: a foundation for using positron emission tomography to efficiently test treatments to prevent Alzheimer's disease. Proc Natl Acad Sci U S A 98:3334–3339, 2001

Riley BP, McGuffin P: Linkage and associated studies of schizophrenia. Am J Med Genet 97:23–44, 2000

Risch N, Botstein D: A manic depressive history. Nat Genet 12:351–353, 1996

Roses AD: Pharmacogenetics and pharmacogenomics in the discovery and development of medicines. Novartis Found Symp 229:63–66, 2000

Rumsey JM, Ernst M: Functional neuroimaging of autistic disorders. Ment Retard Dev Disabil Res Rev 6:171–179, 2000

Sapolsky RM: Glucocorticoids and hippocampal atrophy in neuropsychiatric disorders. Arch Gen Psychiatry 57:925–935, 2000

Sargent PA, Kjaer KH, Bench CJ, et al: Brain serotonin1A receptor binding measured by positron emission tomography with [11C]WAY-100635: effects of depression and antidepressant treatment. Arch Gen Psychiatry 57:174–180, 2000

Saxena S, Brody AL, Maidment KM, et al: Localized orbitofrontal and subcortical metabolic changes and predictors of response to paroxetine treatment in obsessive-compulsive disorder. Neuropsychopharmacology 21:683–693, 1999

Schmauss C, Haroutunian V, Davis KL, et al: Selective loss of dopamine D3-type receptor mRNA expression in parietal and motor cortices of patients with chronic schizophrenia. Proc Natl Acad Sci U S A 90:8942–8946, 1993

Schroder J, Buchsbaum MS, Shihabuddin L, et al: Patterns of cortical activity and memory performance in Alzheimer's disease. Biol Psychiatry 49:426–436, 2001

Schuckit MA: Genetics of the risk for alcoholism. Am J Addict 9:103–112, 2000

Schuckit MA, Smith TL, Kalmijn J, et al: Response to alcohol in daughters of alcoholics: a pilot study and a comparison with sons of alcoholics. Alcohol 35:242–248, 2000

Schwartz JM, Stoessel PW, Baxter LR, et al: Systematic changes in cerebral glucose metabolic rate after successful behavior modification treatment of obsessive-compulsive disorder. Arch Gen Psychiatry 53:109–113, 1996

Schweitzer JB, Faber TL, Grafton ST, et al: Alterations in the functional anatomy of working memory in adult attention deficit hyperactivity disorder. Am J Psychiatry 157:278–280, 2000

Selemon LD, Rajkowska G, Goldman-Rakic PS: Abnormally high neuronal density in the schizophrenic cortex: a morphometric analysis of prefrontal area 9 and occipital area 17. Arch Gen Psychiatry 52:805–818, 1995

Shenton ME, Dickey CC, Frumin M, et al: A review of MRI findings in schizophrenia. Schizophr Res 49(1–2):1–52, 2001

Smeraldi E, Zanardi R, Benedetti F, et al: Polymorphism within the promoter of the serotonin transporter gene and antidepressant efficacy of fluvoxamine (comments). Mol Psychiatry 3:508–511, 1998

Soares JC, Innis RB: Neurochemical brain imaging investigations of schizophrenia. Biol Psychiatry 46(5):600–615, 1999

Staley JK, Malison RT, Innis RB: Imaging of the serotonergic system: interactions of neuroanatomical and functional abnormalities of depression. Biol Psychiatry 44:534–549, 1998

Stanley JA, Pettegrew JW, Keshavan MS: Magnetic resonance spectroscopy in schizophrenia: methodological issues and findings—part I. Biol Psychiatry 48:357–368, 2000

Stanley M, Mann JJ: Increased serotonin-2 binding sites in frontal cortex of suicide victims. Lancet 1:214–216, 1983

Steffens DC, Krishnan KR: Structural neuroimaging and mood disorders: recent findings, implications for classification, and future directions. Biol Psychiatry 43(10):705–712, 1998

Stober G, Saar K, Ruschendorf F, et al: Splitting schizophrenia: periodic catatonia-susceptibility locus on chromosome 15q15. Am J Hum Genet 67:1201–1207, 2000

Stockmeier CA, Dilley GE, Shapiro LA, et al: Serotonin receptors in suicide victims with major depression. Neuropsychopharmacology 16:162–173, 1997

Stoll AL, Renshaw PF, Yurgelun-Todd DA, et al: Neuroimaging in bipolar disorder: what have we learned? Biol Psychiatry 48:505–517, 2000

Strakowski SM, DelBello MP, Adler C, et al: Neuroimaging in bipolar disorder. Bipolar Disorder 3:148–164, 2000

Strausberg RL, Feingold EA, Klausner RD, et al: The mammalian gene collection. Science 286:455–457, 1999

Sullivan PF, Neale MC, Kendler KS: Genetic epidemiology of major depression: review and meta-analysis. Am J Psychiatry 157:1552–1562, 2000

Tang K, Fu DJ, Julien D, et al: Chip-based genotyping by mass spectrometry. Proc Natl Acad Sci U S A 96:10016–10020, 1999

Tarantino LM, Bucan M: Dissection of behavior and psychiatric disorders using the mouse as a model. Hum Mol Genet 9:953–965, 2000

Tillfors M, Furmark T, Marteinsdottir I, et al: Cerebral blood flow in subjects with social phobia during stressful speaking tasks: a PET study. Am J Psychiatry 158:1220–1226, 2001

Todd RT, Botteron KN: Family, genetic and imaging studies of early onset depression. Child Adolesc Psychiatr Clin N Am 10:375–390, 2001

True WR, Xian H, Scherrer JF, et al: Common genetic vulnerability for nicotine and alcohol dependence in men. Arch Gen Psychiatry 56:655–661, 1999

Tuama LA, Dickstein DP, Neeper R, et al: Functional brain imaging in neuropsychiatric disorders of childhood. J Child Neurol 14(4):207–221, 1999

van Beek N, Griez E: Reactivity to a 35% CO2 challenge in healthy first-degree relatives of patients with panic disorder. Biol Psychiatry 47:830–835, 2000

Vawter MP, Cannon-Spoor HE, Hemperly JJ, et al: Abnormal expression of cell recognition molecules in schizophrenia. Exp Neurol 149:424–432, 1998

Vawter MP, Howard AL, Hyde TM, et al: Alterations of hippocampal secreted N-CAM in bipolar disorder and synaptophysin in schizophrenia. Mol Psychiatry 4:467–475, 1999

Venter JC, Adams MD, Myers EW, et al: The sequence of the human genome. Science 291:1304–1351, 2001

Volkow ND, Fowler JS, Wang GJ: Imaging studies on the role of dopamine in cocaine reinforcement and addiction in humans. J Psychopharmacol 13:337–345, 1999

Volkow ND, Ding YS, Fowler JS, et al: Imaging brain cholinergic activity with positron emission tomography: its role in the evaluation of cholinergic treatments in Alzheimer's dementia. Biol Psychiatry 49:211–220, 2001

Weissman MM, Fyer AJ, Haghighi F, et al: Potential panic disorder syndrome: clinical and genetic linkage evidence. Am J Med Genet 96:24–35, 2000

Wickramaratne PJ, Warner V, Weissman MM: Selecting early onset MDD probands for genetic studies: results from a longitudinal high-risk study. Am J Med Genet 96:93–101, 2000

Wolff M, Alsobrook JP, Pauls DL: Genetic aspects of obsessive-compulsive disorder. Psychiatr Clin North Am 23:535–544, 2000

Yates M, Leake A, Candy JM, et al: 5HT2 receptor changes in major depression. Biol Psychiatry 27:489–496, 1990

Yildiz A, Demopulos CM, Moore CM, et al: Effect of lithium on phosphoinositide metabolism in human brain: a proton decoupled ^{31}P magnetic resonance spectroscopy study. Biol Psychiatry 50:3–8, 2001a

Yildiz A, Sachs GS, Dorer DJ, et al: 31P nuclear magnetic resonance spectroscopy findings in bipolar illness: a meta-analysis. Psychiatry Res 106:181–191, 2001b

Zilbovicius M, Boddaert N, Belin P, et al: Temporal lobe dysfunction in childhood autism: a PET study. Am J Psychiatry 157:1988–1993, 2000

CHAPTER 3

Advances in Developmental Science and DSM-V

Daniel S. Pine, M.D., Margarita Alegria, Ph.D., Edwin H. Cook Jr., M.D., E. Jane Costello, Ph.D., Ronald E. Dahl, M.D., Doreen Koretz, Ph.D., Kathleen R. Merikangas, Ph.D., Allan L. Reiss, M.D., Benedetto Vitiello, M.D.

In this chapter we highlight recent progress in developmental neuroscience, genetics, psychology, psychopathology, and epidemiology that will influence psychiatric classification in the next decade. We then outline a research agenda for future studies that will inform developmental aspects of the classification. Given the breadth of this purpose, the chapter cannot include an exhaustive review of all the relevant areas of developmental science (for an overview, see Cairns et al. 1996). Rather, we draw on examples from a range of areas. Because of the rapid changes in behavior, emotion, and cognition that occur during the first two decades of life, we concentrate on this period, although we do provide some discussion of developmental issues as they relate to adulthood.

Our approach to development is encapsulated by the concept of bioecology, as articulated by Uri Bronfenbrenner over the past several decades:

> [Bioecology describes] the progressive, mutual accommodation, throughout the life span, between a growing human organism and the changing immediate environment in which it lives, as this process is affected by relations obtaining within and between these immediate settings, as well as the larger social contexts, both formal and informal, in which the settings are embedded. (Bronfenbrenner 1977, p. 514)

We acknowledge the invaluable assistance of Dr. Mina Dulcan and Natalie Ivanovs.

The individual is seen as existing in, and in some ways the product of, a series of *nested environments or systems.* Development involves interactions between the individual and these nested systems through a transactional process, whereby the individual affects the environment, which, in turn, affects the individual. Broad advances over the past few decades in many areas of developmental science provide a rare opportunity to embrace this perspective. We consider these issues in four stages. First, the bioecological perspective emphasizes aspects of culture and context at every level of interaction. As a result, the initial section of the chapter describes the manner in which contextual, ethnic, and cultural issues affect and are affected by nosology. The issues are relevant across the life course, but they remain particularly significant during childhood. Second, the chapter summarizes key advances and the subsequent questions in four areas of developmental science as they relate to nosology. Seeking the answers to these questions may provide novel opportunities for scientific breakthrough in the coming decades. Third, we outline the manner in which the current nosology in DSM-IV has set the stage for extending these advances, providing a backdrop for the current research agenda. Fourth, we propose a research agenda for the next decade contained within six areas of inquiry.

Culture, Context, and Development

The goal of current taxonomies, exemplified by the systems of DSM and of the World Health Organization's International Classification of Diseases volumes (ICD), has been to provide definitions of mental disorders that, as far as possible, are applicable across age groups, genders, ethnicities, and contexts. Nevertheless, various aspects of psychopathology have been shown to vary by culture and context as well as by developmental stage (Guarnaccia and Rogler 1999; Weisz et al. 1993), emphasizing the potential impact of contextual factors on nosology (see Chapter 6 in this volume for a more detailed discussion about effects of culture on diagnosis). Moreover, framing symptomatic manifestations within culture, context, and developmental stage may also provide clinicians with alternative explanations for behaviors, possible causes of symptoms, and information useful in teasing apart the developmental relationship between symptoms of psychiatric disorders and nondisordered deviance (Bornstein et al. 1998; Lewis-Fernandez and Kleinman 1994). Clinicians should recognize the complexity involved when symptoms can be framed in multiple potentially distinct contextual frames of reference. For example, variations in culture and in environmental disadvantage each represent distinct realms of context that might differentially influence perspectives on symptoms.

Consensus has not emerged on the extent to which considerations of cultural diversity should be incorporated into the assessment of psychopathology (Canino and Lewis-Fernandez 1997). DSM-IV does contain an appendix devoted to culture-bound syndromes, such as *ataque de nervios*, and their association with syndromes, such as panic disorder, that appear in the main text. Moreover, for each disorder in the main text, DSM-IV includes a section "Specific Culture, Age, and Gender Features" that is intended to provide guidance to the clinician concerning variations in the presentation of the disorder that may be attributable to the individual's cultural setting, developmental stage, or gender. Nevertheless, DSM-IV usually treats cultural and contextual factors as relatively removed from symptomatic manifestations and diagnostic formulation, implicitly assuming that the relation between symptoms and illness is universal across contexts or cultures. For some psychiatric disorders, a universal view of illness is consistent with data documenting an impact by context in general and culture in particular on *rates* of illness, as opposed to prototypical manifestations of an illness. For other disorders, however, DSM does not adequately consider the possibility that context affects prototypical manifestations of an illness. In these scenarios, a universal approach to illness in clinical inference may present problems, possibly increasing the chance of misdiagnosis by erroneous inference.

Neighborhood and other environmental contextual factors have long been recognized as mediators of development as well as sources of variation in the nature of youth behaviors and stressors. Concern about rising levels of community violence in the early 1990s led several investigators to document the influence of context, in the form of violence exposure, on the psychosocial development of children and adolescents (Freeman et al. 1993; Gladstein et al. 1992). Other investigators document differences across cultures in rates of various psychiatric symptoms, which may relate to potentially complex interactions among culture, context, and behavior. For example, in a study comparing 11- through 15-year-old Embu youth in Kenya, Thai youth, African American youth, and Anglo youth, Weisz and colleagues (1993) describe variations in behavioral and emotional problems across various cultural groups. These observations are consistent with data comparing the prevalence of conduct disorder, antisocial behaviors, and drug abuse in children ages 9 through 17 years from Atlanta, Georgia; New Haven, Connecticut; San Juan, Puerto Rico; and Westchester County, New York (Shaffer et al. 1996). Significantly lower rates of behavior disorders in Puerto Rican samples than in mainland samples raise questions about the role of cultural factors in behavior disorders, although it is not clear how much of this difference is due to differences in the prevailing culture as opposed to other site difference (e.g., differences in methods of population selection). These data suggest possible protective roles for microenvironmental factors (such as strong familism) or broader contextual factors (such as intense community supervision) in reducing the risk for antisocial and substance use disorders.

A similar role for context emerges from data documenting marked differences in alcohol use by U.S.–born Latino adolescents compared with their recently arrived immigrant counterparts. Gil and colleagues (2000) showed that as traditional values of familism, cohesion, and social control deteriorate over time for U.S.–born Latinos, greater predisposition emerges toward alcohol involvement. Such findings might suggest that a latent predisposition to alcoholism requires environmental provocation. Likewise, studies showing higher rates of conduct disorders among offspring of two parents with a mental disorder versus individuals with only one parent having a mental disorder, irrespective of the specific parental disorders, highlight the importance of the familial environment in the development of behavioral symptoms and disorders (Merikangas et al. 1998).

Finally, contextual factors can also interact with other variables to moderate behavioral outcomes. For example, two studies in rural North Carolina documented the interaction of individual, familial, and environmental factors in the development of psychopathology (Costello et al. 1999c, 2001). These studies demonstrated that growing up in a family living below the federal poverty line was strongly associated with the development of psychiatric disorders in Caucasian children, but not in either American Indian (Costello et al. 1999c) or African American children (Costello et al. 2001), despite the much higher levels of poverty in both minority groups.

In each of these areas, contextual factors have been shown to affect either the expression of particular behaviors or the risk for psychopathology during development. Such effects of context on diagnosis have been found in studies relying on a psychiatric nosology that is designed for use across multiple contexts, and they demonstrate the limitations of a "universal" taxonomy.

Progress in Developmental Science: An Opportunity to Enhance Taxonomy

The past decade of research in the human sciences, particularly in the developmental sciences, has created a unique opportunity to broaden the range of expertise used in refining taxonomies pertinent to developmental psychopathology. Five specific areas of knowledge are briefly reviewed in the following sections. Twenty years ago, these areas barely existed as separate disciplines, but they have now emerged as full-fledged academic specialties, each holding the potential to significantly affect psychiatric nosology. We review scientific advances in these five areas, with an emphasis on questions that follow in the wake of these advances.

Developmental Neuroscience

Symptoms of psychiatric disorders reflect perturbations in brain function. Factors affecting brain function arise from genetic influences, both postnatal and prenatal environmental factors, and gene-environment interactions, all intersecting at the level of neural development and functional neuroanatomy. Although progress in neuroscience research relevant to childhood-onset mental disorders has been rapidly accelerating over the past two decades (Giedd et al. 1999; Kolb et al. 1998; Meaney et al. 1993; Paus et al. 1999; Reiss et al. 2000), much more information will be required before a complete diagnostic system based on brain structure and function can be implemented. However, even before such a comprehensive system can be put in place, classification of psychiatric symptoms should be consistent with current understandings of brain development and function whenever possible.

Appreciating the role that perturbations in brain function play in the expression of psychopathology involves understanding the interplay between person-specific and contextual factors. As an example, genetic or other person-specific factors may predispose individuals to one or another contextual risk factor capable of perturbing brain function (e.g., temperamental factors may predispose to substance use that affects brain development; psychiatric disorders may act as precipitants of life events). Conversely, contextual factors may show similarly complex relationships with person-specific factors (e.g., the environment associated with maternal depression may influence an individual's neurophysiologic response to stress or to early trauma). Recent clinical studies have stimulated interest in developmental approaches to psychopathology that resonate with data from the neurosciences. This interest is reflected in recent research on various syndromes, from the major psychoses (Marenco and Weinberger 2000) to the anxiety disorders (Merikangas et al. 1999). Such an emphasis in clinical research resonates with a recent emphasis on development in neuroscience. Studies throughout the 1980s noted the potentially plastic nature of the mammalian nervous system, demonstrating both "experience-dependent" and "experience-expectant" changes in neural structure and function (Goldman-Rakic 1987; Greenough et al. 1987; Klintsova and Greenough 1999). This was followed by work describing plasticity in somatosensory receptive fields and other aspects of sensory organization

(Buonomano and Merzenich 1998; Kolb et al. 1998).

In the area of emotional regulation, research on hormone-brain interactions stimulated studies revealing long-term impacts of early life experience on brain systems responsible for stress regulation (Liu et al. 1997; McEwen 1998; Meaney et al. 1993). Advances in basic science provided increasingly detailed knowledge about various forms of neural plasticity (Gould et al. 2000; Shors et al. 2001), whereas advances in clinical science offered evidence that the brains of humans exhibit considerable change in structure and function well into the second decade of life (Giedd et al. 1999; Paus et al. 1999). Taken together, such work emphasizes the potential role of brain plasticity in normal as well as pathological development.

Integrating neuroscience advances into taxonomy will require integration between research on mind and on brain. As currently studied by mental health researchers, the mind includes a constellation of cognitive and emotional states that might be induced by one or another specific event. Given the current pace of discoveries in genetics and brain function, future investigations of the mind must emphasize, at every opportunity, the relation to functioning of the brain, as it is capable of being observed and measured with modern techniques in the neurosciences. Neuroscience research is at an exciting, albeit early, stage in describing the development of both typical and atypical brain function in children and adolescents. Because of the categorical nature of the current DSM classification system, findings from neuroscience research, which are often noncategorical in nature, may be difficult to integrate into the current nosology. The degree to which this will be possible in the future may depend on the flexibility of the clinical diagnostic system.

Given the hope of eventually integrating neuroscience and nosology, it is important to encourage a rich and steady dialogue between research domains pertaining to clinical aspects of mental syndromes as well as aspects of basic brain development and function. Such dialogue will eventually provide insights both for classification and for understanding the dimensionality of basic brain function. Three sets of examples illustrate the potential mutual benefit for both clinical and basic areas of research. First, in the area of arousal regulation, research on clinical aspects of narcolepsy outlined a set of basic symptom domains that provided a template for basic research on mechanisms that regulate sleep and arousal (Nishino et al. 2000). This provided the basis for molecular studies delineating the role of specific genes and their products in narcolepsy, which in turn set the stage for novel therapies (Mignot 2000; Nishino et al. 2000). Research on memory provides a second example; clinical studies delineated dissociations between groups of memory functions that were either retained or lost following medial temporal lobe damage. These clinical observations led to basic research on the neural basis and development of such memory functions in animals and humans (Squire and Kandel 1999). Third, particular chromosomal deletion and single-gene disorders are associated with increased risk for neurobehavioral phenotypes that cross the boundaries and dimensions of psychopathology. Examples include an increase in risk for autism-spectrum disorders in maternally inherited 15q11-q13 duplications, Angelman syndrome, MECP2 mutations, fragile X syndrome, and tuberous sclerosis; psychosis in velo-cranial-facial syndrome; reading disorder in Klinefelter's syndrome; compulsive behavior in Prader-Willi syndrome; and attention dysfunction in Turner's syndrome (Eliez et al. 2001; Reiss et al. 2000).

Developmental Genetics

Both clinical and basic research over the past two decades emphasizes the need to expand underlying knowledge in genetics. From the basic science perspective, the sequencing of the human genome raises innumerable questions with respect to behavioral correlates of gene function. From the clinical perspective, the consistent association between mental syndromes in parents and their children raises questions about mechanisms that produce these associations. This enormous and rapidly expanding area of research challenges the current taxonomy. For example, the results of twin studies suggest that it may be necessary to revise the view of relationships between some psychiatric syndromes, such as anxiety and depression, across development (Silberg et al. 1999). Similarly, questions arise from molecular genetic studies that have identified genetic causes of neurodevelopmental and neuropsychiatric syndromes. These studies demonstrate both clinical heterogeneity across individuals with common genetic abnormalities and genetic heterogeneity across individuals with comparable behavioral phenotypes. Such research raises basic questions about the degree to which psychiatric syndromes with similar phenomenology exhibit unique or shared etiologies.

Although genetic epidemiologic study designs may provide a powerful source for validation of diagnostic criteria, studies have not realized their full potential in psychiatry, especially in child psychiatry. The assumption that within-family similarity exceeds between-family similarity is critical to the role of genetics in testing the validity of nosology. Within-family designs minimize the probability of heterogeneity, assuming that the etiology of a disease is likely to be homotypical within families. These designs reduce the danger of genetic heterogeneity, which has been a major impediment to progress in psychiatric genetics. Family studies can be employed to study the validity of diagnostic categories by assessing the specificity of transmission of symptom patterns and disorders within families, as opposed to between families. There have been an increasing number of family studies designed to investigate components of the classification system (i.e., core features, subtypes, thresholds, boundaries/overlap with other syndromes, and underlying components) and mechanisms for comorbidity by examining the strength of the familial relative risk and patterns of co-aggregation of disorders in families (Maier et al. 1993, 1994; Smoller and Tsuang 1998; Swendsen and Merikangas 2000; Tsuang and Faraone 2000; Tsuang et al. 2001). Family studies investigating early signs of disorders among offspring of parents with mental disorders have also informed classification and risk processes. However, this research could be more comprehensively integrated with adult family study research. Future research that generates hypotheses from data in family and twin studies of adults will be an important source of information on the expression of mental disorders across the life span. Longitudinal follow-ups of these samples, such as those by Erlenmeyer-Kimling (2000), Weissman et al. (1999), and Avenevoli et al. (2001), will be highly informative with respect to both the nomenclature and differential expression of underlying diathesis across development.

Twin studies have also provided important data in resolving diagnostic classification issues. A large body of twin research has investigated a range of issues of relevance to psychiatric classification: the definitions of depression (Fava and Kendler 2000; Kendler et al. 1996), comorbidity between major depressive disorder and phobias (Kendler et al. 1993), and common genetic and environmental factors underlying a variety of psychiatric syndromes (Kendler et al. 1995). Twin studies have also examined operational definitions of schizophrenia (McGuffin 1984), as well as questions concerning subtypes or sex differences in substance abuse (Pickens et al. 1991).

Finally, as noted previously, studies in molecular genetics have identified vulnerability genes for a growing number of neurodevelopmental syndromes, such as Rett syndrome (MECP2) (Amir et al. 1999). Such work has begun to facilitate the merging of genetic and neuroscience research programs. Further research on the range of psychiatric syndromes associated with chromosomal disorders may elucidate the range of psychopathology due to genetic, environmental, and stochastic factors, given relatively strong and homogeneous genetic effects. This includes research on velocardiofacial syndrome (VCFS), Williams syndrome, maternal 15q11-q13 duplications, and Turner's syndrome. Despite these important advances, however, their relevance to more common syndromes in children and adolescents, particularly exaggerations of normal development, has yet to be determined.

Developmental Psychology and Developmental Psychopathology

One of the most dramatic developments in psychiatry of the past decade has been the reawakening of interest in basic psychological processes such as attention, memory, learning, and affect regulation. Advances in both neuroscience and developmental theory contributed to this reawakening. Advances in cognitive neuroscience techniques, such as functional magnetic resonance imaging (fMRI), provide a novel opportunity for delineating brain regions engaged by basic psychological processes. Efficient use of these techniques requires thorough understanding of basic psychological processes and their underlying component processes. Such knowledge allows the mapping of brain regions engaged by perceptual, mnemonic, attention-related, or affective processes. The ability to map such processes, in turn, has stimulated interest in their developmental aspects. For example, schizophrenia is increasingly recognized as a neurodevelopmental disorder associated with perturbation in psychological processes, such as working memory, that are subserved by the dorsolateral prefrontal cortex (Callicott et al. 2000; Marenco and Weinberger 2000). These psychological processes mature during adolescence, perhaps linking risk for schizophrenia, aspects of prefrontal maturation, and cognitive processes that engage this brain region. Similarly, studies in depressed adults document abnormalities in the ventral aspects of the prefrontal cortex and associated brain regions involved in hedonic regulation (Drevets 2001). Hedonic regulation shows marked changes during adolescence, particularly during puberty, a time when rates of depression also dramatically increase (Pine et al. 1999).

Emphasis on basic psychological processes also follows from a growing interest in research on the boundaries of normal development. Developmental psychopathology emerged during the past few decades as a scientific area of developmental psychology that used abnormal development as a window into basic processes, while at the same time exploring what our understanding of basic psychological processes could tell us about psychiatric disorders (Cicchetti 1984; Cicchetti and Sroufe 2000; Garber 1984; Rutter and Sroufe 2000; Simonoff et al. 1997; Sroufe and Rutter 1984). In its descriptive work to map the range of behaviors at different life stages, developmental psychopathology has adopted a probabilistic epigenetic approach to development, emphasizing the interplay of internal factors (e.g., genetic, temperamental) and external factors (e.g., major stressors) in the canalization of behavior over time. As a by-product of this approach, the boundaries between normal and abnormal development have at times appeared to blur. For example, symptoms of attention-deficit/hyperactivity disorder, or those of major depressive disorder, may lie on a continuum. Children who do not meet clinical thresholds for these conditions can nevertheless have significant manifestations of their symptoms (Angold et al. 1999). Moreover, such subsyndromal symptoms predict later DSM disorders (Costello et al. 1999c; Pine et al. 1999). Such observations have heightened interest in advancing the knowledge of normal development, in the hopes of facilitating classification approaches to children who cannot be neatly described as either mentally ill or psychiatrically healthy.

Epidemiology of Child and Adolescent Disorders and Services Research

Large-scale psychiatric epidemiologic studies of the 1980s and 1990s documented the relatively high rates of psychopathology among children and adolescents in the community while calling attention to the possible impact that such problems exert on patterns of disease distribution in the adult population (Wadsworth and Kuh 1997). Understanding the relationship between risk and pathophysiology requires epidemiological as well as clinical samples, because apparent associations seen in treatment-seeking samples can be the result of referral biases that bring disproportionate numbers of individuals with certain characteristics (e.g., comorbid disorders) (Berkson 1946) to treatment. Population-based studies also effectively gauge the size of the problem posed by mental illness by documenting the proportion of the population likely to experience a given disorder across age groups. This provides an estimate of the societal burden from disability and the provision of treatment.

During the past two decades, there has been tremendous progress in the development of diagnostic tools and methods for estimating the prevalence of specific mental disorders in the general population. The Epidemiologic Catchment Area study provided estimates of population prevalence of the major DSM-III disorders based on data from five sites in the United States (Robins and Regier 1991). Data from the first nationally representative study employing diagnostic criteria for DSM disorders were provided by the National Comorbidity Survey in 1990 (Kessler et al. 1994). A reinterview of a subsample of this survey, as well as a new nationally representative sample with parallel national surveys of ethnic minorities, including African Americans and Hispanics, is now under way.

Although these studies have generally demonstrated that the age at first onset of the major forms of psychopathology is in childhood or adolescence (Burke et al. 1990), the studies possess limited ability to identify early forms of disorders, contextual factors, and the precise timing during which disorders exhibit an onset. This limitation derives from the retrospective nature of the available information. The results of several prospective longitudinal studies of population-based samples of children and adolescents show that these retrospective adult studies may seriously overestimate the age at onset of many disorders (Brook et al. 1998; Costello et al. 1999b; Giaconia et al. 1994; Lewinsohn et al. 1999, 2000; Pine et al. 1998, 1999). In general, the older the subjects are at the time of the study, the later the onset date that they report for their illness. The field only recently has begun to generate psychometrically acceptable constructs and methods for collecting epidemiologic data on children younger than about age 9, so it is still possible that studies of younger children will show even earlier onsets. Better integration of such prospective and retrospective research would assist in characterizing the life course of psychopathology.

Earlier epidemiologic studies also emphasized the need to view psychiatric disorders in terms of trajectories across development and through adulthood. From this perspective, rates for some syndromes show abrupt changes in prevalence or inflection points during development, as opposed to steady changes in prevalence. For example, rates of depressive symptoms and diagnoses show marked increases during adolescence, particularly during puberty (Angold et al. 1999; Cohen et al. 1993). This suggests that a quantum change may occur in risk, associated with puberty-related processes. This focus on trajectories also calls attention to the roles played by resiliency and protective factors. Many children who either develop in high-risk environments or show initial signs of a mental disorder exhibit good outcomes (Merikangas et al. 1999; Pine et al. 1998). Unique sets of factors may contribute to generally healthy or adverse outcomes over time.

The importance of such work for prevention and treatment is obvious. Namely, studies in developmental epidemiology that have measured need for and use of mental health care have shown that large sections of the juvenile population with psychiatric disorders are not receiving—and often have never received—any treatment (Burns et al. 1995, 1997; Cohen et al. 1991; Costello et al. 1997). These findings also carry many important implications for the taxonomy. First, descriptions of and criteria for a diagnosis clearly cannot be based on knowledge derived exclusively from treated cases, which may represent a small and nonrepresentative subgroup of all cases of a given disorder. Second, differences between the entire population receiving diagnoses, whether in clinical or epidemiologic studies, and the population of those who seek treatment can reveal important gaps in the nosology. The role of impairment in treatment seeking provides a prime example of this. Individuals in need of treatment may lack the skills, desire, or resources to secure such treatment. Third, the fact that few children seek treatment on their own account opens up important questions about the role of adult-child relationships and parental psychopathology in diagnosis and treatment. For example, symptoms of a mood disorder in a parent may increase the degree to which a child's mildly disobedient behavior is perceived by the parent as troublesome. This could lead to referral and evaluation, despite the absence of any other sign of impairment in the child. The current DSM should provide more guidelines for evaluating children in such scenarios. The potential impact of a parent's threshold for seeking treatment also raises general questions about children's status as dependents, in the context of a taxonomy that may implicitly assume most patients seek treatment on their own behalf. Fourth, the clinical professions have to deal with problems that result from a taxonomy that defines large sections of the child population as "disordered" and potentially in need of treatment in the face of limited availability of appropriate services. The use of strict impairment thresholds reduces rates of psychopathology to some degree. Nevertheless, considerable discrepancies remain even when using such strict thresholds between the number of impaired children and the number of available services.

Extending DSM-IV: Setting the Stage for Future Advances

In the decades since the publication of the first DSM, psychiatry has moved away from a psychodynamic concept of development to one based on empiricism operating within the biological and social sciences. This shift has led to a change in taxonomy, from a system based on psychodynamic etiologic principles to one based on symptom clusters derived primarily from clinical observation and epidemiologic research. This shift has in its turn helped to refine basic research questions, setting the stage for subsequent decades of inquiry.

One major advance in successive versions of DSM was the decision to insist on explicit definitions of symptom groups in a taxonomy that could reliably be applied across raters and over time. This advance created a set of common diagnostic criteria that facilitated communication among diverse research groups, allowing considerably greater comparability of research findings across laboratories and even across countries. Emphasis was placed on a descriptive approach to symptoms and the natural history of mental syndromes. Such research has served to strengthen developmental perspectives on many psychiatric disorders; this includes not only disorders explicitly recognized in DSM-IV as developmental conditions, such as pervasive developmental disorder and attention-deficit/hyperactivity disorder (ADHD), but also other syndromes, such as some schizophrenia and major depressive disorder, that may show early prodromes.

Progress in developmental psychopathology demonstrated considerable empirical support for many of the initial symptom groupings defined in earlier versions of DSM. For example, extensive studies have identified basic distinctions between emotional syndromes, characterized by high degrees of mood or anxiety symptoms, and behavioral syndromes, characterized by high degrees of disruptive behavior (Achenbach et al. 1995; Feehan et al. 1993; Ferdinand and Verhulst 1995). This distinction has been identified very early in life, and, with some exceptions, appears to show considerable developmental homotypy across at least the first two or three decades of life (Caspi et al. 1996; Cohen et al. 1993; Costello et al. 1999a; Loeber et al. 1999). Moreover, within these two broad symptom domains, evidence supports the validity for some of the subclassifications made in DSM. For example, the distinction between ADHD and oppositional-defiant/conduct disorder (ODD/CD) receives considerable empirical support, as does that between phobias and depression (Feehan et al. 1993; Loeber et al. 1999; Weissman et al. 1999). Other distinctions in childhood disorders, however, have stood up less well to scrutiny; for example, those between ODD and CD or between major depressive disorder and generalized anxiety disorder appear to be less well supported in both longitudinal community data (Breslau et al. 1987; Costello et al. 1999a; Pine et al. 1998) and family study data (Swendsen and Merikangas 2000). Regardless, a general consensus concerning symptom groupings has facilitated research on patterns of associations among mental syndromes across the life span. For example, consensus on the categorization of depressive symptoms stimulated research on manifestations of the syndrome across development, leading to research on childhood antecedents of some adult mood disorders (Angold et al. 1999; Lewinsohn et al. 2000; Pine et al. 1999; Weissman et al. 1997).

A second major advance reflected in the current nosology resulted from efforts to revise DSM over the past two decades. These efforts emphasized the irreplaceable role to be played by systematically collected, replicable empirical data. As a result, successive editions of DSM have moved further in the direction of a diagnostic system based on observable and testable clusters of symptoms, impairments, and responses to treatment. Like other branches of medicine, psychiatric nosology has become a constantly evolving mixture of etiologic theory and symptomatic description, with the relative contribution of each shifting as knowledge has accumulated. As our understanding of developmental psychopathology increases in coming decades, so will our grasp of the causes of childhood mental illness and their relationship to adult psychopathology. This will likely increase the emphasis on development in ensuing versions of DSM.

Finally, over the past two decades, the development of DSM consistently recognized the need to conceptualize mental syndromes from a developmental perspective. Accordingly, efforts have been made to create a developmentally sensitive taxonomy by defining disorders specific to infancy, others more common in childhood, others with later onset, and yet others with onset throughout the age range. The current DSM also reflects retrospective evidence from epidemiologic studies of the adult population, such as the Epidemiologic Catchment Area study (Burke et al. 1990; Eaton et al. 1991), noting the adolescent onset of several "adult" disorders, including schizophrenia, bipolar disorder, and obsessive-compulsive disorder (Pine et al. 1999; Weissman et al. 1997).

Despite these advances, there are numerous aspects of the multiaxial system that require further investigation. In considering diagnoses among children and adolescents, the current DSM pays relatively little attention to axes other than Axis I. In comparison with the richness of the Axis I taxonomy, concepts pertaining to other axes remain relatively underdeveloped, incompletely operationalized, deficient in assessment methods or instruments, and insufficiently integrated into the diagnostic process. Although similar questions arise in use of each axis among both children and adults, here we point to some of the specific issues that are particularly salient for children and adolescents.

One particularly salient issue relates to the Axis II diagnoses of mental retardation and antisocial personality disorder. Children with mental retardation exhibit very high rates of mental disorders (Borthwick-Duffy 1994; Einfeld and Tonge 1996; Steffenburg et al. 1996). Aman and colleagues (1996) worked to determine norms for dimensional and categorical approaches to diagnosis of psychopathology in patients with mental retardation. DSM-IV gives insufficient guidance on procedures for assessing psychiatric disorders in the presence of mental retardation, or whether the criteria for other disorders should be modified in some way for children with mental retardation. Currently, most studies of developmental psychopathology specifically exclude subjects of all ages with mental retardation. This policy might even be replaced by one of oversampling, rather than excluding subjects with mental retardation. Appropriate modifications of criteria for developmental level and level of language impairment are needed to avoid diagnostic criteria that are either overly inclusive or overly exclusive.

Likewise, antisocial personality disorder needs reformulation in terms of the axial distinction. Earlier versions of DSM have created the somewhat contradictory situation that antisocial personality disorder (ASPD) and CD are both considered instances of problems with behavior involving disregard for others' rights, yet one is on Axis I (for children) while the other is on Axis II (for adults). This conceptualization appears to be inconsistent with evidence for continuity (Kuperman et al. 1999; Langbehn et al. 1998; Myers et al. 1998; Rueter et al. 2000; Simonoff et al. 1998) as well as the requirement in DSM-IV that adults with ASPD "must have had a history of some symptoms of conduct disorder before age 15" (p. 646). There are also inconsistencies between criteria for CD and ASPD symptomatology that are not explained in DSM or supported by data. A decision for DSM-V to assign CD and ASPD to the same or different axes might be based on prospective longitudinal studies that permit both sets of symptoms to be studied in the same people across the period of risk from childhood to early adulthood (Cardon et al. 2000; Langbehn et al. 1998).

The description of Axis IV in DSM-IV (psychosocial and environmental problems) constitutes a page and a half concerning aspects of psychosocial and environmental problems that "may affect the diagnosis, treatment, and prognosis of mental disorders (Axes I and II)" (American Psychiatric Association 1994, p. 29). With the possible exception of educational problems, most of the nine problem categories make little reference to children. Moreover, DSM-IV includes no discussion as to whether psychosocial and environmental problems should be assessed in the same way for children and adults, or should be given the same weight in treatment planning.

With respect to Axis V, DSM-IV includes a recommendation to use the Global Assessment of Functioning (GAF) scale for "reporting the clinician's judgment of the individual's overall level of functioning." The GAF does provide anchors to 10 sets of descriptors or examples (e.g., "41–50 Serious symptoms [e.g., suicidal ideation, severe obsessional rituals, frequent shoplifting]....)." The GAF's examples are sometimes relevant to children. Other child-based scales, such as the Child's Global Adjustment Scale (CGAS), have been developed. Nevertheless, the current consideration of functioning in DSM-IV suffers from two main problems: 1) level of functioning is often confounded with diagnostic symptoms (as in the example just given), and 2) insufficient empirical evidence is presented in the manual concerning the importance of this area for treatment planning and prognosis, independent of symptomatology. In fact, work done in the past decade shows that for children, impairment is often as good a predictor of need for treatment and outcome of treatment as is the nature of symptoms or diagnosis (Costello and Shugart 1992; Costello et al. 1996; Flisher et al. 1997; Simonoff et al. 1997). Many federal, state, and managed care organizations require functional impairment as well as a DSM diagnosis as a condition of access to care. Yet DSM devotes insufficient attention to level of functioning and its assessment (see Chapter 5 in this volume for additional discussion about this issue). These issues emanating from the multiaxial system provide important opportunities for future research to refine the distinctions and assessment of each of the important axes developed in order to provide a more comprehensive classification system, as described in the following sections.

Defining a Research Agenda for the Next Decade

Advances in nosology facilitated by the current DSM have delineated areas in which specific research projects could add to future iterations of DSM, especially the taxonomy for psychiatric disorders of infancy, childhood, and adolescence. Some of this work will be done specifically with a view to informing the taxonomy. An improved taxonomy will also be an additional benefit of work done in pursuit of other scientific goals. Various areas of research have the potential to refine the classification of developmental psychopathology. We concentrate here on work in six areas: 1) developmental neuroscience and genetics; 2) prevention and early intervention; 3) infancy and early childhood; 4) the multiaxial approach; 5) approaches to psychiatric assessment; and 6) developmental epidemiology.

Developmental Neuroscience and Genetics

Flexibility in aspects of DSM will facilitate dialogue between clinical and basic researchers interested in development. For example, some developmental disorders can be viewed as either categorical entities or the tail end of a continuously distributed trait. The view of ADHD as a category, composed of abnormalities in one to three symptom domains, is not consistent with current perspectives on neural regulation of attention or with the overarching cognitive construct of executive function. A continuous perspective on complex mental functions, such as attention, may provide an important avenue for integrating clinical and neuroscientific standpoints. Similarly, knowledge of developmental changes in brain function may shed light on changing symptom manifestations across development. For example, tic disorders show longitudinal associations with obsessive-compulsive disorder (OCD), with tics decreasing and obsessive-compulsive symptoms increasing over time (Peterson et al. 2001). This may result from developmental change in brain circuits that confer susceptibility to both tic disorders and OCD.

It is essential to stimulate and sustain further dialogue between research domains pertaining to clinical aspects of mental syndromes and neuroscientific aspects of basic brain function in children with both typical and atypical development. Dialogue and collaborative research should be encouraged around phenomena such as attention regulation, socialization, the expression of fear, and nurturing behaviors, which can be studied with comparable methodologies in humans and in other species. There is no question that these areas of knowledge will continue to expand rapidly in the next decade, with the potential to revolutionize many areas of psychiatry. Simply integrating this wealth of new knowledge into a revised taxonomy will be a major challenge. However, there are specific programs of research that could be particularly valuable for taxonomic purposes.

Molecular genetic searches for single-gene disorders or chromosomal disorders will continue in uncommon subsets of developmental psychopathology (e.g., a small proportion of cases of autism spectrum disorders). However, aside from Rett syndrome, psychiatric disorders appear to arise from complex molecular genetic factors (i.e., multiple genes) in concert with environmental risk and protective factors. Genetic complexity should not be seen as less reason to determine genetic risk and protective factors in developmental psychopathology. For example, the insulin locus is a genetic risk factor for type I diabetes that has required 15 years to fully confirm. Although the role of insulin in the pathophysiology and treatment of type I diabetes was known before the genetic finding, there are no developmental psychopathological syndromes in which the equivalent of insulin has been identified as a treatment. Research on familial and genetic aspects of developmental psychopathology should proceed in tandem with studies in other areas. This includes research on brain circuitries that underlie physiologic and pathological behavior. For example, studies in animals reveal associations between maternal behavior and hypothalamic-pituitary-adrenal axis regulation. This association is thought to result from effects on a complex neural circuit involving structures implicated in the regulation of emotion across a range of mammalian species (Liu et al. 1997; Meaney et al. 1993). Similarly, prospective follow-up studies may also provide key insights for research on familial and genetic aspects of developmental psychopathology. Long-term follow-up assessments of representative samples of children with well-described behaviors, such as mood instability or inhibited behavior, can help establish continuities or discontinuities between early emotional and behavioral disturbances and later psychopathology in adolescence and adulthood. Researchers conducting such studies might capitalize on the availability of existing longitudinal data sets to identify specific hypotheses before launching new studies. A number of studies have been conducted using clinical samples of convenience, which are not necessarily representative of general psychopathology. Also, these studies have been done mainly to test continuity between adolescent and adult psychopathology. There is also a need to study much younger children, in whom diagnostic nonspecificity may be the rule rather than the exception (see section immediately below). In such efforts, the field will benefit from adopting a broad empirical approach to the nosology of early childhood.

Prevention and Early Intervention

Although DSM was initially created as a tool for clinicians to diagnose specific illnesses, future modifications should acknowledge the growing emphasis on prevention and early intervention in the processes of *developing* an illness—a characteristic of all of medicine in the current era. This emphasis might follow from the observation that the initial signs of many chronic mental disorders emerge during childhood. Routine well-child surveillance, along with the identification and classification of high-risk individuals, high-risk environments, and early signs and symptoms of brain disorders, represent important clinical goals—as important for mental disorders as for cancer or diabetes.

An emphasis on primary and secondary prevention is particularly relevant to classification systems for children and adolescents, in which an overall framework of normal developmental and maturational stages must also be considered. Research studies of early intervention for children and adolescents are needed. In particular, school-based programs that screen for and modify the risk of developing psychiatric disorders (e.g., children with exposure to violence, with low school performance, with poor peer relationships, or with suicidal ideation) are necessary. Numerous examples abound from pediatrics and developmental medicine in which some form of early environmental modification (primary prevention) or intervention (secondary prevention/early detection) acts to reduce the likelihood of disorders later in life. For example, there is emerging evidence that adult osteoporosis can be reduced by interventions during childhood. These include increasing calcium intake and possibly decreasing intake of carbonated phosphate-containing soft drinks during the period of peak bone mass increase (during the late stages of pubertal development) and also include the early identification of individuals at increased genetic risk for osteoporosis (Cardon et al. 2000; Golden 2000). A second example is provided by the dramatic effects on cognitive development of dietary modifications in individuals identified early in life with phenylketonuria (PKU) (Smith et al. 2000; van Spronsen et al. 2001). The ability to screen for and intervene early in these medical disorders required research focused on developmental processes. Routine surveillance, including regular weight checks and dietary counseling to maintain developmentally appropriate growth, are now accepted components of pediatric primary care.

At present, however, many second-party reimbursers require a patient to have symptoms that meet criteria for a *mental disorder* to qualify for treatment. This stands in sharp contrast to well-child care as provided (and reimbursed) under the heading of pediatric primary care. Research in the next decade must pay attention to the costs and benefits of expanding the concept of primary care to include routine surveillance of, and early intervention for, children's emotional and behavioral health. It needs to consider what are the best settings for the delivery of primary mental health care. Educational settings such as Head Start and Early Head Start already provide delivery of some services, whereas primary care pediatricians and family doctors supply other components. However, a move toward primary mental health care for children requires a dramatic rethinking of the role to be played by DSM in mental health care for children and adolescents. DSM will need to provide guidance on the range and limits of normal development, on developmentally safe environments, and on the boundary conditions that are not diseases but are risk markers. For example, just as there is strong rationale for early treatment of borderline hypertension, there may be certain high-risk categories for behavioral and/or emotional symptoms in children that are shown to have improved outcome when given early treatment. The DSM created for primary care practitioners (DSM-PC Child and Adolescent Version) (Wolraich 1997) and taxonomies for infancy such as that developed by the Washington, D.C., group Zero to Three (1994) are examples of moves in this direction.

Although a clear description of the basic requirements for healthy psychological development in humans is still lacking, the expectations of what these requirements might be affect the psychiatric taxonomy, implicitly or explicitly. Research on environments that increase or reduce risk of psychiatric disorder is vital for a prevention-based approach. Environments and their risks exist at every level—from the intrauterine, to physical surroundings with polluted air and contaminated food or water leading to risks of toxin exposure, to the social capital that communities need for healthy child rearing. An integral aspect of this approach is to focus attention on person-specific strengths or other factors that might help promote normal development in at-risk youth. A second dimension is the issue of the timing of screening and intervention—that is, what are the key inflection points and transitions in the developmental trajectories toward disorders (and the mechanisms underlying these periods of vulnerability)? For example, the sharp increase in depression among females in mid-adolescence needs to be understood with respect to pubertal maturation as it affects body composition, with respect to cultural and social factors, and with respect to neurobehavioral systems underpinning motivation and emotion (Angold et al. 1999; Nolen-Hoeksema 1994).

Early detection and treatment of the initial signs of mental disorders may also require monitoring in the "primary care" model. Growing evidence, cited earlier, converges on the view of many adult pathologies as chronic conditions with roots early in life (Wadsworth and Kuh 1997). In the early years, diagnostic specificity is hard to achieve and may sometimes be inappropriate, given that many children show significant functional impairments in the absence of full-blown diagnoses. Research is therefore needed to characterize developing signs, symptoms, and syndromes of psychopathology in children over time, recognizing the wide variability in, and malleability of, child behavior and brain development and the extent to which children are influenced by culture and context. Research is also needed to identify potential risk processes in early development (e.g., poor emotional regulation, attentional difficulties, poor inhibitory control), associated impairments in functioning, and factors that may protect against psychopathology in the face of risk or that may help to differentiate transitory problems from precursors of more serious or persistent psychopathology. Family studies designed to tease apart questions of diagnostic specificity and changing symptom patterns over time are of particular interest and may provide improved phenotypes to be used in the search for genetic vulnerabilities. Finally, studies should also be aimed at identifying the relevant prototypical manifestations of psychiatric illness, determining precise diagnostic criteria applicable to the first two decades of life, and investigating how these vary as a function of culture and context. Cultural and contextual circumstances that may be contributing or mediating factors in symptom definition and in symptom manifestation need to be studied by cross-cultural epidemiologic methods enhanced by clinical and anthropological substudies. One example would be to conduct cross-cultural studies examining symptom definition (by means of cognitive debriefing) and symptom relevance in taxonomy (by how they relate to negative or positive clinical outcomes) across different age groups, cultures, and contexts. Such studies can help elucidate what are and what are not universally valid diagnostic criteria of mental illness, as well as how criteria vary in significance as a function of age, gender, culture, and context.

Developmental epidemiologic studies will be critical for the identification of subgroups with different risk profiles and course of illness, leading to more specific approaches to intervention. Identification of the temporal sequencing of risk and of the course and phases of psychopathology will inform the development of new prevention and early intervention strategies designed to interrupt pathological processes before syndromes become consolidated and more difficult to change (e.g., interrupting smoking behaviors before the development of serious nicotine dependence). Considering that large sections of the juvenile population with psychiatric disorders never receive mental health care, and that many who do get treated do not have a symptom picture that meets the criteria for any specific psychiatric diagnosis, research studies are needed to understand the apparent mismatch between nosology and receipt of care. It would be particularly valuable to have longitudinal studies that can establish differences at the syndrome and criterion level predictive of need for mental health care in the juvenile population. Such studies could identify the crucial manifestations that should be assessed for clinical evaluation and referral to treatment.

Psychiatric Conditions of Infancy and Early Childhood

The importance of establishing a sound research agenda on infancy and early childhood follows from two basic observations. First, with current developmental models of many chronic mental disorders, interest has emerged in implementing preventive interventions as early as possible. Second, many of the key issues currently confronting researchers of psychopathology in infants and young children reflect broader issues pertaining to developmental psychopathology.

In some areas, preschool psychiatric research is now facing issues that confronted researchers studying older children approximately 30 years ago (Angold and Egger 2001). At that time, clinical syndromes such as school phobia, separation anxiety, ADHD, autism, and conduct disorder had been broadly described, but the official DSM and ICD nosologies contained only generic categories and lacked specific rules for determining when diagnostic criteria were met. By 1970, general population studies (Lapouse and Monk 1964; McFie 1934) had begun to document the prevalence of problem behaviors, and factor analytical studies had begun to derive what later emerged as fairly consistent factors from parent-report questionnaires (see Achenbach and Edelbrock 1978). However, only one report, the first Isle of Wight study, had relied on clinician-based diagnoses to define syndromes (Graham and Rutter 1968; Rutter and Graham 1966, 1968).

In that era, clinicians often doubted 1) whether children were developmentally capable of experiencing some disorders (e.g., depression) and 2) whether a categorical approach to diagnosis was appropriate for children, given their rapid development and their dependence on environmental structures, such as the family, which might themselves be pathological. Twenty years later, most clinicians and researchers are generally comfortable with a classificatory system for making diagnoses in school-age children. Even strong supporters of dimensional approaches agree that categorical diagnosis has an important place in psychiatric research and practice (see, e.g., Achenbach 1995).

Although many see the development of categorical diagnosis for preschoolers as a natural outgrowth of earlier work on child diagnosis, others have been wary of down-aging the standard taxonomy (reviewed in Emde et al. 1993). A cautious approach seems advisable when extending adult categories throughout development, particularly in the first years of life. Four major objections have been raised to extending diagnostic conventions and methods that were developed for adults or older children to preschoolers. First, the boundaries between types of emotions and behaviors may be less well defined in preschoolers than in older children or adults, and symptoms and syndromes may be unstable or transient. Therefore, it may not be possible to identify discrete diagnostic categories of disorders. Second, current diagnostic systems may take too little account of the fact that early childhood is a period of rapid development. Third, diagnostic convention emphasizes an individual-based approach in evaluating adult pathology, which does not adequately focus on dyadic dimensions of behavior necessary to evaluate significant relationships of the child from both a categorical and a dimensional perspective. Fourth, it may not be clinically or ethically appropriate or desirable to assign psychiatric diagnoses to young children because it raises the risk of labeling the child, who might be defined or stigmatized in a way that will adversely affect his or her future development (Campbell 1990).

The validity of these concerns is amenable to empirical research and appropriate revision of DSM. In the first case, there is limited evidence to suggest that preschool symptoms and syndromes are less stable than those of older children. In fact, several studies on preschoolers have indicated that broad dimensions of externalizing and internalizing problems remain stable and predict negative outcomes years later (e.g., Campbell and Ewing 1990; Fischer et al. 1984; Ialongo et al. 1996; Keenan and Wakschlag 2000; Lavigne et al. 1998).

On the second point, concerning the rapidity of change during development, the key question concerns the advisability of attempting to extend current data, despite the complexity of the endeavor. Interestingly, although the DSM system has been criticized for having an insufficient focus on development, this limitation largely reflects the lack of sufficient data to support modification of adult-based diagnostic criteria. Where such modifications have been introduced, they have typically reflected the fact that adult criteria were shown to inadequately capture the relevant pathology in children. On the other hand, the application of adult criteria, as in the area of major depressive disorder, sometimes led to the surprising conclusion that they worked much better than expected. Investigating the properties of current criteria sets provides one reasonable strategy for identifying ways in which those criteria need to be modified to take account of developmental phenomena.

The third issue, concerning where to "locate" disorders in infants and young children, requires empirical research. The field now acknowledges that some forms of childhood psychopathology (e.g., autism) are best regarded as characteristics of the child. Evidence also documents relatively stable behavioral and physiologic reaction patterns across toddlerhood and their association with future psychopathology (e.g., Emde et al. 1992; Gersten 1986; Kagan 1994; Rothbart and Mauro 1990), as well as genetic contributions to preschool psychopathology (Kagan 1994; van den Oord et al. 1996). The issue seems less about whether psychopathology resides in the child or the child's social context, and more about how the characteristics of the child and of the social context interact to produce psychopathology. Research designed to resolve these issues extends the bioecological model of development with which we began this chapter (Bronfenbrenner 1977).

Finally, the argument that a diagnostic system for young children would lead to harmful labeling was long ago raised against the use of psychiatric diagnosis for older children and adolescents in general. This argument has been countered by evidence documenting the utility of specific treatments for specific diagnoses. The question is whether application of this argument to preschool diagnosis will suffer the same fate as more is learned about preschool psychopathology. In practice, the decision to provide treatment services must be based on a categorical (yes/no) decision about whether there is something wrong with the child (or the parent-child dyad). The question for research is how to improve the reliability and validity of the "something wrong" level of diagnosis that currently guides treatment decisions for young children in many treatment settings.

The Multiaxial Approach

The distinction between Axes I and II should be a major focus of the next decade of research. There is substantial research on the dimensional components of temperament in children and adolescents, but little systematic research on the longitudinal stability of temperamental traits and their association with mental disorders. Prospective longitudinal studies permit both sets of symptoms to be studied in the same people across the period of risk from childhood to early adulthood (e.g., Cardon et al. 2000; Langbehn et al. 1998). Family and twin studies could also be designed to resolve the distinction between Axis I and Axis II disorders.

A developmentally informative program of research on the links between general medical conditions (Axis III) and mental disorders and symptoms is also an important research priority. Research in medical settings (e.g., primary care and specialty medical clinics) will be important, among other reasons, for studying practitioners' ability to diagnose and treat psychiatric disorders in medically ill children. The importance of independent evaluation of potentially common symptoms is critical, because there has been a tendency to label physical symptoms in children as "psychosomatic" or "stress related" without empirical evidence for doing so. Lessons learned from bacterial causes of ulcers and genetic causes of inflammatory bowel disease should be informative in conceptualizing this research. Familial co-aggregation of mental and physical disorders may be used to address the likely sources of associations between mental and physical conditions, as demonstrated by research showing differential associations between migraine with bipolar and nonbipolar depression.

Future research designed to inform Axis IV classification might involve methods for incorporating the vast literature on contextual risks for the development of psychiatric disorders into a revised DSM. Of particular importance is the integration into the nosology of knowledge on cultural and other contextual influences on the expressions of psychopathology. This revision might also include a synthesis of the key risk factors for specific disorders at specific developmental stages as well as recommendations concerning clinical practices for assessing environmental risk. The first could be done using meta-analysis, with the work of Lipsey and Derzon (1998) on predictors of serious and violent delinquency providing a model for a possible approach. The second would require the collaboration of clinicians, psychosocial researchers, and psychometricians to develop and test appropriate instruments.

With respect to Axis V, it is critical that a revision of DSM provide clinicians and researchers with more help in assessing functioning and integrating functional assessments into diagnostic and treatment decisions. Two levels of research are needed: theoretical, to establish a classification of functional impairment; and methodological, to provide the tools and decision rules needed for clinical and research implementation. Progress has already been made in the first area by the World Health Organization in its recent revision of the *International Classification of Functioning, Disability and Health* (ICF) (World Health Organization 2001). Further work is needed to examine the applicability of this system to child and adolescent psychiatric disorders. In the second area, instrumentation, recent reviews of available measures for children and adolescents (Canino et al. 1999) could provide a basis for developing a consensus process to create the necessary tools.

Finally, beyond research on each individual axis, a program of work is needed to examine the relative usefulness of different kinds of information, from different axes, for treatment planning and preventive interventions. For example, a study comparing the role of diagnosis and impairment in predicting use of mental health services (Angold et al. 2001) showed that Axis V (functional impairment) and Axis IV (impact of the child's problems on the family, including maternal depression) were better predictors of the use of specialty mental health services than was Axis I diagnosis. This has important implications for a system of care set up to treat psychiatric disorder in the child, when in fact what gets children into the system is not the psychiatric disorder but the impact of the disorder on the child's functioning and environment. Yet few treatment trials on clinic samples even examine treatment response in these areas (Costello et al. 1997; Weissman et al. 1974).

Approaches to Psychiatric Assessment

Assessing psychiatric disorders in children and adolescents has become much more accurate in the past decade, thanks to the many new and revised interviews, questionnaires, and computer-based scoring algorithms that have been developed (Angold 2001; Shaffer and Richters 2001). Clinical as well as epidemiologic research now relies heavily on standardized instruments for case finding and treatment studies. The issues concerning proper assessment now relate less to the need for new measures than to the need to translate existing methods from research to clinical practice.

Although the clinical interview will remain at the heart of the diagnostic assessment of children for a long time to come, the past few years have also yielded a great deal of promising information about the role played by different kinds of assessment in predicting the course of illness, and even, in some cases, the best treatment. By *different kinds of assessment* we mean two things: *different ways of conducting the clinical interview*, and *different aspects of the child that can contribute to diagnosis.* In the first case, the weakness has been the growing gap between standards of clinical practice, with heavy reliance on the individual clinician's information-collecting and hypothesis-testing skills, and research practice, which uses a range of empirically tested methods to collect information and make diagnoses. In the second case, we refer to the gap between clinical reliance on a fairly narrow range of information (largely from parent and child interviews, perhaps augmented by a school or social work report) and the rapidly growing range of information on developmental psychopathology available from various techniques. These include psychoeducational and neuropsychological testing, structural and functional brain imaging, genetic testing, and well-researched observational protocols and structured tasks tapping underlying cognitive and emotional functioning. This wave of new research tools may provide a broader perspective on child behavior and potential mental syndromes, forming the basis of a reevaluation of symptom groupings and other aspects of taxonomy. As data culled by these tools accumulate, such a reevaluation of the taxonomy may serve to strengthen confidence in current categories, or it may provide the initiative for reconceptualizations and modifications in developmental diagnoses.

Research comparing the validity and reliability of different ways of obtaining clinically relevant information about children (e.g., Angold 2001) shows that 1) structured interviews are more reliable than unstructured clinical assessments; 2) structured interviews are superior on several measures of validity; 3) different informants (parents, teachers, children) contribute different, often nonoverlapping, information; and 4) the same methodology is not necessarily the best for all diagnoses. By this we mean that, for example, parent-report questionnaires about conduct disorder symptoms appear to be as reliable and valid as diagnostic interviews on the same diagnosis, while being much less onerous. On the other hand, questionnaires and even some structured interviews can generate large numbers of false-positive cases of specific phobias and psychotic disorders (Breslau 1987). Audio computer-assisted methods (Audio-CASI), in which the child responds in private to a response-dependent series of probes, may elicit more, and more reliable, information than do clinical interviews about sensitive topics such as drug use (Metzger et al. 2000). A research agenda focused on the best ways to integrate information from different approaches, for different clinical and research situations, is very much needed. For example, more information on the receiver-operated characteristic curve linking sets of screening instruments (such as the Children's Depression Inventory, Beck Depression Inventory, Center for Epidemiologic Studies Depression Scale, and the Mood and Feelings Questionnaire [MFQ] for depression) and a state-of-the art, best-estimate psychiatric assessment of depression would permit researchers, clinicians, and administrators to decide how best to allocate resources to self-report screens versus interviews with clinicians to arrive at diagnoses most efficiently in various settings.

Practice guidelines from the American Academy of Child and Adolescent Psychiatry and the American Psychiatric Association encourage the clinician to integrate different kinds of information into the diagnostic process. However, in practice, clinicians often make diagnoses based on relatively few items of information (Cantwell and Rutter 1994). Other sources of information, while individually reliable and valid, often show little agreement among themselves. For example, neurocognitive testing of executive function can have strong theoretical links to ADHD and show excellent psychometric properties, without mapping cleanly onto the diagnosis (Denckla 1996; Koziol and Stout 1992). A great deal of research is needed to establish both the best combinations of different measures and the most cost-efficient way of combining them.

Genetic measures can also contribute both to the diagnosis of the child and to refining the taxonomy. Identification of vulnerability genes though molecular genetic methods has already begun. Rett syndrome has been found in a large majority of patients to be due to point mutations in a single gene (MECP2) (Amir et al. 1999). For other disorders, genetic contributions may confer a susceptibility or protective effect, in the face of environmental variability. In these instances, psychopathology might be more reflective of gene-environment interplay, as opposed to the overriding effects of genetic contributions. Animal models may assist in identifying the relationship between genotype, environment, and phenotypes during development (Young et al. 1999). Research programs capable of moving between animal and human models and methods will be central to understanding brain-environment interactions in normal and abnormal development.

Developmental Epidemiology

In this chapter we have referred several times to the need for longitudinal, community-based data to illuminate aspects of psychiatric classification. In recent years, some of the most powerful findings concerning developmental aspects of mental illness derive from research in representative population-based samples of children studied from birth, or even earlier, through adulthood (Arseneault et al. 2000; Caspi et al. 1996; Neeleman et al. 1998; Power et al. 1997; Tiihonen et al. 1997). This raises questions on the need for a "developmental Framingham" study, referring to the seminal study of heart disease risk factors that has been ongoing for more than 50 years (Robins and Regier 1991). Although such a large-scale study could be enormously influential, considerable debate remains concerning the advantages and disadvantages of this approach, as opposed to smaller, more intensive analytical epidemiologic studies.

To properly conduct a large-scale study, the following issues would require careful consideration and possible preliminary work over the next several years: 1) To be truly representative of the changing United States population, such a study would need to be very large, include several minority groups, and oversample minority children. 2) The marked difference between inner-city and other minority children demonstrate the need to sample both urban and rural areas (Costello et al. 1999c; Tolan and Henry 1996). 3) Given differences in rates of depression, substance abuse, and other disorders across recent decades (O'Malley et al. 1988; Takei et al. 1996; Wickramaratne et al. 1989), such a study would probably need to recruit multiple cohorts over several years. 4) We have noted the importance of integrating symptom data with biological, neuropsychological, and family-based measures; researchers conducting such a study would need to consider including a range of such variables to test key developmental hypotheses. 5) Such a study would need to include data from a range of informants, including parents, children, teachers, and peers. 6) Finally, a program of psychometric work would be needed. Given concerns highlighted in this chapter regarding major limitations in the classification and assessment of children, satisfactorily addressing the research recommendations described herein would represent an important prerequisite to the development of a large, expensive benchmarking study of youth.

Conclusion

We have begun the process of evaluating developmental aspects of the current psychiatric nomenclature, DSM-IV, by summarizing recent advances in developmental research and by identifying questions that have emerged from such research. In general, much of the research in mental health sciences surrounding DSM-IV has illuminated developmental processes in mental illness. This chapter summarizes research areas most in need of further scrutiny. In some areas, complementary questions arise concerning aspects of nosology in children and in adults. In other areas, unique questions arise pertaining to early developmental aspects of the psychiatric nosology. In closing, we describe four areas of research where focused inquiry could significantly inform efforts to revise the psychiatric nomenclature.

First, collaborative research among clinicians, developmentalists, and epidemiologists is needed to refine psychiatric assessment techniques best suited for identifying pathological symptoms and symptom clusters across developmental stages. Two aspects of research on assessment techniques appear particularly important. The field needs to evaluate the degree to which information beyond symptom reports can meaningfully inform the diagnostic process and affect the taxonomy. This might include data from direct observations, neuropsychological probes, or family history/genetic assessments. The field also needs to refine methods for integrating developmental assessments of functioning and symptom-based data into the diagnostic process. Although considerable research already describes cross-sectional clustering of these constructs, efforts are needed to describe the prospective relationships among observational data, symptom reports, and functioning at different developmental stages. Finally, research in this area must consider the degree to which findings can be generalized across context, gender, ethnicity, and other factors, given prior evidence that diagnosis, symptom ratings, and impairment can each vary widely from one ethnic or cultural group to another (Canino et al. 1999; Weisz et al. 1989).

Second, advances in neuroscience generate considerable enthusiasm for their potential impact on psychiatry. Nevertheless, considerable deficiencies in essential knowledge so far preclude the use of neuroscience to inform psychiatric diagnosis. Prior advances in related areas of medicine have resulted from a close dialogue between researchers working in clinical and basic areas. It is essential to stimulate such dialogue in research on the biological aspects of mental illness. In particular, research should be pursued that studies components of psychological processes across developmental periods using comparable methodologies in humans and other species. This research might begin by examining relatively well-understood phenomena, such as attention regulation, socialization, and the expression of fear or nurturing behaviors.

Third, developmental perspectives on many chronic mental disorders emphasize the need for research on prevention. In one set of studies, potent risk factors for later psychiatric disorders have been identified among children whose symptoms do not meet current criteria for any categorical DSM-IV diagnoses. A few controlled prevention studies have begun to target such risk factors, but as knowledge of risk factors and their amenability to intervention increase, controlled prevention trials should also increase. In another set of studies, some of the proposed new psychiatric assessment tools described earlier in this chapter might be embedded within research designs where there is knowledge of the genetics. This could provide knowledge on other potential risk markers to be targeted in future prevention trials. Although prior studies established the familial nature of many mental syndromes, integrating diverse measures into future studies may elucidate mechanisms through which risk, protection, and diagnoses are transmitted from parents to children.

Fourth, developmental perspectives have also heightened interest in procedures for making diagnoses among preschoolers. Studies are needed to evaluate procedures for applying current criteria sets to this population, for evaluating the properties of these criteria sets, and for considering alternative procedures or potential alternative criteria for use in this population.

In closing, understanding of psychopathology has advanced enormously during the past two decades. Refinements in DSM have played an integral role in such advances. Moreover, the fields related to developmental psychopathology have witnessed particularly marked advances. The fact that DSM was been revised periodically has proved particularly valuable in this respect. This chapter reviews the nature of advances in relevant developmental science, and it outlines a set of central questions that follow from such advances. By addressing these questions, a systematic series of research endeavors might encourage the continual advance of the psychiatric nosology as captured in DSM.

References

Achenbach TM: Diagnosis, assessment, and comorbidity in psychosocial treatment research. J Abnorm Child Psychol 23:45–65, 1995

Achenbach TM, Edelbrock CS: The classification of child psychopathology: a review and analysis of empirical efforts. Psychol Rev 85:1275–1301, 1978

Achenbach TM, Howell CT, McConaughy SH, et al: Six-year predictors of problems in a national sample of children and youth, I: cross-informant syndromes. J Am Acad Child Adolesc Psychiatry 34:336–347, 1995

Aman MG, Tasse MJ, Rojahn J, et al: The Nisonger CBRF: a child behavior rting form for children with bahavioral difficulties. Res Dev Disabil 17:41–57, 1996

American Psychiatric Association: Diagnostic and Statistical Manual of Mental Disorders, 4th Edition. Washington, DC, American Psychiatric Association, 1994

Amir RE, Van den Veyver IB, Wan M, et al: Rett syndrome is caused by mutations in X-linked MECP2, encoding methyl-CpG-binding protein 2. Nat Genet 23:185–188, 1999

Angold A: Assessment in child and adolescent psychopathology, in The New Oxford Textbook of Psychiatry. Edited by Gelder M, Lopez-Ibor J, Andreason N. Oxford, Oxford University Press (in press)

Angold A, Egger HL: Psychiatric diagnosis in preschool children, in Handbook of Infant and Toddler Mental Health Assessment. Edited by del Carmen-Wiggins R, Carter A. New York, Oxford University Press (in press)

Angold A, Costello EJ, Worthman CM: Pubertal changes in hormone levels and depression in girls. Psychol Med 29:1043–1053, 1999

Angold A, Erkanli A, Farmer EM, et al: Caring for Children in the Community: a study of psychiatric disorder, impairment and service use in rural African American and white youth. Arch Gen Psychiatry (in press)

Arseneault L, Moffitt TE, Caspi A, et al: Mental disorders and violence in a total birth cohort: results from the Dunedin Study. Arch Gen Psychiatry 57(10):979–986, 2000

Avenevoli S, Stolar M, Li J, et al: Comorbidity of depression in children and adolescents: models and evidence from a prospective high-risk family study. Biol Psychiatry 49(12):1071–1081, 2001

Berkson J: Limitations of the application of fourfold table analysis to hospital data. Biometrics Bulletin 2:47–52, 1946

Bornstein MH, Haynes OM, Azuma H, et al: A cross-national study of self-evaluations and attributions in parenting: Argentina, Belgium, France, Italy, Japan, and the United States. Dev Psychol 34(4):662–676, 1998

Borthwick-Duffy SA: Epidemiology and prevalence of psychopathology in people with mental retardation. J Consult Clin Psychol 62:17–27, 1994

Breslau N: Inquiring about the bizarre: false positives in Diagnostic Interview Schedule for Children (DISC) ascertainment of obsessions, complusions, and psychotic symptoms. J Am Acad Child Adolesc Psychiatry 26:639–644, 1987

Breslau N, Davis GC, Prabucki K: Searching for evidence on the validity of generalized anxiety disorder: psychopathology in children of anxious mothers. Psychiatry Res 20:285–297, 1987

Bronfenbrenner U: Ecology of childhood. Child Dev 45:1–5, 1974

Bronfenbrenner U: Toward an experimental ecology of human development. American Psychologist 32:513–531, 1977

Brook JS, Cohen P, Brook DW: Longitudinal study of co-occurring psychiatric disorders and substance use. J Am Acad Child Adolesc Psychiatry 37:322–330, 1998

Buonomano DV, Merzenich MM: Cortical plasticity: from synapses to maps. Annu Rev Neurosci 21:149–186, 1998

Burke KC, Burke JD Jr, Regier DA, et al: Age at onset of selected mental disorders in five community populations. Arch Gen Psychiatry 47:511–518, 1990

Burns BJ, Costello EJ, Angold A, et al: Children's mental health service use across service sectors. Health Aff (Millwood) 14:147–159, 1995

Burns BJ, Costello EJ, Erkanli A, et al: Insurance coverage and mental health service use by adolescents with serious emotional disturbance. Journal of Child and Family Studies 6:89–111, 1997

Cairns RB, Elder GH, Costello EJ: Developmental Science. New York, Cambridge University Press, 1996

Callicott JH, Bertolino A, Mattay VS, et al: Physiological dysfunction of the dorsolateral prefrontal cortex in schizophrenia revisited. Cereb Cortex 10(11):1078–1092, 2000

Campbell SB: Behavior Problems in Preschool Children: Developmental and Clinical Issues. New York, Guilford, 1990

Campbell SB, Ewing LJ: Follow-up of hard-to-manage preschoolers: adjustment at age 9 and predictors of continuing symptoms. J Child Psychol Psychiatry 6:871–889, 1990

Canino G, Lewis-Fernandez B: Methodological challenges in cross-cultural mental health research. Transcultural Psychiatry 34(2):163–184, 1997

Canino G, Costello EJ, Angold A: Assessing functional impairment for child mental health services research: a review of measures. Journal of Mental Health Services Research 1:93–108, 1999

Cantwell DP, Rutter M: Classification: conceptual issues and substantive findings, in Child and Adolescent Psychiatry: Modern Approaches. Edited by Rutter M, Taylor E, Hersov L. Cambridge, Blackwell Scientific, 1994, pp 3–21

Cardon LR, Garner C, Bennett ST, et al: Evidence for a major gene for bone mineral density in idiopathic osteoporotic families. J Bone Miner Res 15(6):1132–1137, 2000

Caspi A, Moffitt TE, Newman DL, et al: Behavioral observations at age 3 years predict adult psychiatric disorders: longitudinal evidence from a birth cohort. Arch Gen Psychiatry 53:1033–1039, 1996

Cicchetti D: The emergence of developmental psychopathology. Child Dev 55:1–7, 1984

Cicchetti D, Sroufe LA: The past as prologue to the future: the times, they've been a-changin'. Dev Psychopathol 12(3):255–264, 2000

Cohen P, Kasen S, Brook JS, et al: Diagnostic predictors of treatment patterns in a cohort of adolescents. J Am Acad Child Adolesc Psychiatry 30:989–993, 1991

Cohen P, Cohen J, Kasen S, et al: An epidemiological study of disorders in late childhood and adolescence, I: Age- and gender-specific prevalence. J Child Psychol Psychiatry 34(6):851–867, 1993

Costello EJ, Shugart MA: Above and below the threshold: severity of psychiatric symptoms and functional impairment in a pediatric sample. Pediatrics 90:359–368, 1992

Costello EJ, Angold A, Burns BJ, et al: The Great Smoky Mountains Study of Youth: functional impairment and severe emotional disturbance. Arch Gen Psychiatry 53(12):1137–1143, 1996

Costello EJ, Farmer EM, Angold A, et al: Psychiatric disorders among American Indian and white youth in Appalachia: The Great Smoky Mountains Study. Am J Public Health 87:827–832, 1997

Costello EJ, Angold A, Keeler GP: Adolescent outcomes of childhood disorders: the consequences of severity and impairment. J Am Acad Child Adolesc Psychiatry 38:121–128, 1999a

Costello EJ, Erkanli A, Federman E, et al: Development of psychiatric comorbidity with substance abuse in adolescents: effects of timing and sex. J Clin Child Psychol 28:298–311, 1999b

Costello EJ, Farmer EMZ, Angold A: Same place, different children: white and American Indian children in the Appalachian Mountains, in Where and When: Historical and Geographical Aspects of Psychopathology. Edited by Cohen P, Robins L, Slomkowski C. Hillsdale, NJ, Erlbaum, 1999c, pp 279–298

Costello EJ, Keeler GP, Angold A: Poverty, race/ethnicity, and psychiatric disorder: a study of rural children. Am J Public Health 91(9):1494–1498, 2001

Denckla MB: Biological correlates of learning and attention: what is relevant to learning disability and attention-deficit hyperactivity disorder? Journal of Developmental and Behavioral Pediatrics 17:114–119, 1996

Drevets WC: Neuroimaging and neuropathological studies of depression: implications for the cognitive-emotional features of mood disorders. Curr Opin Neurobiol 11(2):240–249, 2001

Eaton WW, Dryman A, Weissman MM: Panic and phobia, in Psychiatric Disorders in America: The Epidemiologic Catchment Area Study. Edited by Robins LN, Regier DA. New York, Free Press, 1991, pp 155–179

Einfeld SL, Tonge BJ: Population prevalence of psychopathology in children and adolescents with intellectual disability, II: rationale and methods. J Intellect Disabil Res 40(2):99–109, 1996

Eliez S, Antonoarakis SE, Morris MA, et al: Parental origin of the deletion of 22q11.2 and brain development in velocardiofacial syndrome: a preliminary study. Arch Gen Psychiatry 58:64–68, 2001

Emde RN, Plomin R, Robinson J, et al: Temperament, emotion, and cognition at fourteen months: the MacArthur Longitudinal Twin Study. Child Dev 63:1437–1455, 1992

Emde RN, Bingham RD, Harmon RJ: Classification and the diagnostic process in infancy, in Handbook of Infant Mental Health. Edited by Zeanah CH Jr. New York, Guilford, 1993, pp 225–235

Erlenmeyer-Kimling L: Neurobehavioral deficits in offspring of schizophrenic parents: liability indicators and predictors of illness. Am J Med Genet 97(1):65–71, 2000

Fava M, Kendler KS: Major depressive disorder. Neuron 28(2):335–341, 2000

Feehan M, McGee R, Williams SM, et al: Mental health disorders from age 15 to age 18 years. J Am Acad Child Adolesc Psychiatry 32:1118–1126, 1993

Ferdinand RF, Verhulst FC: Psychopathology from adolescence into young adulthood: an eight-year follow-up study. Am J Psychiatry 152:1586–1594, 1995

Fischer M, Rolf JE, Hasazi JE, et al: Follow-up of a preschool epidemiological sample: cross-age continuities and predictions of later adjustment with internalizing and externalizing dimensions of behavior. Child Dev 55:137–150, 1984

Flisher AJ, Kramer RA, Grosser RC, et al: Correlates of unmet need for mental health services by children and adolescents. Psychol Med 27:1145–1154, 1997

Freeman LN, Mokros H, Poznanski EO: Violent events reported by normal urban school-aged children: characteristics and depression correlates. J Am Acad Child Adolesc Psychiatry 32(2):419–423, 1993

Garber J: Classification of childhood psychopathology: a developmental perspective. Child Dev 55:30–48, 1984

Gersten M: The contribution of temperament to behavior in natural contexts. Unpublished doctoral dissertation, Harvard University Graduate School of Education, Cambridge, MA, 1986

Giaconia RM, Reinherz HZ, Silverman AB, et al: Ages of onset of psychiatric disorders in a community population of older adolescents. J Am Acad Child Adolesc Psychiatry 33:706–717, 1994

Giedd JN, Blumenthal J, Jeffries NO, et al: Brain development during adolescence: a longitudinal MRI study. Nat Neurosci 10:861–863, 1999

Gil AG, Wagner EF, Vega WA: Acculturation, familism, and alcohol use among Latino adolescent males: longitudinal relations. Journal of Community Psychology 28(4):443–458, 2000

Gladstein J, Rusonis EJ, Heald FP: A comparison of inner-city and upper-middle class youths' exposure to violence. J Adolesc Health 13(4):275–280, 1992

Golden NH: Osteoporosis prevention: a pediatric challenge. Archives of Pediatrics and Adolescent Medicine 154(6):542–543, 2000

Goldman-Rakic PS: Development of cortical circuitry and cognitive function. Child Dev 58:601–622, 1987

Gould E, Tanapat P, Rydel T, et al: Regulation of hippocampal neurogenesis in adulthood. Biol Psychiatry 48(8):715–720, 2000

Graham P, Rutter M: The reliability and validity of the psychiatric assessment of the child, II: interview with the parent. Br J Psychiatry 114:581–592, 1968

Greenough WT, Black JE, Wallace CS: Experience and brain development. Child Dev 58:539–559, 1987

Guarnaccia PJ, Rogler LH: Research on culture-bound syndromes: new directions. Am J Psychiatry 156(9):1322–1327, 1999

Ialongo N, Edelsohn G, Werthamer-Larsson L, et al: The course of aggression in first-grade children with and without comorbid anxious symptoms. J Abnorm Child Psychol 24:445–456, 1996

Kagan J: Galen's Prophecy: Temperament in Human Nature. New York, Basic Books, 1994

Keenan K, Wakschlag LS: More than the terrible twos: the nature and severity of behavior problems in clinic-referred preschool children. J Abnorm Child Psychol 28:33–46, 2000

Kendler KS, Neale MC, Kessler RC, et al: Major depression and phobias: the genetic and environmental sources of comorbidity. Psychol Med 23(2):361–371, 1993

Kendler KS, Walters EE, Neale MC, et al: The structure of the genetic and environmental risk factors for six major psychiatric disorders in women. Phobia, generalized anxiety disorder, panic disorder, bulimia, major depression, and alcoholism. Arch Gen Psychiatry 52(5):374–383, 1995

Kendler KS, Eaves LJ, Walters EE, et al: The identification and validation of distinct depressive syndromes in a population-based sample of female twins. Arch Gen Psychiatry 53(5):391–399, 1996

Kessler RC, McGonagle KA, Zhao S, et al: Lifetime and 12-month prevalence of DSM-III-R psychiatric disorders in the United States. Arch Gen Psychiatry 51:8–19, 1994

Klintsova AY, Greenough WT: Synaptic plasticity in cortical systems. Curr Opin Neurobiol 9:203–208, 1999

Kolb B, Forgie M, Gibb R, et al: Age, experience, and the changing brain. Neurosci Biobehav Rev 22:143–159, 1998

Koziol LF, Stout CE: Use of a verbal fluency measure in understanding and evaluating ADHD as an executive function disorder. Percept Mot Skills 75:1187–1192, 1992

Kuperman S, Schlosser SS, Lidral J, et al: Relationship of child psychopathology to parental alcoholism and antisocial personality disorder. J Am Acad Child Adolesc Psychiatry 38:686–692, 1999

Langbehn DR, Cadoret RJ, Yates WR, et al: Distinct contributions of conduct and oppositional defiant symptoms to adult antisocial behavior: evidence from an adoption study. Arch Gen Psychiatry 55:821–829, 1998

Lapouse R, Monk MA: Behavior deviations in a representative sample of children: variation by sex, age, race, social class and family size. Am J Orthopsychiatry 34:436–446, 1964

Lavigne JV, Arend R, Rosenbaum D, et al: Psychiatric disorders with onset in the preschool years, I: stability of diagnoses. J Am Acad Child Adolesc Psychiatry 37:1246–1254, 1998

Lewinsohn PM, Rohde P, Klein DN, et al: Natural course of adolescent major depressive disorder, I: continuity into young adulthood. J Am Acad Child Adolesc Psychiatry 38:56–63, 1999

Lewinsohn PM, Rohde P, Seeley JR, et al: Natural course of adolescent major depressive disorder in a community sample: predictors of recurrence in young adults. Am J Psychiatry 157:1584–1591, 2000

Lewis-Fernandez R, Kleinman A: Culture, personality, and psychopathology. J Abnorm Psychol 103(1):67–71, 1994

Lipsey MW, Derzon JH: Predictors of violent or serious delinquency in adolescence and early adulthood: a synthesis of longitudinal research, in Serious and Violent Juvenile Offenders. Edited by Loeber R, Farrington DP. Thousand Oaks, CA, Sage, 1998, pp 86–105

Liu D, Diorio J, Tannenbaum B, et al: Maternal care, hippocampal glucocorticoid receptors, and hypothalamic-pituitary-adrenal responses to stress. Science 277:1659–1662, 1997

Loeber R, Stouthamer-Loeber M, White HR: Developmental aspects of delinquency and internalizing problems and their association with persistent juvenile substance use between ages 7 and 18. J Clin Child Psychol 28:322–332, 1999

Maier W, Lichtermann D, Minges J, et al: Continuity and discontinuity of affective disorders and schizophrenia: results of a controlled family study. Arch Gen Psychiatry 50:871–883, 1993

Maier W, Lichtermann D, Minges J: The relationship between alcoholism and unipolar depression—a controlled family study. J Psychiatr Res 28:303–317, 1994

Marenco S, Weinberger DR: The neurodevelopmental hypothesis of schizophrenia: following a trail of evidence from cradle to grave. Dev Psychopathol 12(3):501–527, 2000

McEwen BS: Protective and damaging effects of stress mediators. N Engl J Med 338:171–179, 1998

McFie BS: Behavior and personality difficulties in school children. British Journal of Educational Psychology 4:34, 1934

McGuffin P, Farmer AE, Gottesman II, et al: Twin concordance for operationally defined schizophrenia. Confirmation of familiality and heritability. Arch Gen Psychiatry 41(6):541–545, 1984

Meaney MJ, Bhatnagar S, Diorio J, et al: Molecular basis for the development of individual differences in the hypothalamic pituitary-adrenal stress response. Cell Mol Neurobiol 13:321–347, 1993

Merikangas KR, Dierker LC, Szatmari P: Psychopathology among offspring of parents with substance abuse and/or anxiety: a high risk study. J Child Psychol Psychiatry 39:711–720, 1998

Merikangas KR, Avenevoli S, Dierker L, et al: Vulnerability factors among children at risk for anxiety disorders. Biol Psychiatry 46(11):1523–1535, 1999

Metzger DS, Koblin B, Turner C, et al: Randomized controlled trial of audio computer-assisted self-interviewing: utility and acceptability in longitudinal studies. Am J Epidemiol 152:99–106, 2000

Mignot E: Perspectives in narcolepsy and hypocretin (orexin) research. Sleep Med 1:87–90, 2000

Myers M, Stewart D, Brown SA, et al: Progression from conduct disorder to antisocial personality disorder following treatment for adolescent substance abuse. Am J Psychiatry 155:479–485, 1998

Neeleman J, Wessely S, Wadsworth M: Predictors of suicide, accidental death, and premature natural death in a general-population birth cohort. Lancet 351(9096):93–97, 1998

Nishino S, Riehl J, Hong J, et al: Is narcolepsy a REM sleep disorder? analysis of sleep abnormalities in narcoleptic Dobermans. Neurosci Res 38:437–446, 2000

Nolen-Hoeksema S: An interactive model for the emergence of gender differences in depression in adolescence. Journal of Research on Adolescence 4:519–534, 1994

O'Malley PM, Bachman JG, Johnston LD: Period, age, and cohort effects on substance use among young Americans: a decade of change, 1976–86. Am J Public Health 78(10):1315–1321, 1988

Paus T, Zijdenbos A, Worsley K, et al: Structural maturation of neural pathways in children and adolescents: in vivo study. Science 283:1908–1911, 1999

Peterson BS, Pine DS, Cohen P, et al: Prospective, longitudinal study of tic, obsessive-compulsive, and attention-deficit/hyperactivity disorders in an epidemiological sample. J Am Acad Child Adolesc Psychiatry 40(6):685–695, 2001

Pickens R, Svikis D, McGue M, et al: Heterogeneity in the inheritance of alcoholism: a study of male and female twins. Arch Gen Psychiatry 48:19–28, 1991

Pine DS, Cohen P, Gurley D, et al: The risk for early adulthood anxiety and depressive disorders in adolescents with anxiety and depressive disorders. Arch Gen Psychiatry 55:56–66, 1998

Pine DS, Cohen E, Cohen P, et al: Adolescent depressive symptoms as predictors of adult depression: moodiness or mood disorder. Am J Psychiatry 156:133–135, 1999

Power C, Hertzman C, Matthews S, et al: Social differences in health: life-cycle effects between ages 23 and 33 in the 1958 British birth cohort. Am J Public Health 87(9):1499–1503, 1997

Reiss AL, Eliez S, Schmitt JE, et al: Brain imaging in neurogenetic conditions: realizing the potential of behavioral neurogenetics research. Ment Retard Dev Disabil Res Rev 6:186–197, 2000

Robins LN, Regier DA (eds): Psychiatric Disorders in America. New York, Free Press, 1991

Rothbart MK, Mauro JA: Temperament, behavioral inhibition, and shyness in childhood, in Handbook of Social and Evaluation Anxiety. Edited by Leitenberg H. New York, Plenum, 1990, pp 139–160

Rueter MA, Chao W, Conger RD: The effect of systematic variation in retrospective conduct disorder reports on antisocial personality disorder diagnoses. J Consult Clin Psychol 68:307–312, 2000

Rutter M, Graham P: Psychiatric disorder in 10- and 11-year-old children. Proceedings of the Royal Society of Medicine 59:382–387, 1966

Rutter M, Graham P: The reliability and validity of the psychiatric assessment of the child, I: interview with the child. Br J Psychiatry 114:563–579, 1968

Rutter M, Sroufe LA: Developmental psychopathology: concepts and challenges. Dev Psychopathol 12:265–296, 2000

Shaffer D, Richters J (eds): Assessment in Child and Adolescent Psychopathology. New York, Guilford, 2001

Shaffer D, Fisher P, Dulcan M, et al: The NIMH Diagnostic Interview Schedule for Children (DISC 2.3): description, acceptability, prevalences, and performance in the MECA study. J Am Acad Child Adolesc Psychiatry 35(7):865–877, 1996

Shors TJ, Miesegaes G, Beylin A, et al: Neurogenesis in the adult is involved in the formation of trace memories. Nature 410(6826):372–376, 2001

Silberg J, Pickles A, Rutter M, et al: The influence of genetic factors and life stress on depression among adolescent girls. Arch Gen Psychiatry 56:225–232, 1999

Simonoff E, Pickles A, Meywr JM, et al: The Virginia Twin Study of adolescent behavioral development: influences of age, sex and impairment on rates of disorder. Arch Gen Psychiatry 54:801–808, 1997

Simonoff E, Pickles A, Meyer J, et al: Genetic and environmental influences on subtypes of conduct disorder behavior in boys. J Abnorm Child Psychol 26:495–509, 1998

Smith ML, Saltzman J, Klim P, et al: Neuropsychological function in mild hyperphenylalaninemia. Am J Ment Retard 105(2):69–80, 2000

Smoller JW, Tsuang MT: Panic and phobic anxiety: defining phenotypes for genetic studies. Am J Psychiatry 155(9):1152–1162, 1998

Squire LR, Kandel ER: Memory: From Mind to Molecules. New York, Scientific American Press, 1999

Sroufe LA, Rutter M: The domain of developmental psychopathology. Child Dev 55:17–29, 1984

Steffenburg S, Gillberg C, Steffenburg U: Psychiatric disorders in children and adolescents with mental retardation and active epilepsy. Arch Neurol 53:904–912, 1996

Swendsen JD, Merikangas KR: The comorbidity of depression and substance abuse disorders. Clin Psychol Rev 20(2):173–189, 2000

Takei N, Lewis G, Sham PC, et al: Age-period-cohort analysis of the incidence of schizophrenia in Scotland. Psychol Med 26(5):963–973, 1996

Tiihonen J, Isohanni M, Rasanen P, et al: Specific major mental disorders and criminality: a 26-year prospective study of the 1966 northern Finland birth cohort. Am J Psychiatry 154:840–845, 1997

Tolan PH, Henry D: Patterns of psychopathology among urban poor children: comorbidity and aggression effects. J Consult Clin Psychol 64(5):1094–1099, 1996

Tsuang MT, Faraone SV: The future of psychiatric genetics. Curr Psychiatry Rep 2:133–136, 2000

Tsuang MT, Stone WS, Faraone SV: Genes, environment and schizophrenia. Br J Psychiatry 178:S18–S24, 2001

van den Oord EJCG, Verhulst FC, Boomsma DI: A genetic study of maternal and paternal ratings of problem behaviors in 3-year-old twins. J Abnorm Psychol 105:349–357, 1996

van Spronsen FJ F, van Rijn M M, Bekhof J, et al: Phenylketonuria: tyrosine supplementation in phenylalanine-restricted diets. Am J Clin Nutr 73(2):153–157, 2001

Wadsworth MEJ, Kuh DJL: Childhood influences on adult health: a review of recent work from the British 1946 national birth cohort study, the MRC National Survey of Health and Development. Paediatr Perinat Epidemiol 11:2–20, 1997

Weissman MM, Klerman GL, Paykel ES, et al: Treatment effects on the social adjustment of depressed patients. Arch Gen Psychiatry 30(6):771–778, 1974

Weissman MM, Warner V, Wickramaratne P, et al: Offspring of depressed parents, 10 years later. Arch Gen Psychiatry 54:932–940, 1997

Weissman MM, Wolk S, Goldstein RB, et al: Depressed adolescents grown up. JAMA 281:1707–1713, 1999

Weisz JR, Suwanlert S, Chaiyasit W, et al: Epidemiology of behavioral and emotional problems among Thai and American children: teacher reports for ages 6–11. J Child Psychol Psychiatry 30(3):471–484, 1989

Weisz JR, Sigman M, Weiss B, et al: Parent reports of behavioral and emotional problems among children in Kenya, Thailand, and the United States. Child Dev 64(1):98–109, 1993

Wickramaratne PJ, Weissman MM, Leaf PJ, et al: Age, period and cohort effects on the risk of major depression: results from five United States communities. J Clin Epidemiol 42(4):333–343, 1989

Wolraich ML: Diagnostic and Statistical Manual for Primary Care (DSM-PC) Child and Adolescent Version: design, intent, and hopes for the future. J Dev Behav Pediatr 18(3):171–172, 1997

World Health Organization: International Classification of Functioning, Disability and Health—ICF. Geneva, World Health Organization, 2001

Young LJ, Nilsen R, Waymire KG, et al: Increased affiliative response to vasopressin in mice expressing the V1a receptor from a monogamous vole. Nature 400:766–768, 1999

Zero to Three: Diagnostic Classification, 0–3: Diagnostic Classification of Mental Health and Developmental Disorders of Infancy and Early Childhood. Arlington, VA, Zero to Three/National Center for Clinical Infant Programs, 1994

CHAPTER 4

Personality Disorders and Relational Disorders

A Research Agenda for Addressing Crucial Gaps in DSM

Michael B. First, M.D., Carl C. Bell, M.D., Bruce Cuthbert, Ph.D., John H. Krystal, M.D., Robert Malison, M.D., David R. Offord, M.D., David Reiss, M.D., M. Tracie Shea, Ph.D., Tom Widiger, Ph.D., Katherine L. Wisner, M.D., M.S.

In this chapter we focus on two of the most important gaps in the current DSM-IV: the categorical method of diagnosing personality disorders and their relationship with Axis I disorders and 2) the limited provision for the diagnosis of relational disorders. Although the developers of DSM-IV (American Psychiatric Association 1994) were aware of the limitations in the diagnostic system with regard to personality disorders (see the discussion in Widiger 1996) and relational disorders (see the discussion in Frances et al. 1996), there was an insufficient empirical database to permit the implementation of the major changes that would have been required to correct the problems. In this chapter we review both the current status and problems in each of these areas and offer suggestions for a possible research agenda that might provide the empirical base to allow a solution to the problems and gaps that have been identified.

Personality Disorders and Traits

Personality disorders have been included in the DSM since its first edition in 1952, reflecting the strong interest in treatment of personality disorders by psychoanalytically trained psychiatrists. Although the number and types of disorders have changed over the various editions of the DSM, the basic conceptual principle (i.e., that they are lifelong, deeply ingrained maladaptive patterns of behavior) has been carried through. Starting with DSM-III (American Psychiatric Association 1980), the personality disorders were given increased prominence in the diagnostic system (along with developmental disorders) by placing them on a separate axis to "ensure that consideration is given to the possible presence of disorders that are frequently overlooked."

There are a number of reasons for continuing to include in the DSM a section for personality disorders. Maladaptive personality traits can have a significant impact on other mental disorders and on physical disorders, and might themselves result in clinically significant impairments to social or occupational functioning or personal distress (Livesley 2001; Millon et al. 1996). For example, one of the more well-validated personality disorders is the antisocial or psychopathic personality disorder (Stoff et al. 1997). Persons who have a personality disturbance that meets the various diagnostic criterion sets for this personality disorder have been shown to be at significant risk for unemployment, impoverishment, injury, violent death, substance and alcohol abuse, incarceration, recidivism (parole violation), and significant relationship instability (Hart and Hare 1997; L.N. Robins et al. 1991).

Despite the compelling impact of maladaptive personality traits, there is notable dissatisfaction with the current conceptualization and definition of the DSM-IV-TR (American Psychiatric Association 2000) personality disorders. Problems identified by both researchers and clinicians include confusion regarding the relationship between the DSM-IV-TR personality disorders and certain Axis I disorders (especially those that are chronic and have their onset in childhood or adolescence); excessive comorbidity among the DSM-IV-TR personality disorders; arbitrary distinction between normal personality, personality traits, and personality disorder; lack of empirically documented clinical utility for treatment decisions for most of the personality disorders; and limited coverage (the most commonly diagnosed personality disorder is the residual diagnosis of personality disorder not otherwise specified).

This section focuses on two related issues around which confusion and lack of clarity exists: one is how best to describe and conceptualize the maladaptive personality patterns themselves; the other is the nature of the relationship between maladaptive personality patterns/traits/disorders and Axis I disorders.

Dimensional Models of Personality

"The diagnostic approach used in [DSM-IV-TR] represents the categorical perspective that Personality Disorders are qualitatively distinct clinical syndromes" (American Psychiatric Association 2000, p. 689). However, a variety of studies using diverse methodologies have raised compelling concerns regarding the validity of this assumption of distinct diagnostic categories (Clark et al. 1997; Livesley 1998; Widiger 1993; Widiger and Sanderson 1995). There does not appear to be a qualitative distinction between normal personality functioning and personality disorder, nor does there appear to be a qualitative distinction among the individual personality disorders.

Limitations of the Categorical Model

Maser et al. (1991) surveyed 146 psychologists and psychiatrists in 42 countries with respect to their satisfaction with DSM-III-R (American Psychiatric Association 1987). They reported that "the personality disorders led the list of diagnostic categories with which respondents were dissatisfied" (Maser et al. 1991, p. 275). The personality disorders were considered to be problematic by 56% of the respondents. The second most frequently cited category were the mood disorders, cited by only 28%. In response to an optional, write-in question, "35 of 101 respondents (35%) chose to write in personality disorders 'most in need of revision' (p. 275). Much of this dissatisfaction could be secondary to the inadequacies, limitations, and problems generated by the categorical model of classification.

Boundary with normal personality functioning. Researchers have been unable to identify a qualitative distinction between normal personality functioning and personality disorder (e.g., Kass et al. 1985; Livesley et al. 1992; Nestadt et al. 1990; Zimmerman and Coryell 1990). DSM-IV provides specific and explicit rules for distinguishing between the presence and absence of each of the personality disorders (e.g., five of eight specified criteria are necessary for the diagnosis of histrionic personality disorder), but the thresholds for diagnosis provided in DSM-IV are largely unexplained and are weakly justified (Clark 1992; Tyrer and Johnson 1996; Widiger and Corbitt 1994). The DSM-III schizotypal and borderline personality disorder diagnoses are the only two for which a published rationale has ever been provided. No explanation, rationale, or justification has been provided for any of the other diagnostic thresholds, and the justification for the thresholds for the borderline and schizotypal diagnoses may no longer apply (Widiger 2001). The DSM-III thresholds for the diagnosis of the borderline and schizotypal personality disorders were selected on the basis of maximizing agreement with the thresholds provided by a large sample of clinicians (Spitzer et al. 1979). However, there have been so many revisions, deletions, and additions to the criteria sets for these personality disorders provided by DSM-III-R and DSM-IV that the current diagnostic thresholds may no longer apply (Blashfield et al. 1992; Morey 1988). For example, Blashfield et al. (1992) reported a κ of only –0.025 for the agreement between the DSM-III and DSM-III-R criterion set for schizotypal personality disorder, with a reduction in prevalence from 11% to 1%.

The maladaptive personality traits included within the diagnostic criteria for the DSM-IV personality disorders appear to be present within members of the general population who would not be diagnosed with a DSM-IV personality disorder (Widiger and Costa 1994). Much (if not all) of the fundamental symptomatology of the DSM-IV personality disorders can be understood as maladaptive variants of personality traits evident within the normal population (Widiger et al. 1994). For example, much of the symptomatology of borderline personality disorder can be understood as extreme variants of the angry hostility, vulnerability, anxiousness, depressiveness, and impulsivity included within the broad domain of neuroticism (identified by others as negative affectivity or emotional instability) that is evident within the general population (Clarkin et al. 1993; Morey and Zanarini 2000; Trull 1992; Wilberg et al. 1999). Similarly, much of the symptomatology of antisocial personality disorder appears to be extreme variants of low conscientiousness (rashness, negligence, hedonism, immorality, undependability, and irresponsibility) and high antagonism (manipulativeness, deceptiveness, exploitativeness, aggressiveness, callousness, and ruthlessness) that have long been evident within the general population (Miller et al. 2001; Trull 1992).

The structure and heritability of personality disorder symptoms also appear to be just as evident within general community samples of persons without the DSM-IV personality disorders as it is in persons who have been diagnosed with these disorders (Tyrer and Alexander 1979). Livesley and colleagues (1998) compared the phenotypic and genetic structure of a comprehensive set of personality disorder symptoms in samples of 656 personality disorder patients, 939 general community participants, and 686 twin pairs. Principal components analysis yielded four broad dimensions (emotional dysregulation, dissocial behavior, inhibitedness, and compulsivity) that were replicated across all three samples. Multivariate genetic analyses also yielded the same four factors. The researchers concluded that "the stable structure of traits across clinical and nonclinical samples is consistent with dimensional representations of personality disorders" (Livesley et al. 1998, p. 941). Livesley et al. (1998) and Widiger (1998) also noted the remarkable consistency of the four broad domains of personality disorder with four of the five broad domains consistently identified in studies of general personality functioning. Livesley et al. (1998) concluded that "the higher-order traits of personality disorder strongly resemble dimensions of normal personality" (p. 941).

Boundaries among the personality disorders. Research has also failed to support the existence of qualitatively distinct boundaries among the personality disorder diagnostic categories. In fact, research has consistently indicated the presence of excessive diagnostic co-occurrence (Bornstein 1998; Lilienfeld et al. 1994; Widiger 1993). For example, Oldham et al. (1992) administered two different semistructured interviews for diagnosis of the DSM-III-R personality disorder diagnostic categories to 100 applicants to a long-term inpatient clinic for severe personality disorders (one interview was administered in the morning, the other in the afternoon). They reported that administration of one of the interviews resulted in the diagnosis of 290 personality disorders in the 100 patients; administration of the other interview resulted in 249 diagnoses. Fewer than 15% of the patients had a personality disturbance that met the criteria for just one personality disorder.

Widiger and Trull (1998) reported co-occurrence rates for the DSM-III-R personality disorder diagnoses obtained for the construction of the DSM-IV criteria sets from unpublished data provided by six research sites (four of which used semistructured interviews). They reported, "If one takes a rate of 33.3% as indicating problematic co-occurrence (i.e., at least a third of the persons meet the criteria for another personality disorder), then there is problematic co-occurrence for each personality disorder" (Widiger and Trull 1998, p. 362). These findings were consistent with previously published comorbidity studies (Widiger et al. 1991) and with more recent research using the DSM-IV criteria sets (e.g., McGlashan et al. 2000).

O'Connor and Dyce (1998) explored whether the covariation among the personality disorders reported in nine previously published studies could be explained adequately by alternative dimensional models of personality functioning. They conducted independent principal-axes confirmatory factor analyses for alternative dimensional models on 12 correlation matrices provided in the nine studies. The personality disorder matrices were rotated to a least-squares fit to the target matrices generated by the alternative dimensional models. Highly significant congruence coefficients were obtained for all 12 correlation matrices for two of the dimensional models. "The highest and most consistent levels of fit were obtained for the five-factor model and for Cloninger and Svrakic's (1994) seven-factor model" (O'Connor and Dyce (1998, p. 14). O'Connor and

Dyce (1998) concluded that "the personality disorder configurations that were most strongly supported ... were the two that are based on attempts to identify basic dimensions of personality that exist in both clinical and nonclinical populations" (p. 15).

Lynam and Widiger (2001) explored in more detail whether the comorbidity among the personality disorders could be explained from the perspective of the five-factor model (FFM) of general personality functioning. These investigators had personality disorder researchers describe prototypical cases of each of the DSM-IV personality disorders in terms of the 30 facets of the FFM. They then obtained the correlations among the DSM-IV personality disorders with respect to these FFM descriptions, and they empirically compared these correlations to the co-occurrences among the personality disorders reported in nine previously published DSM-III studies aggregated by Widiger et al. (1991) and the six unpublished DSM-III-R data sets aggregated by Widiger and Trull (1998). The agreement between the co-occurrence predicted by the FFM and the co-occurrence reported by the two data sets generally matched and at times even equaled the agreement between the co-occurrence rates provided by the two aggregated data sets. Lynam and Widiger (2001) concluded that "the conceptual overlap among FFM profiles reproduced well the covariation obtained for the schizoid, schizotypal, antisocial, borderline, histrionic, narcissistic, and compulsive personality disorders aggregated across several sets of studies" (p. 410) and suggested that the diagnostic co-occurrence that is obtained among the personality disorders is consistent with an understanding of the DSM-IV personality disorders as constellations of personality traits present within general personality functioning.

Clinical application of diagnostic categories. The apparent imposition of arbitrary categorical distinctions on what might instead be dimensions of personality functioning appear to have contributed to a number of diagnostic quandaries, frustrations, and dilemmas for the practicing clinician, including the presence of overly heterogeneous diagnostic categories, inadequate coverage of clinically significant maladaptive personality traits, problematic differential diagnoses, and confusing multiple diagnoses (Clark et al. 1997; Lilienfeld et al. 1994; Westen 1997; Widiger 1993).

The DSM-III criteria sets for many of the personality disorders were monothetic, in that all of the diagnostic criteria were required. These monothetic criteria sets would presumably identify relatively homogeneous groups of persons (i.e., all of the persons with the same diagnosis would have the same personality disorder symptoms). However, it quickly became evident that the reality did not match the assumption of diagnostic homogeneity. The vast majority of persons with personality disorders do not match prototypical cases (i.e., they do not have all of the symptoms or traits of a hypothetical prototypical case). Therefore, all of the personality disorder criteria sets were modified to a polythetic format for DSM-III-R, in which a set of optional diagnostic criteria are provided and only a subset are needed for diagnosis (Spitzer and Williams 1987; Widiger et al. 1988). The polythetic format is more consistent with clinical reality but it also results in substantial diagnostic heterogeneity (Clarkin et al. 1983; Shea 1992; Widiger and Sanderson 1995). There is considerable variability among patients with the same personality disorder diagnosis, which contributes to inconsistent clinical description and research findings. In some instances, patients can even have the same personality disorder diagnosis but have none of the same diagnostic criteria.

Nevertheless, the broader polythetic diagnostic criteria sets have still failed to result in an adequate coverage of clinical cases. Clinicians provide a diagnosis of personality disorder not otherwise specified (NOS) when they determine that a person has a personality disorder that is not adequately represented by any one of the 10 officially recognized diagnoses (American Psychiatric Association 2000). Personality disorder NOS is often the single most frequently used personality disorder diagnosis in clinical practice (Fabrega et al. 1991; Koenigsberg et al. 1985; Loranger 1990; Morey 1988), which is itself a testament to the inadequate coverage that is provided by the existing diagnostic categories. Clinicians must often rely on the diagnosis of personality disorder NOS to diagnose the presence of maladaptive personality traits that are not covered by the existing diagnostic categories (Clark et al. 1995; Westen and Arkowitz-Westen 1998).

Clinicians also fail to recognize the entire array of personality disorder symptoms that are typically present in their patients. Despite the fact that most patients have a personality disturbance that will meet the DSM-IV diagnostic criteria for more than one personality disorder (Bornstein 1998; Lilienfeld et al. 1994), clinicians typically apply only one diagnosis to each patient (Gunderson 1992). Clinicians tend to diagnose personality disorders hierarchically. Once a patient is identified as having a particular personality disorder (e.g., borderline), the clinician often fails to assess whether additional personality traits are present (Herkov and Blashfield 1995). Adler et al. (1990) provided 46 clinicians with case histories of a patient that met the DSM-III criteria for four personality disorders (i.e., histrionic, narcissistic, borderline, and dependent). "Despite the directive to consider each category separately … most clinicians assigned just one [personality disorder] diagnosis" (Adler et al. 1990, p. 127). Sixty-five percent of the clinicians provided only one diagnosis, 28% provided two, and none provided all four.

Comorbidity is a pervasive phenomenon that can have substantial importance to clinical research and treatment (Clark et al. 1995; Lilienfeld et al. 1994; Widiger and Clark 2000), yet comorbidity may be grossly underrecognized in general clinical practice (Zimmerman and Mattia 1999). The reason that clinicians provide only one personality disorder diagnosis per patient is unclear. One possibility is the failure to conduct systematic or comprehensive assessments; another possibility is that the presence of multiple personality disorder diagnoses is confusing and inconsistent with clinical theory. Patients have just one personality (excluding those with a dissociative disorder); it is inconsistent with most clinical theory to suggest that a person has two, three, or even five qualitatively distinct personality disorders, each with its own particular etiology and pathology (Lilienfeld et al. 1994; Widiger 1993). It might be more consistent with clinical theory to indicate that a patient has one personality disorder, characterized by the presence of a variety of maladaptive personality traits (Widiger and Costa 1994).

Alternative Dimensional Models of Personality Disorder

An alternative to the categorical approach of DSM-IV-TR is to consider the maladaptive behavior patterns covered by the DSM-IV-TR personality disorder diagnoses to be maladaptive variants of general personality functioning (Cloninger et al. 1993; Livesley 1998; Trull 2000; Watson et al. 1994; Widiger and Costa 1994). Dimensional models of personality that are more directly related to general personality functioning were considered for inclusion in DSM-IV (Widiger 1996) and the text of DSM-IV-TR now acknowledges explicitly that "an alternative to the categorical approach is the dimensional perspective that Personality Disorders represent maladaptive variants of personality traits that merge imperceptibly into normality and into one another" (American Psychiatric Association 2000, p. 689).

The dimensional models cited within the text of DSM-IV are those within the FFM (Costa and Widiger 1994), the Temperament and Character Inventory (TCI) (Cloninger et al. 1993), the Dimensional Assessment of Personality Pathology–Basic Questionnaire (DAPP-BQ) (Livesley et al. 1998), the Schedule for Nonadaptive and Adaptive Personality (SNAP) (Clark 1993), the Interpersonal Circumplex (IPC) (Benjamin 1993; Wiggins and Pincus 1992), and polarities suggested by Millon et al. (1996). An additional dimensional model published subsequently to DSM-IV is the Shedler-Westen Assessment Procedure (SWAP-200) (Westen and Shedler 1999a, 1999b).

The presence of alternative dimensional models of personality disorder is itself an indication of the theoretical, scientific, and clinical interest in the development of this alternative method for diagnosis and classification. The viability of a dimensional model of personality disorder is becoming increasingly recognized by theorists and researchers (Oldham and Skodol 2000; Widiger 1992), and one expected response would be the development of alternative models. Some of the proposed models have been developed largely on the basis of theoretical reasoning informed by research (e.g., TCI and Millon's polarities), whereas others have been developed largely through factor analyses of systematic and reasonably comprehensive sets of personality traits or symptoms (e.g., DAPP-BQ, FFM, IPC, SNAP, and SWAP-200). The models can also be differentiated with respect to whether they are confined largely to personality disorder symptomatology (e.g., DAPP-BQ, Millon's polarities, and SNAP) or whether they intend to cover the full range of normal and abnormal personality functioning (e.g., FFM, IPC, TCI, and SWAP-200). An additional alternative is to simply indicate that each of the DSM-IV personality disorders be considered along a continuum with normal personality functioning (Oldham and Skodol 2000).

The generation of alternative dimensional models may continue until an authoritative or governing body imposes or compels a uniform classification of general personality functioning. The classification of mental disorders was notoriously inconsistent across nations, states, and clinical settings before the emergence of the authority of the ICD and DSM classifications and would likely continue to be inconsistent in the absence of the authoritative impact of the World Health Organization and the American Psychiatric Association (Blashfield 1984; Kendell 1975; Widiger 2001). No comparable authority or control is present in the classification and assessment of general personality functioning.

Table 4–1 lists the dimensional models of general personality functioning included within the FFM, TCI, DAPP-BQ, and SNAP. It is apparent from simply scanning the constructs presented in Table 4–1 that there should be substantial convergence among these alternative dimensional models. The domains of functioning that they cover overlap substantially, and the ways in which these models cover these domains are in some cases quite comparable. A substantial amount of data have been published regarding the convergence and divergence among the FFM, DAPP-BQ, and SNAP dimensional models (Clark and Livesley 1994; Clark et al. 1996; Livesley et al. 1998; Schroeder et al. 1992; Widiger 1998).

An important and fundamental question is the extent to which alternative dimensional models of general personality functioning would or could adequately represent the personality disorder psychopathology diagnosed by the existing diagnostic categories. The existing diagnostic categories evolved to meet the need of clinicians to adequately describe personality

TABLE 4–1. FFM, TCI, DAPP-BQ, and SNAP dimensional models of general personality functioning

FFM	TCI	DAPP-BQ	SNAP
Neuroticism	Harm avoidance	Anxiousness	Mistrust
Anxiousness	Anticipatory worry	Compulsivity	Manipulation
Angry hostility	Fear of uncertainty	Conduct problems	Aggression
Depressiveness	Shyness	Diffidence	Self-harm
Self-consciousness	Fatigability	Identity problems	Eccentric perceptions
Impulsivity	Novelty seeking	Insecure attachment	Dependency
Vulnerability	Exploratory excitability	Intimacy problems	Exhibitionism
Extraversion	Impulsiveness	Narcissism	Entitlement
Warmth	Extravagance	Suspiciousness	Detachment
Gregariousness	Disorderliness	Affective lability	Impulsivity
Assertiveness	Reward dependence	Passive opposition	Propriety
Activity	Sentimentality	Cognitive distortion	Workaholism
Excitement seeking	Sociability	Rejection	
Positive emotions	Attachment	Self-harm behaviors	
Openness	Dependence	Restricted expression	
Fantasy	Persistence	Social avoidance	
Aesthetics	Eagerness of effort	Stimulus seeking	
Feelings	Work hardened	Interpersonal disesteem	
Actions	Ambitiousness		
Ideas	Perfectionism		
Values			

TABLE 4–1. FFM, TCI, DAPP-BQ, and SNAP dimensional models of general personality functioning *(continued)*

FFM	TCI	DAPP-BQ	SNAP
Agreeableness	Self-directedness		
Trust	Responsibility		
Straightforwardness	Purposefulness		
Altruism	Resourcefulness		
Compliance	Self-acceptance		
Modesty	Congruent second nature		
Tendermindedness	Cooperativeness		
Conscientiousness	Social acceptance		
Competence	Empathy		
Order	Helpfulness		
Dutifulness	Compassion		
Achievement striving	Pure heartedness		
Self-discipline	Self-transcendence		
Deliberation	Self-forgetfulness		
	Transpersonal identification		
	Spiritual acceptance		
	Enlightened		
	Idealistic		

Note. FFM=Five Factor Model (Costa and McCrae 1992); TCI=Tridimensional Character Inventory (Cloninger et al. 1994); DAPP-BQ=Dimensional Assessment of Personality Psychopathology–Basic Questionnaire (Livesley and Jackson, in press); SNAP=Schedule for Nonadaptive and Adaptive Personality (Clark 1993).

disorder symptomatology. Most of the DSM-IV personality disorders were developed originally by psychodynamically oriented clinicians, but the existing diagnostic categories now represent a quite diverse set of theoretical perspectives and are used now by clinicians with cognitive-behavioral, neurobiological, and interpersonal theoretical perspectives (Frances and Widiger 1986; Livesley 1998, 2001). If dimensional models of personality disorder were to replace the existing diagnostic categories, it would be important to indicate that the symptomatology and traits covered by the existing categories would still be covered by the dimensional model.

One would expect that the DAPP-BQ, SNAP, and SWAP-200 dimensional models would provide adequate coverage because these dimensional models explicitly included all of the DSM-IV personality disorder symptomatology (Clark 1993; Livesley et al. 1998; Westen and Shedler 1999a). Studies have also indicated substantial convergence among the FFM, DAPP-BQ, IPC, and SNAP dimensional models (e.g., Clark and Livesley 1994; Clark et al. 1996; Schroeder et al. 1992), and there is empirical support for the ability of the TCI and the FFM to account for personality disorder symptomatology (e.g., Ball et al. 1997; Goldman et al. 1994; Soldz et al. 1993; Svrakic et al. 1993; Trull et al. 2001). O'Connor and Dyce (1998) conducted a series of confirmatory factor analyses that compared the ability of the TCI, FFM, IPC, and Millon et al. (1996) dimensional models to predict the structural relationships among the personality disorders as reported in nine previously published studies using a variety of samples and assessment instruments. They concluded that "the highest and most consistent levels of fit were obtained for the five-factor model and for Cloninger and Svrakic's (1994) seven-factor model" (O'Connor and Dyce 1998, p. 14). In sum, the maladaptive personality traits included within the DSM-IV personality disorder diagnostic criteria do appear to be included within the alternative dimensional models of general personality functioning, but future research should explore whether there are important, fundamental components of a personality disorder that could not be represented by a dimensional model of general personality functioning.

On the other hand, there is currently no compelling rationale for why the 10 personality disorders included in DSM-IV would necessarily constitute a comprehensive or even adequate coverage of maladaptive personality (Frances and Widiger 1986; Livesley 1998). Four new personality disorders (borderline, schizotypal, avoidant, and narcissistic) were added to DSM-III, one of which (narcissistic) is still not included in ICD-10. Two personality disorders (sadistic and self-defeating) were added to a DSM-III-R appendix for proposed diagnostic categories but were deleted in DSM-IV (Pincus et al. 1992; Widiger 1995), and one (passive-aggressive) that had been in every edition of the diagnostic manual was downgraded to inclusion in a comparable appendix in DSM-IV. Nevertheless, compelling criticisms of the decision to downgrade the passive-aggressive personality disorder diagnosis to the appendix have been raised (Wetzler and Morey 1999), proposals for a depressive personality disorder diagnosis have been offered (Huprich 1998; Phillips et al. 1995; Ryder and Bagby 1999), and clinicians and researchers have argued that the current set of 10 diagnostic categories fails to provide adequate coverage of maladaptive personality functioning (Westen and Arkowitz-Westen 1998). An important question for future research is how best to obtain a scientifically based decision for what constitutes a necessary or adequate coverage of maladaptive personality functioning. With respect to the alternative dimensional models, future research should address the question of which model best provides the fundamental biobehavioral dimensions that constitute temperament and personality. The existing dimensional models do offer theoretical and empirical arguments for what are proposed by these models to be the fundamental biobehavioral dimensions of personality functioning (Benjamin 1993; Clark et al. 1996; Cloninger 2000; Livesley and Jang 2000; Millon et al. 1996; Westen and Shedler 1999b, 2000; Widiger 2000). An important scientific and clinical question is which model best accounts for the behavioral, neurobiological, genetic, and epidemiologic data. The decision of which dimensional model is to be used in clinical practice should be informed by scientific research that compares the alternatives with respect to clinical utility and predictive validity, as well as other forms of construct validity, rather than leaving any such future decisions to subjective or arbitrary decisions that are only weakly guided by empirical data.

An equally important question is whether and how alternative dimensional models could be used to provide clinically useful diagnoses of personality disorder. If the distinction between normal and abnormal personality functioning is indeed arbitrary (Strack and Lorr 1994), can a reliable, meaningful, and justifiable distinction be made? Clinicians should be provided with a more explicit and scientifically compelling rationale for determining what constitutes a disorder of personality. Several approaches have been taken to try to delineate personality disorder from normal personality traits using a dimensional system. For example, Cloninger (2000) suggested that personality disorder in a particular patient would be indicated by clinically low levels of cooperativeness, self-transcendence, and, most importantly, self-directedness (the ability to control, regulate, and adapt behavior); the specific variants of personality disorder are said to be governed by the temperaments of novelty seeking, harm avoidance, reward dependence, and persistence (Cloninger and Svrakic 1994). Alternatively, Widiger et al. (2002) suggested a four-step procedure for the diagnosis of personality disorder consistent with the hypothesis that personality disorders are maladaptive variants of common personality traits (Widiger 2000). The first step is a description of an individual's personality structure in terms of the FFM; the second is the identification of problems and impairments associated with these personality traits (a comprehensive list of problems and impairments associated with each facet of the FFM is provided); the third is a determination of whether these impairments reach a specified level of clinical significance (e.g., whether the traits significantly interfere with work or social functioning, modeled after Axis V of DSM-IV); and the fourth is a matching of the personality profile to prototypical cases to determine whether a single, parsimonious diagnostic label can be applied.

An additional focus of future research would be the field testing of clinical applications of dimensional models of personality disorder. Prior research has indicated that the excessive diagnostic co-occurrence, heterogeneity within diagnostic categories, inadequate coverage of clinically significant maladaptive personality traits, and weakly justified diagnostic thresholds are problematic for clinical treatment decisions. Proponents of dimensional models of personality disorder indicate how their dimensional models would presumably address these problems (Cloninger 2000; Livesley and Jang 2000; Oldham and Skodol 2000; Widiger 2000), but the clinical utility of these models has not yet been adequately demonstrated. For example, a substantial proportion of clinicians might find the personality disorder constructs within some of these models (e.g., reward dependence and closedness to experience) to be so unfamiliar that they are unable to use them to effectively guide their clinical decisions. Cutoff points will be necessary along dimensions of personality functioning to guide diagnostic and treatment decisions, but the clinical utility of these cutoff points has not yet been adequately specified or tested empirically. For example, it remains unclear if simply an elevation on a particular personality scale would warrant a diagnosis (e.g., self-directedness or neuroticism), whether a disorder could be suggested instead by particular constellations of maladaptive personality traits (e.g., high antagonism and low conscientiousness), and whether a separate, independent assessment of social and occupational functioning or personal distress should be required. In sum, the reliability, validity, and clinical utility of alternative diagnostic procedures for rendering a personality disorder diagnosis from the perspective of dimensional models should be field tested in future research.

The Nomological Network of Personality Disorder

If a dimensional model of personality functioning is to replace the existing personality disorder diagnostic categories, it will also be important for such a model to also account for the nomological (theoretical) network of relationships associated with the personality disorders. Substantial amounts of clinical theory and literature concerning the DSM-IV personality disorders have been developed since the diagnostic categories were first developed (Clarkin and Lenzenweger 1996; Livesley 2001; Millon et al. 1996). This literature concerns fundamental components of the concept of a personality disorder—such as temporal stability, heritability, neurochemical correlates, and childhood development—and implications for future physical health, mental health, and treatment. It would be difficult to replace the existing diagnostic categories with a dimensional model of personality (e.g., to have the model accepted by practicing clinicians) if the model was inconsistent with or failed to provide useful clinical information with respect to these fundamental validators of a personality disorder diagnosis. Issues of particular importance for future clinical research are the longitudinal course of personality dispositions, their development through childhood and adolescence, their biological mechanisms, and their implications for the development and treatment of general medical conditions and other mental disorders.

Longitudinal course. Fundamental to the validity of a personality disorder is documentation that "the pattern is stable and of long duration, and its onset can be traced back at least to adolescence or early adulthood" (American Psychiatric Association 2000, p. 689). The temporal stability of only one personality disorder diagnosis (borderline) has received much attention, and the findings have been mixed (McDavid and Pilkonis 1996; Zimmerman 1994).

Temporal stability has been studied for only a few of the alternative dimensional models of general personality functioning, but the results of this research are encouraging (Costa and McCrae 1994). Temporal stability coefficients across 6–9 years for self and spousal ratings of the FFM and SNAP higher-order constructs (e.g., neuroticism or negative affectivity) have ranged from 0.75 to 0.85 (Costa and McCrae 1985, 1994; Costa et al. 2000); temporal stability across 25 years has ranged from 0.51 to 0.68 (Costa and McCrae 1994; Helson and Klohnen 1998). There is only a minor decrease in temporal stability for lower-order facets (the vast majority obtain temporal stability coefficients across 6–9 years above 0.70).

Of particular importance for future research will be the demonstration of temporal stability within clinical populations. The instability of personality disorder diagnoses might not only be due to the arbitrariness or unreliability of the diagnostic categories; it may also be the result of the effect of fluctuating mood states on the assessment of personality traits (McDavid and Pilkonis 1996; Widiger et al. 1999; Zimmerman 1994). It is unclear whether the dimensional models of general personality functioning will demonstrate adequate levels of temporal stability within clinical populations (Bagby et al. 1995; Morey and Zanarini 2000).

Biological mechanisms. Fundamental to the validity of any mental disorder diagnosis, including the personality disorders, is establishment of its heritability, the biological mechanisms for this heritability, and current pathology (E. Robins and Guze 1970). Biogenetic and heritability research has been confined largely to antisocial, borderline, and schizotypal personality disorders, with very little research specifically concerning dependent, narcissistic, histrionic, and other personality disorders (McGuffin and Thapar 1992; Nigg and Goldsmith 1994). There is considerable support from twin, family, and adoption studies for a genetic contribution to the etiology of antisocial personality disorder, and this research is now focusing on isolating the precise genetic and neuropsychological mechanisms (Carey and Goldman 1997; Newman 1997; Patrick et al. 1993). Schizotypal personality shares much of its heritability with schizophrenia (Siever 1992). There is some evidence that borderline personality disorder might breed true, but there are also indications that this personality disorder shares much of its heritability with mood, impulse dyscontrol, and other personality disorders (Gunderson and Zanarini 1989; Torgersen 1992). The implications of the heritability research for the understanding and classification of schizotypal and borderline personality disorders is unclear (Gunderson 1992; Paris 1999).

There has been considerable biogenetic and heritability research on dimensional models of personality functioning (Plomin and Caspi 1999). The heritability of neuroticism is typically estimated to be approximately 50%; the heritability of extraversion is estimated at 60%; and the domains of agreeableness, openness, and conscientiousness are estimated to have a heritability of 40% (Loehlin 1992; Plomin and Caspi 1999). Heritability at the level of the 30 facets of the FFM has been demonstrated in twin studies by Jang et al. (1996, 1998). Empirical support for the heritability of the 18 DAPP-BQ dimensions has been demonstrated in studies by Livesley et al. (1998), and support for heritability of the four temperaments of the TCI has been demonstrated in studies by Heath et al. (1994) and Stallings et al. (1996).

The fundamental nature of dimensions of personality is also suggested by their utility in the classification of behavior patterns across animal species. Gosling and John (1999) reviewed the published studies for 12 nonhuman species (e.g., chimpanzee, hyena, rat, dog, and octopus) and reported support for three of the domains of the FFM (neuroticism, extraversion versus introversion, and agreeableness versus antagonism). The anatomy and physiology of humans are quite similar to those of animals, and research on the neurobiology of animal behavior can contribute to an understanding of the neurophysiology of human personality functioning (Cloninger 1998; Depue 1996; Gosling 2001). For example, the personality domain of extraversion (positive emotionality) is quite analogous to the search, foraging, and approach system studied in various animal species, at times more globally referred to as a behavioral facilitation system (BFS). Depue and his colleagues are exploring the neurobiology of the personality domains of positive affectivity (extraversion), negative affectivity (neuroticism), and constraint (conscientiousness) through pharmacologic challenge studies (e.g., Depue et al. 1994).

"One of the more exciting directions for genetic research on personality involves the use of molecular genetic techniques to identify some of the specific genes responsible for genetic influence on personality" (Plomin and Caspi 1999, p. 261). This research may ultimately lead to an understanding of the causal pathways from cells to social systems that will elucidate how genes affect personality development (Hyman 1998). For example, novelty seeking is hypothesized by Cloninger (1998) to involve genetic differences in dopamine transmission. Individuals with the long-repeat DRD4 allele are thought to be dopamine deficient and seek novelty to increase dopamine release (Cloninger et al. 1996a). Support for hypotheses concerning the personality traits within the TCI and FFM dimensional models has been obtained (e.g., Ebstein et al. 1996, 1997; Lesch et al. 1996; Osher et al. 2000), but just as many failures to replicate have also occurred (e.g., Gelernter et al. 1998; Hamer et al. 1999; Herbst et al. 2000). The possible reasons for the failures to replicate are many (Greenberg et al. 2000; Hamer et al. 1999). The effect sizes for broad personality dispositions provided by single genes are likely to be quite small and perhaps difficult to replicate (Plomin and Caspi 1999). Greater specificity of relationships might be obtained through studies of the more specific facets of personality functioning (Jang et al. 1998; Livesley et al. 1998).

A related area of future research is the clarification of the physiologic substrates underlying these personality dimensions (Cloninger 1998; Depue 1996). For example, clinical studies have suggested that low 5-hydroxytryptamine (5-HT or serotonin) activity might be related to angry, hostile, and aggressive behavior. This research has included populations with personality disorders (e.g., antisocial and borderline), but "one of the most remarkable aspects of this literature is the general consistency of these findings across different study samples and using various assessments of 5-HT function" (Coccaro 1998b, p. 2). In other words, the 5-HT findings have not been specific to any particular mental disorder but are associated instead with more fundamental dimensions of impulsivity and aggression that cut across diagnostic categories.

The neurobiology of personality is not necessarily nor solely a study of the genetic bases of personality. "To provide a more comprehensive foundation for future research on the neurobiology of personality disorders, the functional principles of the neurobiological variables must be derived (i.e., the manner in which they influence behavior), as must the way in which the variables interact with salient environmental stimuli to produce behavior" (Depue and Lenzenweger 2001, p. 137). The past two decades of research on fear circuits in the brain have provided a much better understanding of how defensive behavior and avoidance are learned and implemented. Studies that combine leading-edge behavioral and physiologic measures of personality and temperament are vitally needed to unravel the complicated relationships between activity of various brain systems and observed behavior.

Childhood development. Fundamental to the concept and diagnosis of personality disorder is its development during childhood and emergence in adolescence. However, one of the more remarkable gaps in knowledge is the childhood antecedents for personality disorders (Widiger and Clark 2000). Included in DSM-III were four childhood antecedents of the personality disorders: identity disorder as an antecedent of borderline personality disorder, avoidant disorder as an antecedent of avoidant personality disorder, oppositional-defiant disorder for passive-aggressive personality disorder, and conduct disorder for antisocial personality disorder. Only the childhood antecedents for antisocial personality disorder remain. Empirical support for the childhood antecedents of antisocial personality disorder and psychopathy have been so compelling that evidence of their presence is required for the diagnosis of antisocial personality disorder (Lynam 1996; L.N. Robins et al. 1991), but it is unclear why there would be so much empirical support for one personality disorder with almost no data on the childhood antecedents for most of the other personality disorders (Widiger and Sankis 2000).

"Goals of temperament researchers have traditionally been to identify the psychological processes by which individual differences arise, the neuropsychological systems underlying these psychological processes, the developmental course of these processes, and the interaction of these processes and the environment" (Ahadi and Rothbart 1994, pp. 189–190). There has been little research on the relationship of temperament to the DSM-IV personality disorders, but there is an increasing amount of research on the relationship of temperament to more general models of personality functioning (Clark and Watson 1999; Halverson et al. 1994). The FFM, for example, has been effective at providing an integrative structure for the classification and understanding of commonly studied childhood temperaments (Ahadi and Rothbart 1994; Angleitner and Ostendorf 1994;

John et al. 1994; R.W. Robins et al. 1994; Shiner 1998).

Prospective longitudinal studies from childhood into adulthood are needed to provide empirical documentation of how maladaptive personality traits are developed, sustained, altered, or remitted in their presentation across the life span (Caspi 1998; Lynam 1996; Sher and Trull 1996; Widiger and Sankis 2000). Ideally, the personality dispositions studied in adulthood would have conceptually meaningful and empirically valid relationships to the behavior patterns and temperaments studied in childhood, and this integration might be achieved by a more dimensional model of personality functioning (Digman 1994). For example, research has suggested that individuals with antisocial personality disorder demonstrate a hyporeactive electrodermal response to stress that is associated with a commonly studied domain of normal personality functioning, neuroticism, or negative affectivity (Patrick 1994; Patrick et al. 1993). This research might be consistent with the developmental research on the interaction of parenting and fundamental temperaments (e.g., low anxiousness and low inhibition) on the development of a moral conscience (Kochanska 1991). From this perspective, the pathology of psychopathy might not be a deficit that is qualitatively distinct from general personality functioning (Widiger and Lynam 1998). "The observed absence of startle potentiation in psychopaths (Patrick et al. 1993) may reflect a temperamental deficit in the capacity for negative affect" (Patrick 1994, p. 325).

There has been substantial research on the contributions of sexual and psychological abuse to the etiology of borderline personality disorder (Gunderson and Sabo 1993; Zanarini 2000). Linehan (1993) has hypothesized that borderline personality disorder is the result of a heritable temperament of emotional instability interacting with a severely invalidating (e.g., abusive) environment. However, the broad diagnostic category of borderline personality disorder may not capture well the specific traits or temperament that is especially vulnerable to abusive and stressful experiences. Perhaps this research could be integrated with existing developmental studies of the interaction of parenting and temperament (e.g., Kochanska 1991; Rothbart and Ahadi 1994).

Morey and Zanarini (2000) reported better temporal stability over a 4-year period for the personality dimensions of the FFM in comparison to the symptomatology of borderline personality disorder. They suggested that the latter is "a disorder that waxes and wanes in severity over time, whereas neuroticism reflects a putatively stable trait configuration" (p. 737). On the other hand, they also indicated that borderline personality disorder was more highly and specifically related to childhood sexual abuse than were the personality trait dimensions of the FFM. "From this perspective, the FFM could indicate a temperamental vulnerability to a disorder that is then triggered by developmental events (such as childhood neglect or abuse), resulting in functional levels that may be quite variable in response to situational elements even while the underlying traits remain relatively stable" (p. 737).

The neurobiology of trauma appears to involve primarily the hypothalamic-pituitary-adrenal (HPA) axis, which is the central neuroendocrine stress-response regulator (Yehuda 1998). Initial research on patients with personality disorder symptoms has suggested HPA axis findings that closely resemble those typically found in patients with posttraumatic stress disorder, namely decreased basal cortisol and cortisol hypersuppression associated with abuse and increased lymphocyte glucocorticoid receptor density (Siever et al. 1998). Siever et al. suggest that decreased basal cortisol and cortisol hypersuppression might be a trait marker for more enduring borderline personality traits, whereas decreased glucocorticoid receptor density might be a state measure associated with more acute responsivity to stress.

Physical health. "The relationship between personality and [physical] health is currently a topic of considerable scientific interest" (Contrada et al. 1999, p. 576). This research has included the contribution of personality traits to the onset of disease and to maladaptive responses to the occurrence of illness (Contrada et al. 1999; Wiebe and Smith 1997). For example, Friedman et al. (1993, 1995) indicated that personality trait data obtained through parent and teacher ratings of children at approximately age 11 predicted longevity over the next 70 years. In particular, conscientiousness as assessed in childhood predicted survival into middle and old age. A 20-year-old within the top quartile of conscientiousness could expect to live 2 years longer than someone within the bottom quartile.

Many studies have indicated that angry hostility is a significant risk factor for cardiovascular disease (Wiebe and Smith 1997). Concurrent and future research is concerned with explicating the specific pathophysiological mechanisms for this association. Angry hostility as a stable personality trait may contribute to a gradual progression of coronary heart disease through an increase in sympathetic nervous activity, hyperlipidemia, and hypertension that result in the development of atherosclerosis, and may also provide an acute risk of cardiac ischemia, arrhythmia, plaque rupture, and thrombosis associated with specific episodes of angry outbursts (Kop 1999; Rozanski et al. 1999). Another active area of investigation is the effect of personality traits on the immune system (Segerstrom 2000). For example, Cole and colleagues (1997) examined the relationship between human immunodeficiency virus (HIV) progression and rejection sensitivity, a personality dimension related closely to introversion. Consistent with experimental cold virus research, higher rejection sensitivity predicted accelerated HIV progression as indicated by time to critically low T (CVD4) cell count, acquired immune deficiency syndrome (AIDS), and death in gay men.

Treatment. Personality disorders are at times misperceived as being untreatable conditions. This reputation is due in part to the temporal stability of personality (Costa and McCrae 1994) and to the decreased effectiveness of the treatment of mood, anxiety, substance, and other Axis I disorders that occur in the presence of a comorbid personality disorder (Shea et al. 1992; Widiger et al. 1999). Personality disorders are among the most difficult of mental disorders to treat, but there are data to indicate that meaningful responsivity to treatment does occur (Kapfhammer and Hippius 1998; Perry et al. 1999; Sanislow and McGlashan 1998).

There is considerably more systematic research on the treatment of the DSM-IV personality disorders than on the treatment of general personality functioning (Perry et al. 1999; Sanislow and McGlashan 1998). Nevertheless, the available data do suggest that clinically meaningful changes in general personality functioning might also be obtained (Cloninger and Svrakic 1997; Coccaro 1998a; Piedmont 1998). For example, B. Knutson and colleagues (1998) administered in a double-blind manner paroxetine, a selective serotonin reuptake inhibitor (SSRI), for 4 weeks to 23 of 48 ostensibly normal volunteers; the other participants received a placebo. The researchers reported that SSRI administration (relative to placebo) increased social facilitation (assessed in a blind laboratory task of cooperation) and reduced self-reported levels of negative affectivity (neuroticism) and hostility. The magnitude of changes was even correlated with plasma levels of SSRI within the SSRI group. "This is the first empirical demonstration that chronic administration of a selective serotonin reuptake blockade can have significant personality and behavioral effects in normal humans in the absence of baseline depression or other psychopathology" (B. Knutson et al. 1998, p. 378).

A fully comprehensive model of personality functioning might also include aspects of personality that might facilitate treatment responsivity, as well as identifying maladaptive personality traits that would undermine or complicate treatment. "The last 40 years of individual differences research require the inclusion of personality trait assessment for the construction and implementation of any treatment plan that would lay claim to scientific status" (Harkness and Lilienfeld 1997, p. 349). As dimensional models of normal (adaptive) as well as abnormal personality functioning, the TCI and FFM might be of particular benefit to those researching treatment outcome (Cloninger 1998; Piedmont 1998; C. Sanderson and Clarkin 1994).

Conclusions and Proposed Research Agenda

In sum, if a dimensional model of personality disorder is ever to replace the existing diagnostic categories, future research will need to determine whether a dimensional model can in fact resolve the many problems that occur with the existing diagnostic categories (e.g., inadequate coverage, heterogeneity of classification, excessive diagnostic co-occurrence, and arbitrary diagnostic boundaries), provide theoretically and clinically useful information that is currently provided by the existing diagnostic categories, and go beyond the existing diagnostic system in offering a compelling scientific rationale for the fundamental biobehavioral dimensions of personality functioning. This information should include a validation of the childhood developmental antecedents of personality disorder; the biological mechanisms for heritability, learning, and pathology; temporal stability; and implications for health and treatment.

Research that would be particularly relevant and informative to a decision on whether to replace the DSM-IV personality disorder diagnostic categories with a dimensional model of personality functioning would be studies that:

- *Identify the fundamental biobehavioral dimensions of temperament and personality that would best account for existing behavioral, neurobiological, genetic, and epidemiologic data, and that would also determine whether there are clinically important aspects of a personality disorder that are not or could not be adequately represented by dimensional models of general personality functioning.* Many studies have indicated substantial convergence of dimensional models of general personality functioning with the DSM-IV personality disorders. There does appear to be considerable overlap. Future research should address such questions as whether dimensional models of classification do in fact improve the coverage of personality disorder symptomatology and whether there are particular components or aspects of the DSM-IV personality disorders that are not adequately represented within or covered by existing dimensional models (e.g., identity disturbances, attachment conflicts, cognitive aberrations, or perceptual abnormalities). In addition, this research should determine whether these components could or should be incorporated within dimensional models of general personality functioning. Do such individual symptoms of personality disorder in fact represent components of personality functioning that are qualitatively distinct from general personality functioning (and from Axis I disorders), or could they be understood as maladaptive variants of general personality functioning with minor revisions or extensions of a dimensional model?

- *Determine whether and how a particular dimensional model would provide a clinical diagnosis of personality disorder in a manner that would be more reliable, specific, and clinically informative than the existing diagnostic categories.* Proposals for the diagnosis of personality disorder using general models of personality functioning are being developed. These proposals need to be field tested within clinical populations. It is possible, for example, that clinicians may find the clinical concepts within some dimensional models to be too unfamiliar for clinical practice and would be uncertain how to use them to guide clinical decisions. The thresholds recommended for respective dimensional models should be compared to the thresholds for the existing DSM-IV personality disorder diagnoses. Can a scientifically and clinically meaningful boundary with normal personality functioning be identified that will have clinical utility for diverse social and clinical decisions? Researchers might explore the utility of different cutoff points on scales of personality functioning for different social and clinical decisions.
- *Determine whether and how dimensional models of personality functioning can be used to effectively guide treatment decisions in a manner that would be more reliable and clinically informative than the existing diagnostic categories.* Clinicians are currently guided in their treatment decisions by the DSM-IV personality disorder diagnostic categories. Research is needed that compares dimensional models of general personality functioning with the existing diagnostic categories with respect to clinically relevant treatment process and outcome issues (e.g., treatment responsivity).
- *Determine whether dimensional models of personality functioning obtain adequate levels of temporal stability within clinical settings.* Existing research has suggested inadequate temporal stability of personality disorder diagnostic categories. It is unclear whether this reflects limitations of assessment instruments that fail to provide adequate differentiation from Axis I disorders or more fundamental limitations of the diagnostic categories. Good to excellent temporal stability has been obtained using dimensional models of general personality functioning within general community populations. However, it is unclear whether the dimensional models will be as successful within settings that involve persons who are characterized in part by the instability of their functioning and who are involved in treatment interventions that are intended to make changes to emotional, cognitive, and interpersonal functioning. In addition, it is still unclear how much stability and change in maladaptive personality functioning is normative across the life span. Future research needs to determine the factors that affect the stability of personality functioning over time, and how long-term temporal fluctuations affect an understanding of the impairments that may be associated with personality disorder.

- *Conduct research to study how dimensions of personality as studied through behavioral and self-report measures may be related to the broad motivational and cognitive systems of the brain, such as those involved with appetitive and consummatory behavior, or defense and avoidance.* Furthermore, elucidate the heritability of those various systems, and how genetic factors may both determine personality factors and also constrain the effects of various environmental impacts on central nervous system plasticity. This research would facilitate the development of a neurophysiologic understanding of maladaptive personality traits that may ultimately lead to the development of more valid laboratory techniques for diagnosis and methods of treatment.
- *Provide a longitudinal understanding of the interaction between temperaments and environment that result in the development of personality disorder, and allow a more refined conceptualization of what is meant by a personality disorder.* The effect of the interaction of biogenetic temperaments with traumatic experiences that eventually results in the development of maladaptive personality traits and the diagnosis of personality disorders needs to be explored longitudinally. The relative importance of the genetic dispositions and traumatic experiences to the development of maladaptive personality traits should be addressed through longitudinal studies of persons at high risk for the development of maladaptive personality traits.
- *Explicate the social, cultural, and neurophysiologic mechanisms that explain the impact of maladaptive (and adaptive) personality traits on physical disease (and physical health).* Dimensional models of personality functioning have been of considerable utility for general medicine, whereas the DSM-IV personality disorder diagnostic categories have generally received less interest from primary care physicians and other practitioners within general medicine. The potential utility to general medicine of a dimensional model of personality disorders should be explored in future research. Dimensional models of personality disorder might facilitate the integration and application of the psychiatric nomenclature to the practice of primary care physicians and other specialists within general medicine. The explication of the social, cultural, and neurophysiologic mechanisms that explain the vulnerability for and resilience against the development of physical diseases provided by personality traits could be of considerable interest and use to the DSM-V work groups as they attempt to identify a meaningful boundary between normal and abnormal personality functioning.

Personality Traits/Disorders and Their Relationship to Axis I Disorders

The preceding section was devoted to a detailed consideration of the problems with the current definitions of personality disorders, and the possibility that dimensional models of personality could offer a superior approach both in clinical utility and in linking to large literatures from basic personality research and neurobiology, which could further inform new developments. In this regard, the focus remained on aspects of functioning traditionally ascribed to the personality disorders, that is, those that appear to represent relatively sustained patterns of behavior and modes of interacting with the environment. However, another issue that has also received increasing discussion concerns the relationships between personality disorders and Axis I disorders. This section addresses research considering the Axis I–Axis II distinction. This interface represents an important component of the contemporary challenge in redefining the notions of how to conceptualize not merely personality disorders, but the fundamental nature of all mental disorders.

The extremely high rates of concurrent Axis I disorders in individuals with personality disorder diagnoses—as well as the reverse, high rates of Axis II disorders in individuals with Axis I disorders—raise questions regarding the independence and distinctiveness of these disorders. For example, in one study of 2,344 patients with Axis II diagnoses, 79% also met criteria for an Axis I disorder (Fabrega et al. 1990). A recent report from the Collaborative Longitudinal Personality Study (Gunderson et al. 2000) showed similar findings (McGlashan et al. 2000). Such findings have been reported in diverse samples assessed by different methods (Dolan et al. 2001). In addition to high rates of Axis II disorders, samples of individuals with Axis I disorders have also been characterized by high levels of dysfunctional personality traits such as neuroticism, introversion, dependency, and/or perfectionism (e.g., Barnett and Gotlib 1988; Clark et al. 1996). Such findings have led to questions regarding the meaning of these associations, including the conceptual differences between the disorders on Axis I and on Axis II.

Several models or hypotheses have been described in the literature to account for different possible temporal and/or causal relationships between personality disorders and Axis I disorders (Klein et al. 1993). Some of the more prominent types of models include common cause, spectrum or subclinical, predisposition or vulnerability, pathoplasty or exacerbation, and complication or scar (Klein et al. 1993). Briefly, common cause models assume that the Axis I and II disorders, although distinct phenomenologically, are each determined by the same underlying process or core liability.

The causal factor could involve biological and/or environmental mechanisms. The closely related spectrum model assumes that the Axis I and II disorders are different manifestations or phases of the same underlying disease processes; one disorder is a manifestation or variant of the other. Disorders associated within a disease spectrum might share some, but not all, genes conveying risk or modifying the expression of a disease (Peltonen and McKusick 2001). The two disorders may share some clinical features but differ in severity, or one may be an early stage or less fully developed form of the other. Predisposition or vulnerability models assume that when one condition exists, it is a risk factor for the other. In contrast to the spectrum model, two different pathological processes or disorders are assumed. The pathoplasty or exacerbation models assume that the Axis I and II disorders are causally distinct, but that the presence of one influences the presentation (pathoplasty) or severity/outcome (exacerbation) of the other through additive or interactive effects. Finally, the complication or scar models suggest that one disorder or condition develops as a result of or in the context of another preceding disorder and continues after the initial disorder remits. There is considerable conceptual overlap among these models, and distinguishing them empirically is difficult. However, they highlight the different ways that the high rates of co-occurrence among Axis I and Axis II disorders may be viewed.

Personality Traits/Disorders as Spectrum Conditions of Axis I Disorder

Of the models described above, the spectrum model may be the most relevant to addressing some of the current problems with the boundaries between Axis I and Axis II disorders. One of the more comprehensive spectrum models that has been proposed (Siever and Davis 1991) postulated four basic psychobiological dimensions of temperament and behavior that may underlie and cut across the Axis I and II disorders: cognitive/perceptual aberrations, affective regulation, impulse control, and anxiety modulation. These four dimensions are conceptualized as core causal factors that contribute, singly or in combination, to the development of personality traits, personality disturbances or disorders, or their more severe Axis I counterparts. Core temperamental vulnerabilities along these dimensions are proposed to interact with early environmental experiences, resulting in the development of psychopathology that spans the Axis I and II disorders as currently defined.

Most evidence supporting a spectrum model exists for psychotic psychopathology (cognitive perceptual aberrations). Early observations of the family members of patients with schizophrenia, including those made by both Bleuler and Kraepelin, strongly suggested the presence of peculiar personality traits and characteristics that were clinically suggestive of schizophrenia. Such individuals, although often not displaying psychosis themselves, nonetheless demonstrated odd or eccentric behaviors that were qualitatively like those of the full psychotic syndrome. Such observations formed the basis for the concept of schizotaxia, a spectrum of psychotic-realm behaviors that were familial in origin with common pathogenetic origins (Meehl 1945). In fact, the initial appearance of schizotypal personality disorder in DSM-III was conceived on this basis, and its criteria were derived from case histories of a Danish adoption study of the biological relatives of schizophrenic patients (Kety 1975; Kety et al. 1994). Over the past two decades, a large body of phenomenological, genetic, biological outcome, and treatment research has provided significant support for the close relationship between schizotypal personality disorder and the Axis I diagnosis of schizophrenia (Goldberg et al. 1986; Kendler 1985; Kendler et al. 1995; McGlashan 1986; Serban and Siegel 1984; Siever 1994; Siever et al. 1993; Stein 1992). Because of this, questions remain as to the advantages and disadvantages of its current classification as a personality disorder on Axis II rather than its being grouped with other Axis I psychotic disorders. In particular, the issue of whether schizotypal personality disorder should be reclassified as an Axis I psychotic-spectrum disorder (as are the analogous mood disorders dysthymia and cyclothymia) merits particular attention given currently available research.

Perhaps nearly as strong as evidence favoring a continuum for the psychotic spectrum have been data on the relationship between the Axis I construct of social phobia and the Axis II construct of avoidant personality disorder. In contrast to schizotypal personality disorder, however, the introduction of avoidant personality disorder in DSM-III occurred in the relative absence of a significant clinical tradition or literature. Thus, empirical observations of overlapping diagnostic criteria and frequently high rates of comorbidity (20%–90%) have given rise to the ongoing nosologic debate about the validity of clinical distinctions between the two disorders (Brooks et al. 1989; Holt et al. 1992; Jansen et al. 1994; W.C. Sanderson et al. 1994; Schneier et al. 1991, 1992; Skodol et al. 1995; Turner et al. 1991). Treatment studies showing the pharmacologic responsiveness of avoidant personality traits in persons with social phobia provide support for the continuity between the disorders (Reich et al. 1989). More compelling, however, is the documented familial aggregation of the disorders and comparably elevated relative risks (i.e., 2–3 fold) for both social phobia and avoidant personality disorder among the relatives of affected probands (Tillfors et al. 2001). Taken together, such data argue in favor of the widely held view that both avoidant personality disorder and social phobia represent dimensions of social anxiety rather than separate disorders.

Although they are less well established, similar spectrum relationships have been posited for other Axis I and II disorders based on the dimension of affect regulation. For example, investigators in the area of bipolar disorder have posited relationships among personality and subthreshold disorders characterized by affective instability (Akiskal 1994; Cassano et al. 1999). At or before the onset of the full syndrome, individuals presenting with manic-like symptoms, particularly children and adolescents, are often diagnosed with conduct disorders or with borderline personality disorder or other cluster B personality disorders. Thus, subsyndromal disturbances in behavior or mood that may reflect an underlying bipolar diathesis are often viewed or diagnosed (misdiagnosed) as personality disorders. For borderline personality disorder, such a relationship has received empirical support from polysomnographic (Akiskal et al. 1985) and psychopharmacologic response (Pinto and Akiskal 1998) data. In contrast, family history and biological data have tended not to favor a mood spectrum (Coccaro 1998a; Silverman et al. 1991). Some evidence suggests that borderline personality disorder may have a greater familial relationship to two distinct dimensions of affective instability and impulsivity than to major affective disorders (Silverman et al. 1991). Although numerous reasons may underlie the apparent disparity in the limited evidence acquired to date, it is likely that borderline personality disorder is not a unitary construct and that clinical heterogeneity underlies current difficulties in its reconceptualization (e.g., mood disorder vs. dimensions of affective instability or impulsivity).

In contrast, significant research has focused on the relationship between subsyndromal affective states (and personality traits) and Axis I major depressive disorder. Overall, the most robust findings are for neuroticism, which has been shown to be a risk factor for depression and to be associated with a more chronic course (Angst and Clayton 1986; Boyce et al. 1991; Clayton et al. 1994; Hirschfeld et al. 1989; Kendler et al. 1993; Nystrom and Lindegard 1975). However, these findings also raise the question of the distinction between the personality dimension of neuroticism and the clinical disorder of depression. The spectrum interpretation posits that neuroticism is a subclinical or prodromal manifestation of depression, rather than a distinct personality trait. Within Axis I, recent research has suggested little longitudinal stability in categorical diagnoses of depressive subtypes (Angst et al. 2000), which is consistent with the notion of the highly variable, spectrum nature of affective disorder syndromes. In fact, dimensional approaches to the classification of depressive disorders are currently under evaluation and suggest that depression may be better represented on a continuum as opposed to discrete categories, with symptom number, frequency, and duration of episodes providing more valid classification criteria (Angst and Merikangas 1997). Such findings raise broader questions concerning the nature and meaningfulness of the conceptual distinctions between the constructs of mood and personality (Klein et al. 1993). Affective styles (or temperament) are central to both personality and depression. Positive and negative affect can be understood as mood states included within broader personality dispositions of positive affectivity (extraversion) and negative affectivity (neuroticism), with both states and traits being integrally related to basic affective and motivational systems (Clark et al. 1994; Tellegen 1985). The literature thus reveals a close relationship between traditional constructs of personality traits and disorders and Axis I disorders, manifested cross-sectionally and longitudinally. A key question is how best to conceptualize these associations—that is, as representing manifestations of common underlying psychopathological processes (spectrum), or as distinct dimensions that interact in clinically significant ways.

Proposed Research Agenda for Clarifying Spectrum Relationships

We propose that the research agenda should emphasize two high-priority areas from the spectrum perspective: schizophrenia and mood disorders.

1. *Schizophrenia-spectrum disorders:* The prospects for an integrated and valid diagnostic schema for schizotypal personality disorder and schizophrenia depend on further elucidation of the specific nature of the etiologic and pathophysiological processes (e.g., genetic and nongenetic) accounting for the commonalities and distinctions between these diagnoses. The research agenda includes a more detailed characterization of cellular and molecular mechanisms that might define the associations and boundaries of schizophrenia and schizotypal personality disorder, as might be generated by postmortem study of brain tissue from individuals who have undergone careful antemortem assessment. Additional information about circuitry structure and function will be generated through in vivo structural, functional, and neurochemical neuroimaging; by additional cognitive neuroscience approaches; and by experimental psychopharmacologic research. These tools may promote the development of endophenotypes that facilitate the identification of disease and disease-modifying genes that have both diagnostic and prognostic value. Human molecular genetic (parametric and nonparametric linkage approaches, as well as case-control and family based association methods) also show promise in this regard.
2. *Mood disorders:* The relationship between affectively unstable temperaments, such as borderline personality disorder (and related personality traits and disorders), and bipolar disorder deserves additional study.

> Empirical research in the area of family studies will initially be important for establishing the relative risk of developing borderline personality disorder or for the dimensions of affective instability and/or impulsivity among the relatives of bipolar disease probands. Should such studies provide substantive support for the spectrum model, prospective studies on the defining characteristics of such bipolar-spectrum subjects will then be required to better distinguish those individuals' descriptively similar, albeit etiologically distinct, personality disorder subtypes. In parallel with descriptive studies, neurobiological studies, including neuroimaging and molecular genetic methods, might play a role in defining neural circuitry alterations or neuronal dysfunctions that might link borderline personality disorder or subsyndromal mood disturbance to other mood disorder–spectrum disorders.

Similar issues face the boundary of personality traits and disorders and the nonbipolar depressive disorders. In particular, research clarifying the relationship of low positive affectivity and high negative affectivity (neuroticism) to acute and chronic depressive disorders is needed. Longitudinal studies examining individual differences in the degree and persistence of positive and negative affectivity and depressive symptoms, as well as the specific concordance of each with disturbances in neurobehavioral motivational systems, would be valuable.

Cross-Cultural and Gender Issues Regarding Personality Disorders and Traits

The issues regarding how personality interfaces with culture are extremely complex. Behavior is multidetermined, and, accordingly, many factors (biological, psychological, and social/cultural) shape personality development and psychopathology. The purpose of this section is to highlight how culture and acculturation influence the domains of personality traits and personality disorders.

There is a fair amount of cross-cultural research that suggests that the five-factor model (neuroticism, extroversion, openness to experiences, agreeableness, and conscientiousness) developed by Costa and McCrae (1985) is applicable cross-culturally (Katigbak et al. 1996; McCrae and Costa 1997; McCrae et al. 1999; Trull and Geary 1997). In addition, Cloninger's (1998) work on the tridimensional (i.e., harm avoidance, reward dependence, and novelty seeking) TCI also supports the notion that similar personality traits cross all cultural, ethnic, and racial lines. Although there is not consensus regarding how to categorize personality traits (Herbst et al. 2000), there is sufficient evidence that there must be some universal set of basic personality traits. Furthermore, there appear to be pan-cultural patterns of age and gender difference (McCrae et al. 1999). This consistency in the development of personality traits lends extra credence to the idea that there are some basic personality traits that are universal in nature and extend across cultural, ethnic, and racial groups. It is likely that these traits and their covariates are to a considerable extent genetically based.

Despite these cross-culture similarities in personality structure there are also differences between cultures (e.g., cultures differ in the mean level of self-reported traits). It is not clear, however, whether these differences are real or an artifact of self-reporting. Furthermore, if the differences are real, it is not clear whether they are due to a cultural effect, a difference in gene pools, or both. For example, Asian American women have significantly lower narcissism scores than do Anglo American women (Smith 1990). Is this due to different ethnic response sets or the influence of traditional Asian cultures, which are antithetical to narcissism and include modesty, respect for authority, and valuing relationship over individualism? Support for the hypothesis that these variations in the results of personality inventories may be cultural in origin has been found in studies that measure personality traits in subjects with different levels of acculturation. For example, Chinese students show increased openness, cheerfulness, and prosocial behavior and attitudes with exposure to Canadian culture (McCrae et al. 1998). Acculturation also affects bias in certain personality measures. For example, scores by Mexican Americans on the Minnesota Multiphasic Personality Inventory (MMPI) vary according to their level of acculturation. Subjects of European descent had significantly different scores from those of Mexican American subjects on 10 of 13 MMPI scales. With acculturation and age statistically controlled, European Americans and Mexican Americans differed only on the Lie (L) and Masculinity/Femininity (MF) scales. However, the personality differences identified by the L and MF scales may reflect genuine characteristics of the Mexican American culture. (Montgomery and Orozco 1985). Thus, differences between European Americans and Mexican Americans as identified by the MMPI may be due to culture or acculturation (Montgomery and Orozco 1985).

Cloninger and Svrakic (2000) reported that the Millon Clinical Multiaxial Inventory–II (MCMI-II) (Millon 1987), the NEO Personality Inventory (Costa and McCrae 1985), the TCI (Cloninger et al. 1994), and DAPP are the most frequently used dimensional tests of personality disorders. Unfortunately, these measurement tools for personality traits, temperament, and personality disorders have not, in general, been normed on groups with different cultural and ethnic backgrounds, which calls into question the applicability of findings using these instruments to those groups. There have been several studies that have demonstrated the inappropriateness of administering European American personality assessment tools on different ethnic and cultural populations. For example, the MMPI finds psychopathology in clinically normal African American men (Adebimpe et al. 1979; Gynther et al. 1971). The bias contained in the MMPI can also be influenced by acculturation (see above). On the MCMI, African Americans score significantly higher than Caucasians on Narcissistic, Aggressive, Paranoid, Drug, and Psychotic-Delusional subscales (Hamberger and Hastings 1992). The MCMI-II reveals different profiles for Alaskan Native and nonnative incarcerated offenders, which suggests that culture and cultural styles may contribute to a significantly different type of "criminal personality" seen in forensic settings (Glass et al. 1996).

Because personality traits are systematically related to personality disorders, it would seem that if personality traits were universal, then by corollary personality disorders might be similarly universal. There is some evidence to suggest that this may be the case. The International Personality Disorder Examination has proved to be acceptable to clinicians and has demonstrated an interrater reliability and temporal stability similar to instruments used to diagnose other disorders (Loranger et al. 1994). On the other hand, because cultures differ in the mean level of self-reported traits (e.g., the mean level of neuroticism in Japan, Spain, and Russia are among the highest, and the levels in India, the United States, and the Netherlands are among the lowest [McCrae, personal communication, November 2000]), rates of borderline personality, for example, also would likely vary along the same lines. However, if the rates of such disorders do not vary along the same lines, the differences may be due to features of culture. For example, the same countries cited above vary in levels of uncertainty avoidance measures, which is a dimension of culture in which rules and routines are used to limit stress. Perhaps this is an effective strategy that reduces the influence of neuroticism in developing psychopathology.

Whether a personality trait is maladaptive or causes functional impairment or subjective distress is related to the cultural context. Personality traits unique to individuals in other cultures may at times result in impairment in those cultural contexts but not meet full criteria for any specified DSM personality disorder. These traits might be classified as personality disorders not otherwise specified or as culture-bound syndromes. For example, Type A behavior patterns (i.e., perceptions of chronically struggling against time, frustrations experienced in failing to achieve goals, hyperaggressiveness and ambition, workaholism, impatience in interpersonal relations) may be an example of a Western culture-bound syndrome, which may not be viewed as maladaptive or causing functional impairment or subjective distress within the United

States but may be seen as very pathologic in other cultures.

Furthermore, considering that personality disorder diagnoses might be made in a cross-cultural context—given that the diagnosis of personality disorder requires that the maladaptive traits deviate markedly from the expectation of the individual's culture (according to DSM-IV general criteria for personality disorder)—how is the clinician or researcher supposed to apply the criteria in actual settings without being familiar with the cultural expectations?

Gender Issues and Personality

As stated in DSM-IV-TR, certain personality disorders are diagnosed more frequently in men and others more frequently in women. Paranoid, schizoid, schizotypal, antisocial, narcissistic, and compulsive personality disorders are more commonly diagnosed in males. Dependent, histrionic, and borderline personality disorders are more commonly diagnosed in women. Although DSM-IV-TR directs clinicians to be cautious not to overdiagnose or underdiagnose certain personality disorders in females or in males because of stereotypes about gender roles and behaviors, this advice can be applied only if information about diagnostic thresholds (e.g., What do *overdiagnosis* and *underdiagnosis* mean? Are the normal personalities of men and women different?) is made available for clinical use.

The terms *sex* and *gender* were clarified by the Institute of Medicine (2001) in *Exploring the Biological Contributions to Human Health: Does Sex Matter? Sex* is a classification (male or female) according to the reproductive organs and functions that derive from the chromosomal complement. *Gender* refers to a person's self-representation as male or female, or how that person is responded to by social institutions on the basis of the individual's gender presentation. This very definition of gender emphasizes its importance in conceptualizing personality. In addition to culture as an important contextual framework in which to understand behaviors that constitute personality disorder, gender is also a basic contextual variable that must be considered. Gender affects every aspect of personality. The role of gender in the expression, natural history, relationship to Axis I and III comorbidities, and treatment response of personality disorders represents an area of opportunity for investigation.

The Institute of Medicine (2001) also emphasized that variations between the sexes are a rich source of information about similarities and differences that provide critical details about physiological processes at the cellular level. These differences occur in nonreproductive as well as reproductive tissues. The variability of incidence and severity of diseases between the sexes may be related to differences in exposures, routes of entry and the processing of foreign agents, and cellular responses. Although reproductive hormones play a role in the behavioral and cognitive sex differences, they are not solely responsible.

We are tackling basic conceptual issues related to the diagnosis of disordered personality to advance our field's classification system. Personality is essentially a stable and enduring pattern of inner experience and behavior. A fundamental question is the degree to which self-representation and its behavioral sequelae are dictated by sex (and rapidly by gender). When a child is born, the immediate question is about its sex, which is symbolized by color (blue or pink) to elicit expected reactions in others. This single variable launches a continuum of lifetime expectations and risks from the moment of birth: educational level, career choice and wages, probability of sexual abuse, risk for specific psychiatric disorders, environmental exposures, and lifespan itself are only a few examples. Observations about gender differences will help reshape and redefine our conceptualizations of personality. The opportunity to address this fundamental question in preparation for DSM-V is timely.

Proposed Research Agenda

There are several important issues that should be a focus of a research agenda for studying cross-cultural and gender implications of personality traits and disorders.

1. There may be different genetic pools in different cultures leading to different levels of personality traits in different groups. Research relating genetics and temperament must take this into account. However, different cultures may suppress or encourage genotypic expression, resulting in different phenotypic outcomes of the same genotypic patterns. Thus, the variable of how culture influences genotypic personality expression should be studied.
2. Systematic research needs to be done to quantify cultural variation in the application of the criteria for personality disorders and to discover some of the culture-specific reasons underlying these differences. How much does cultural context—which determines the culture's receptivity to various personality styles—influence the level of dysfunction necessary to be considered a personality disorder?
3. Some cultural/ethnic groups tend to live in environments that put individuals at greater risk of experiencing trauma. Do these different sociological contexts contribute to different levels of personality dysfunction? Specifically, does culturally related differential exposure to trauma (via HPA axis mechanisms) generate certain personality char-

acteristics? On the other hand, do certain culturally related aspects act as protective factors when an individual from that culture is in a stressful environment? For example, the very low rates of suicide among African American women are believed to be related to the systems of social support they find within the African American church (Taylor et al. 1991).

4. Research needs to be done to determine the degree of cultural bias associated with the existing personality measures and to determine its effect on their validity. Can new methods be developed that might allow for the measurement of personality traits independent of culture, perhaps with biomarkers?
5. It is important to investigate whether there is a core group of DSM personality disorders that are seen as pathological or dysfunctional in diverse ethnic groups. Furthermore, it should be determined whether there are personality disorders that exist in certain ethnic groups and cultures that are not contained in standard DSM nosology. As research focusing on the alternative models for personality discussed in previous sections is undertaken, it will be important to investigate how these conceptualizations of personality vary across diverse ethnic groups as well. For example, do certain characteristic dimensional patterns occur more frequently in one culture than in another?
6. Whether categorical or dimensional definitions of personality disorder are used, gender must be an important consideration. To clarify the finding of sex differences in the differential prevalence of personality disorders, Widiger (1998) proposed several areas of potential bias in research: diagnostic constructs, thresholds for diagnosis, application of diagnostic criteria, sampling of populations, assessment instruments, and the diagnostic criteria themselves. Thus, potential gender bias must be considered during the design of any research studies investigating personality traits or disorders. A model of incorporation of gender and culture into domains of psychiatric research is presented in Chapter 6 in this volume.

Relational Disorders

Relational disorders are painful, persistent behavioral problems that seriously affect adjustment and should be considered for inclusion in the next edition of the DSM. However, including these disorders would require a conceptual shift in the DSM's exclusive focus on the diagnosis of individual patients. In contrast, relational disorders always involve two or more individuals. It is the juncture or bond between or among the members of a relationship that is disordered. The disorder cannot be reduced to an

TABLE 4–2. Eight characteristics of relational disorders that are similar to disorders in DSM-IV-TR

Characteristic of relational disorder	Example	References
Has distinctive features for classification	Established clinical interview strategies and clinically useful standardized test instrument	Messer and Reiss 1999
Causes severe emotional, social, and occupational impairment	Marital and child abuse disorders lead to high physical morbidity and death.	J.F. Knutson and Schartz 1997; O'Leary and Cascardi 1998
Has recognizable clinical course	Early signs of marital dissolution are established and replicated in longitudinal studies.	Gottman 1994; Karney and Bradbury 1995
Has recognized patterns of comorbidity	Comorbidity of depression and alcoholism with marital disorders is well documented and has significant implications for treatment.	Beach et al. 1994; Steinglass et al. 1987
Has patterns of family aggregation	Genetic epidemiology has shown familial patterns of parenting and marital difficulties, suggesting genetic influence on both.	Kendler 1996; McGue and Lykken 1992
Etiology involves both biological and psychosocial factors	Genetic studies and measures of autonomic responses have elucidated the development and persistence of relational disorders.	Gottman 1994; Gottman et al. 1995; Reiss et al. 2000
Respond to specific treatments	The efficacy of therapy addressing relational problems has been demonstrated in numerous controlled, clinical trials.	Bray and Jouriles 1995; Pinshof and Wynne 1995
Can be prevented	Controlled trials have demonstrated prevention of marital disorders and parent-child disorders.	Markman et al. 1993; Olds et al. 1986

individual diagnosis of any member and its consequent impact on others. For example, a parent may be withdrawn from and neglectful of one child but not another. The parent-child relational disorder is between the *particular* parent and child, and according to the concept being elaborated here, it cannot be adequately understood or characterized as a secondary consequence of a psychiatric disorder of either the parent alone or the child alone. Despite this distinctive feature, relational disorders share at least eight features with disorders now included in the DSM. These characteristics are listed in Table 4–2.

These similarities between relational disorders and DSM disorders, noted in Table 4–2, suggest that they can be defined and assessed using concepts and research strategies that have been used for individual-based psychiatric disorders. In all, four steps can be recognized. These are summarized in Figure 4–1.

Clinical Importance of Relational Disorders

First, as noted in Table 4–2, relational disorders are serious behavioral disturbances that can lead to major impairments in physical health and psychological adjustment. Second, research shows repeated instances of the impact of relational problems on the course of Axis I disorders and on medical conditions. One example is the well-known work on expressed emotion. A review of 27 longitudinal studies by Butzlaff and Hooley (1998) showed that marital or parental hostility and overinvolvement predict an adverse clinical course of schizophrenia and have even stronger predictive associations on relapse in major depressive disorder and eating disorders. Other research on families of psychiatric patients suggests that hostility and overinvolvement are understandable consequences of living with a severely ill individual. However, there are substantial differences among families in this regard. These differences influence the clinical course of patients, particularly those with chronic disorders. As an example of data in the medical realm, marital difficulties have been shown to adversely influence the course of renal disease, particularly in women (Kimmel et al. 2000), with the magnitude of the risk being equivalent to those of well-known medical risk factors such as diabetes. Third, as outlined below, problematic relationships are well-known risk factors for the development of a range of psychiatric disorders.

Fourth, in the last decade a broad range of animal and human studies is clarifying the role of parent-child and marital disorders in the expression of biological influence on psychiatric disorders. For example, women who were adopted soon after birth and who are at high genetic risk for depression show no evidence of the disorder if they are reared in adoptive families

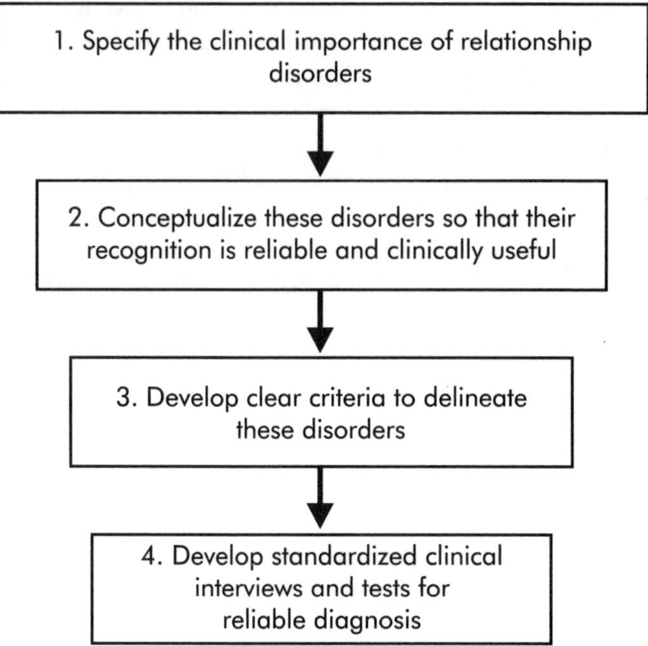

FIGURE 4–1. Four steps for a research program on relationship disorders.

without marital difficulties or psychopathology in the rearing parents (Cadoret et al. 1996). Similar findings have been reported for schizophrenia (Tienari et al. 1994). Even more important recent data suggest that relational behavior in humans is under substantial genetic influence. For example, heritable characteristics of adolescents can elicit hostile and critical behavior in fathers, which precedes the evolution of antisocial behavior in teenagers and may be a crucial mechanism for the influence of genetic factors on adolescent antisocial behavior (Reiss et al. 2000). Conversely, recent animal data suggest that poor maternal care by rat dams of their pups within the first 10 days of life influences gene expression. Specifically, poor maternal care leads to increased hippocampal glucocorticoid receptor messenger RNA expression and enhanced glucocorticoid feedback sensitivity. This appears to be the basis for lifetime sensitivity to stress of the maltreated pups (Liu et al. 1997).

Issues in the Conceptualization of Relational Disorders

First, it is important to distinguish between explicit and embedded relational disorders. Explicit relational disorders are those in which the relational problem is a prime or exclusive clinical concern. Marital violence is an obvious example. Embedded disorders are relational problems that are implanted in already defined syndromes of individual psychopathology. Examples are feeding disorders and conduct disorders in children and are discussed in more detail below.

Second, the number of individuals that might be involved in the relational disorder must be clarified. Family therapists can delineate patterns of disordered relationships that link marital and parent-child relationships and may involve members of the extended family as well. Although a range of research efforts have measured these familywide patterns of relational problems (Conger and Rueter 1996; Hetherington and Clingempeel 1992; Reiss 1981; Tienari et al. 1994), it seems unlikely that these efforts will be ready for routine clinical use in the near future.

The majority of research on relational disorders concerns three relationship systems: adult children and their parents (e.g., work on expressed emotion, on elder abuse, and on children as caregivers for their aging parents), minor children and their parents, and the marital relationship. There is also an increasing body of research on problems in dyadic gay relationships (C.J. Patterson 2000; Waldner-Haugrud 1999) and on problematic sibling relationships (Cicirelli 1982; Dunn 1988; Dunn and Munn 1986; Stocker et al. 1989), which suggests the clinical importance of disorders in these relationships. More research on disorders of these relationships is strongly encouraged.

We note here that focusing on two-person relationships may not be equally appropriate for all cultures. For example, Jackson (1993) emphasizes that in many African American families there are multiple caregivers for any one child. Thus, concepts and measures are needed that assess the quality of these multiple caregiving relationships. Within these families, a single mother-child relationship may capture only a sliver of the child's rearing experience.

Relational disorders are persistent and painful patterns of feelings, behavior, and perceptions involving two or more partners in an important personal relationship. In contrast to variations in healthy relationships, they are marked by distinctive, maladaptive patterns that show little change despite a great variety of challenges and circumstances. Relational disorders can be distinguished from a broad range of interpersonal difficulties by four prominent features. First, clear, repeated, fixed patterns of painful and destructive patterns of feelings, behavior, and perceptions can be clearly recognized. There is little flexibility or change in these patterns, and the dyad responds to a range of stresses and challenges with the same distinctive and maladaptive patterns. Second, and following from the first, the patterns are of long standing and are not a response to a recent stressful event. Third, the corrosive patterns of the relationship are unresponsive to supportive features that may occur naturally in the social environment, which include religious, social, and family networks. Fourth, there is clear evidence of a major impact of these patterns on psychological functioning, physical health, social adaptation, and/or occupational effectiveness in one or both partners.

These characteristics of relational disorders, as well as those enumerated in Table 4–2, provide a guideline for future research on relational disorders but do not resolve all conceptual difficulties about their boundaries. For example, folie à deux, the phenomenon of delusions shared by two or more members of a relationship, is recognized in the clinical literature. This may arise in situations in which one member of a relationship is frankly paranoid and the other is suggestible. As noted below, research is needed to clarify the ways in which assessing a relational disorder improves clinical treatment. In instances in which successful treatment of the psychotic disorder brings prompt resolution of the folie à deux, there may be little need of an additional diagnosis. However, shared delusions may become deeply embedded in a relationship and may lead a couple to resist treatment or may blunt efforts at treating the psychotic member. In such cases, relational diagnoses are crucial for proper treatment. Also at the border of definition are phenomena of social contagion. These have been reported, for example, in the outbreaks of adolescent suicide in the same locations or following each other in very short time periods. In most cases, these fall outside the focus here. First, the co-occurrence of contagious suicide may not reflect a persistent relationship problem among the victims themselves. (For an interesting exception see Reiss's [1968] account of suicidal adolescent groups.) Further, as noted above, relational disorders in dyads—rather than in more complex groups—are a useful focus for the initial efforts at including these disorders in the DSM nosology. Finally, relational problems may be considered as risk factors for the onset of and relapse from serious mental disorders. The same, of course, may be said of many well-established mental disorders. Anxiety disorders and antisocial personality disorder are risk factors for substance use disorders, which are themselves risk factors for relapse and suicidality in bipolar disorders. A more refined question is whether relational disorders are merely risk factors or whether clinical evidence justifies regarding them as disorders in their own right. Below, we recommend research to clarify this issue. However, as summarized in this section, the evidence is already persuasive that these are common, severe disorders for which there are already effective treatments. Regarding them as merely risk factors, of importance only as they affect the course of established disorders, may seriously impair effective clinical treatment.

Empirical Delineation of Syndromes: Explicit Relational Disorders

In this section we provide three examples of relational disorders: marital conflict disorder, marital abuse diorder, and parent-child abuse disorder. Data outlined here provide only a starting point for delineating these disorders from normal variations in relationships. In the case of the marital disorders, this section suggests ways of distinguishing between relational disorders. As is noted, more research is needed

Marital Relational Disorders: General Features

Couples with marital disorders come to clinical attention for a variety of reasons, but four predominate. First, a couple recognize long-standing dissatisfaction with their marriage and come to the clinician on their own initiative or are referred by an astute health care professional. Second, there is serious violence in the marriage—usually the husband battering the wife. The emergency room or a legal authority often is the first to notify the clinician. Third, marital difficulties are noted as part of a comprehensive assessment of an Axis I or Axis II disorder in one of the marital partners—most frequently depression or alcohol or substance abuse. Fourth, marital difficulties are frequently noted as part of a thorough evaluation of a child with a psychiatric problem; in most of these cases, marital difficulties are linked with problems in parent-child relationships. It is likely that clinicians would be aided by valid and reliable criteria for identifying these marital difficulties and differentiating them from less severe marital problems. One standard for differentiating disorder from normality is whether there is a serious disorder in the relationship that definitely merits treatment (i.e., what clinical manifestations have been identified that suggest there is an underlying and serious disorder that would definitely merit treatment?).

Several characteristics of marital relational disorders need to be clarified by further research. First, do manifestations of marital disorder tend to cluster or aggregate in recognizable patterns in the same way that the symptoms of individual psychiatric disorders cluster in identifiable syndromes? If they do, this might be particularly useful in helping clinicians to distinguish a serious disorder from a more transitory disturbance. Second, are there important distinctions among manifestations of particular marital disorders? For example, what distinguishes marital conflict disorders without and with violence? On clinical grounds, the Committee on the Family (1995) of the Group for the Advancement of Psychiatry (GAP) proposed these two as distinct diagnostic entities. Is the latter just a more severe version of the former, or is there evidence that marital disorder with violence is a sufficiently distinctive type of relationship to merit a separate category?

Third, what is the clinical utility of making these classificatory distinctions? Are there different treatment approaches to each of these conditions?

Marital Conflict Disorder Without Violence

Clinical research on marital disorders to date has not focused on defining cases. As with parent-child relationships, the major emphasis has been on defining and measuring continuous dimensions that distinguish between problematic and successful relationships. The development of useful and valid procedures for defining cases requires combining or clustering these dimensions to make meaningful distinctions between noncases and cases and, where appropriate, to distinguish among different types of cases. Recent clinical research does suggest that severely disturbed relationships can be identified by an *aggregate* of manifestations. Although the data do not currently exist to determine how many of these manifestations must be present to indicate a severe disturbance, if several are present it does boost the clinician's confidence that there is a severe relational disorder. Longitudinal studies effectively define characteristics of marriages experiencing sustained difficulties and point to clinical indicators that the relationship is at high risk for deteriorating further if no treatment is instituted. In addition, analysis of research exploring the clustering of clinical manifestations and of research that helps distinguish among relationship disorders has led to the development of seven criteria that define a case. Table 4–3 summarizes these empirical criteria and compares them with those proposed by the GAP. The table is divided into three sections based on the approach the clinician can take to determine the presence or absence of particular features. Interaction patterns need to be directly observed. Standardized interviews or questionnaires can determine the subjective experience of partners. Finally, to apply the last criterion, a complex clinical judgment is required. Ascertainment of the seventh characteristic, impact of marital disorder on psychological adaptation, must be done with care. Problems in adjustment, such as depression or alcoholism, may precede rather than follow the development of marital disorders, or marital disorders and psychological problems may both be consequences of a common risk process. The GAP proposal suggests additional features of disordered marriages that need to be verified by more research.

Table 4–3 serves only as a schematic impetus to research. Some research suggests amendments to this scheme. With respect to criteria, for example, some data suggest adding to the list the entrenched and serious negative attributions that partners in distressed marriages hold toward each other (Bradbury 1990). In addition, important clinical data can be included in diagnostic evaluations of marriages with the use of specifiers, rather than

TABLE 4–3. Comparison of empirically derived and consensus criteria for marital conflict disorder

Empirically derived characteristics[a]	Consensus-derived criteria (GAP)
Interaction patterns between partners	
Failure to control anger and other negative affect *(observation)* (Gottman 1994; Karney and Bradbury 1995)	Emotional climate is hostile or indifferent
Partners appear defensive in response to potential attacks or are unresponsive to other's initiative in the interaction *(observation)* (Gottman 1994)	Repeated instances of one or both partners cheating, humiliating, exploiting, or deceiving the another
Subjective experience of partners	
Partners feel flooded with negative feelings about the other spouse *(questionnaire)* (Gottman 1994)	(No corresponding feature)
Partners feel alone and give up working on problems with spouse *(questionnaire)* (Gottman 1994)	(No corresponding feature)
Sexual dissatisfaction *(questionnaire)* (Snyder and Smith 1986)	Impaired sexual relationship over a 6-month period
Deficit in problem-solving communication *(questionnaire)* (Snyder and Smith 1986)	Inability to communicate effectively
Integrative evaluation	
Impairments in psychological adjustment, physical health, or occupational and social adjustment of at least one partner that is temporally subsequent to marital discord *(several methods)* (Burman and Margolin 1992; Gove et al. 1983; Kimmel et al. 2000; Segraves 1980)	Alcoholism and depression are listed as associated features
(No corresponding feature)	Presence of intergenerational coalitions

Note. GAP=Group for the Advancement of Psychiatry.
[a]Methods used to ascertain the characteristics in the empirically derived syndrome are listed in italics within parentheses.

with additional clinical criteria. Many clinicians, for example, would note the presence or absence of pathological alliances within the family (e.g., mother allied with daughter against the father) or the presence or absence of an ongoing extramarital relationship. With respect to assessment, other methods, such as interviews or questionnaires, might detect clinical features that are indicated in Table 4–3 as being observable by direct observation. For example, rapid escalation of anger, which is listed in Table 4–3 as being observable primarily through direct observation, might also be addressed using questionnaires or a standard interview. Indeed, assessment of relational disorders would be advanced by a standard assessment module that uses at least two different methods of observation for assessing each of the major diagnostic criteria (see research recommendations below).

Marital Abuse Disorder (Marital Conflict Disorder With Violence)

There is wide clinical consensus that the most important distinction among marital relationship disorders is to distinguish between those with and without physical aggression. There are two important clinical reasons for making this distinction. First, and most important, marital violence is a major risk factor for serious injury and even death. Although both husbands and wives can be violent with each other, women in violent marriages are at much greater risk of being seriously injured or killed (National Advisory Council on Violence Against Women 2000). Second, there is evidence that marriages with violence have distinctive features that set them apart from marriages without violence.

The most pertinent feature of marital abuse disorder is physical aggression on the part of one or both marital partners, which can include hitting, threatening with a weapon, physical confinement of a spouse, or marital rape. Clinicians assessing any marriage should include the assessment of actual or potential violence as regularly as they assess the potential for suicide in depressed patients. Clinicians should not relax their vigilance after a battered wife leaves her husband, because some data suggest that the period immediately following a marital separation is the period of greatest risk for the women (Wilson et al. 1993). Many men will stalk and batter their wives in an effort to get them to return or punish them for leaving. Initial assessments of the potential for violence in a marriage can be supplemented by standardized interviews and questionnaires, which have been reliable and valid aids in exploring marital violence more systematically (O'Leary et al. 1992; Straus 1979). Table 4–4 summarizes empirically derived criteria for marital abuse disorder. Again, this table should be regarded as a schematic initiative. There is current considerable controversy over whether male-to-female marital violence is best regarded as a reflection of male psychopathology and control or whether there is an empirical base and clinical utility for conceptualizing these patterns as relational. We return to this issue in research recommendations.

TABLE 4–4. Empirically derived criteria for marital abuse disorder[a]

Interaction patterns between partners

Hitting, marital rape, threatening with a weapon *(husband's and wife's reports)*

Husbands are domineering and critical *(observation)* (Cordova et al. 1993; Jacobson et al. 1994)

Unusual degree of provocative belligerence and contempt from both partners *(observation)* (Cascardi et al. 1995; Jacobson et al. 1994)

Wives appear sad and frightened *(observation)* (Cascardi et al. 1995; Jacobson et al. 1994)

Subjective experiences of partners

Husbands report that wives withdraw after husbands are demanding *(interview)* (Babcock et al. 1993; Holtzworth-Munroe et al. 1998)

Husbands show unusual jealousy and preoccupation with their wives *(interview)* (Holtzworth-Munroe et al. 1997)

Integrative evaluation

Defining especially high-risk variant: husbands show antisocial personality, violence occurs outside the home, and—in interaction with their wives—husbands are frankly intimidating *(clinician integration and judgment)* (Gottman et al. 1995; Holtzworth-Munroe and Stuart 1994)

[a]Methods used to ascertain the characteristics of the disorder are listed in italics within parentheses.

Clinical Utility of Classifying Marital Relational Disorders

To treat or not to treat? Even though effective family interventions for relational disorders tend to be brief (Bray and Jouriles 1995), they nonetheless represent significant investments of time and energy by the family and clinician. Responsible clinicians would urge treatment only if they thought it unlikely that the relational disorder would spontaneously remit. Sufficient data to understand the clinical course of untreated marital disorders have been available only recently. Indeed, as noted, these longitudinal data validate many of the manifestations of marital disorders that are highlighted above (e.g., Gottman 1994; Karney and Bradbury 1995). Recent data on couples who show those features of marital conflict disorders confirm that they are at much greater risk of divorce than couples who do not have these characteristics. Indeed, the risk of separation and divorce is more than three times higher in the disordered group with these features over a period of 3 years (Gottman 1994).

There is also very recent information on the course of violent marriages. Data suggest that over time a husband's battering may abate somewhat, but perhaps because he has successfully intimidated his wife. The risk of violence remains strong in a marriage in which it has been a feature in the past (Jacobson et al. 1996). Thus, treatment is essential here; the clinician cannot just watch and wait.

It remains unclear, however, whether diagnostic thresholds must be achieved to facilitate treatment decisions by mental health clinicians. Earlier in this chapter, we described the rationale for using dimensions to characterize disorders of personality. A similar argument could be made for some or all of the relational disorders. For example, in marital disorders the constructs of *escalation of anger* or *provocative belligerence* can be assessed using dimensions or using categories, and it remains for systematic research to clarify the relevant clinical utility of each approach.

Distinctions among disorders and the selection of treatment. A variety of effective treatments, most involving conjoint therapy with the couple, have been tested in controlled clinical trials for marital conflict disorders without violence and have shown to be effective (Bray and Jouriles 1995; Pinshof and Wynne 1995). There may be conditions under which analogous techniques can be used for violent couples (Goldner 1998). The treatment of marital abuse disorders has a different set of priorities and strategies. The most urgent clinical priority is the protection of the spouse at risk, most frequently the wife. Indeed, some forms of marital therapy that may be effective in other circumstances, such as supporting assertiveness by a battered wife in the face of husband's threats, may lead to more severe beatings (O'Leary et al. 1985) or even death.

Parent-child abuse disorder. Research on parent-child abuse bears some similarity to that on marital violence. The defining characteristic of this disorder, of course, is physical aggression by the parent toward a child. This disorder, often concealed by parent and child, may come to the attention of the clinician in many ways, from emergency room medical staff to reports from child protective services. However, the available research suggests that the abusive behavior is part of a broader disorder in parent-child relationships. Table 4–5 lists several features that emerged from studies in which observations of interactions between abusing parents and their children were compared with similar observations of nonabusing parents and their children. In general, these studies use different procedures for coding interaction between parent and child, have small samples, and do not distinguish clearly between abuse and neglect or between abuse and other forms of parenting problems. Thus, the list in Table 4–5 should be regarded as a starting point for research that needs to be more ambitious using larger samples, more uniform measures, and more exacting controls. For example, parent-child abuse might reflect a broader coercive disorder of parent-child relationships. In that instance, the presence or absence of abuse might be regarded as a specifier in this more comprehensive diagnostic category.

TABLE 4–5. Some features of abusive parent-child relationships

Parent is physically aggressive with a child, often producing physical injury.
Parent-child interaction is coercive. Parents are quick to react to provocations with aggressive response, and children often reciprocate aggression (Wolfe 1985).
Parents do not respond effectively to positive or prosocial behavior in the child (Dolz et al. 1997, in a study of infants and mothers at risk for abuse).
Parents do not engage in discussion about emotions.
Parent engages in deficient play behavior: ignores child, rarely initiates play, and does little teaching (Wasserman et al. 1983).
Children are insecurely attached (Egeland and Sroufe 1981) and, where mothers have a history of physical abuse, show distinctive patterns of disorganized attachment (Lyons-Ruth and Block 1996; Lyons-Ruth et al. 1989).
Parents' relationship shows coercive marital interaction patterns (Wolfe 1985).

Empirical Delineation of Embedded Relational Disorders in Syndromes of Childhood and Adolescence

As noted, relational problems can be either explicit and the central focus of clinical concern or they can be embedded in syndromes that are partially defined by characteristics of the child. Defining the relational aspects of these childhood disorders can have important consequences. For example, in the case of early appearing feeding disorders, attention to relational problems may help delineate different types of clinical problems within a broad, poorly defined category. In the case of conduct disorder, the relational problems may be so central to the maintenance, if not the etiology, of the disorder that effective treatment may be impossible without recognizing and delineating it.

Provided below are only two examples of embedded relational disorders. Many others are amenable to similar analyses. These might include separation anxiety disorder, reactive attachment disorder in children, and several of the sexual dysfunctions in adults.

Feeding disorder of infancy or early childhood. The category of feeding disorder of infancy or early childhood was introduced in DSM-IV, but no effort was made to distinguish among various important subtypes. Preliminary evidence suggests that several important variants present themselves in early childhood. For example, children may refuse to eat after experiencing a serious trauma involving the upper gastrointestinal tract, or their food refusal may reflect an interplay of their own temperament and an anxious, intrusive feeding pattern by their principal caregiver. Direct observation of caregiver-infant feeding patterns holds considerable promise in making these distinctions. For example, feeding disorders secondary to trauma reveal a child's high level of anxiety and difficulty in swallowing very early in a feeding episode, whereas disorders secondary to temperament or relationship interplay are clearly revealed in confliction patterns of attempting feeding by the caregiver and food refusal by the child. To verify these results, further research is needed that uses larger samples and improved methods for validating these different forms of eating problems (Chatoor et al. 1997, 1998b, 2001).

Conduct disorder or antisocial behavior. There is consistent evidence from numerous studies that a coercive, hostile, punitive parenting style is associated with a markedly increased risk of developing antisocial behavior (Loeber and Stouthamer-Loeber 1986; McCord 1991; G. Patterson 1982; G.R. Patterson and Forgatch 1995; G.R. Patterson et al. 1992; Sampson and Laub 1993). Observational data indicate that the parents' desperate efforts to control a child, who is essentially socially unskilled, consist of threats, scolding, and demands (Stoolmiller et al. 1997). However, the punishments they use are ineffective. The child's counterattacks to the parents' coercion are in the form of aggressive behaviors. The parent backs off and ceases to require the child's compliance. This sequence of events occurs time and again, maintaining, and perhaps escalating the child's antisocial behavior. As a recent review notes, scores of controlled outcome studies confirm the efficacy of treatments aimed at improving parent-child relationship for childhood conduct disorders, although the results for adolescents are less certain (Kazdin 1997). Probably no other approach to treating these children has compiled an equally impressive scientific record.

However, despite this impressive evidence, caution must be used in interpreting the association of disturbances in the parent-child relationship with the development of conduct disorder. For example, Rutter et al. (1998) provided a critical review of the role of disordered parenting, especially of the coercive type, in antisocial behavior. They point out that it is possible that some of the effects of the ineffective parenting on the offspring are genetically mediated. That is, parents and children share 50% of their individual difference genes. Genes that influence coercive behavior in the parent may be the same genes that influence the antisocial behavior in children. Reiss and colleagues (2000) provided evidence for this. Furthermore, Rutter et al. (1998) suggested that not all of the effects involved in the relationship between coercive parents and antisocial children are in one direction, namely, from the parent to the child. Clearly, there are child effects in which the child evokes ineffective parenting. Evaluating the relative effectiveness of intervention studies focusing on different aspects of the parenting process is a worthwhile strategy to resolve this dilemma.

Reliable and Valid Assessments of Relational Disorders for Clinical Use

Diagnoses are practical only if clinicians can make them reliably. Two different clinicians seeing the same patient should reach the same classificatory conclusions. Likewise, it is crucial that epidemiologists and other researchers and research assistants, particularly nonprofessional interviewers, can be trained to reach classification decisions reliably. Important research, particularly with the large samples ordinarily required for good epidemiologic studies, would be too expensive if it required fully trained clinicians for collecting data. We briefly review these two related issues in turn.

Both clinicians and researchers must accomplish three interlocked tasks in reaching a reliable and valid diagnosis. First, they must observe critical interaction patterns between the two people involved. Second, they must discover subjective perceptions that each participant holds of the relationship. Third, they must integrate additional information about the dyad—for example, in the case of marital conflict disorder, they must make a judgment whether or not the relational disturbance has adversely affected the adaptation of at least one partner. Current evidence suggests that well-trained clinicians who are given clear definitions of relationship problems cannot, without training, reach satisfactory levels of reliability (Shaffer et al. 1991). However, with adequate training, clinicians can be taught to make reliable discrimination between disorders and nondisorders either from structured interviews (Hayden et al. 1998) or, as noted, from observing quotidian interactions such as mothers feeding their young children (Chatoor et al. 1997, 1998a, 1998b, 2000).

However, even these carefully constructed assessment procedures, coupled with training of clinicians, do not cover the full range of clinical manifestations of relational disorders. One suggestion for establishing an accurate assessment procedure for relationship classification consists of three parts: 1) standardized procedures for evoking and observing interaction within the dyad; 2) questionnaires for each member to delineate his or her individual perceptions of the relationship, including its level of violence; and 3) a structured clinical interview to supplement questionnaires and observations and integrate additional clinical information. Reliable methods for evoking, recording, and coding interactions in dyads have been carefully reviewed for researchers (Grotevant and Carlson 1989) and clinicians (Bray 1995). Clinicians can be trained to reliably code family interaction evoked by standard stimuli, such as asking a family to discuss a recent argument. Typically these discussions are video recorded and coded. These coding procedures are sensitive to individual differences among families and their response to treatment (Szapocznik et al. 1991). The procedure of making video recordings of interactions and systematically coding these recordings is eminently suitable for use in population-based epidemiologic studies. Two studies, using national samples in the United States (Reiss et al. 2000) and Sweden (Reiss et al. 2001), have shown that most families contacted by research staff will agree to have their interaction videotaped. Coding of videotaped interactions in these population-based samples is reliable and valid (Reiss et al. 2000). Valid and reliable questionnaires for assessing marital and parent-child relational problems that are suitable for both clinicians and researchers have recently been reviewed (Messer and Reiss 1999). Some reports suggest that practical assessments combining many of these methods can be designed and routinely conducted in clinical settings (Floyd et al. 1989). However, these assessments can take 2 hours or longer.

Cultural and Racial Issues in Conceptualizing and Assessing Relational Disorders

Culture has a profound effect on the quality and development of family relationships. These cultural issues are important both for conceptualizing and assessing relational disorders and for their clinical evaluations. We cite but two of many examples. First, there are important cultural differences in the degree to which family members are obligated to one another across the life span. In collectivistic (non-European) cultures, there is a marked difference between the in-group and the out-group, with people strongly devoted to their in-group but largely indifferent to out-groups. In individualistic cultures (European/American), the distinction is blurred, and the more central difference is between self and others. This may have important implications for the classification, identification, and treatment of relational problems. For example, in the United States, if an adult does not get along with his or her parents, he or she usually has the option of avoiding them, but in much of the rest of the world this is not an option. Thus, in collectivistic societies it may be crucial to focus on parent-offspring disorders that involve both child and adult offspring. In individualistic societies, the clinical priorities focus on these disorders when the offspring is a child or when the offspring is an adult caregiver who is crucial for the well-being of an aged, demented, or severely ill parent.

A second example concerns domestic violence. For example, domestic homicide has historically been a significant problem in the African American community, but it rarely occurs in the Latin American community. This clue suggests that the characteristics of marital violence, as well as its determinants, might be different across these cultures, and future research should be sensitive to this possibility.

In addition to these family and social norms that exert influence on all the members of a given culture, a number of differences between individuals may also contribute to the formation and course of disordered relationships. These include differential behavior toward others on the basis of such factors as culture, race, sex, age, sexual orientation, and religious status. In considering such factors, it may be useful to differentiate between two broad classes of relationships. One comprises those within the family, such as the parent-child and spousal relationships discussed above. The other class consists of relationships outside the family, and particularly work groups.

Although families were formerly more uniform with respect to all of these social variables, marriages and spouse-equivalent relationships have increasingly transcended boundaries of religion and ethnicity over the last few generations. However, the attractions that result in the formation of long-term romantic relationships may not necessarily completely undo the attitudes and modes of behavior that had become inculcated in preceding years. Accordingly, cultural, religious, and other differences may be important considerations in contributing to the emergence and maintenance of difficulties in relationships—even in circumstances where, by definition, both partners have initially committed to the relationship and express the desire to maintain it if possible. Similar effects can occur for the children of an ongoing relationship. These might become relevant either for adoptive children of a different ethnic background from that of the parents, or may evolve as children grow up and develop attitudes and behaviors that vary from those of their parents in areas such as religion or sexual orientation. Thus, once again, although individuals may strongly express the desire to foster a highly affiliated family relationship, these differences can strongly contribute to relationship stress or dissolution.

In contrast, relationships outside the family pose a somewhat different set of considerations. In circumstances such as in the workplace and in other organized groups, standards of professional deportment exist, but friendship or other attachment is not required. Although ethnic or religious strains in a family play out in the context of the cumulative duration of family history and ties, these considerations are not so relevant for the workplace, where merely professional civility and courtesy represent acceptable normative behavior. Workplace standards require tolerance of others and nondiscrimination in all aspects of behavior but do not mandate affiliation or affection. Nonetheless, violation of these behavioral norms remains an all-too-frequent occurrence and can generate significant distress in work and similar relationships. In the United States this has historically been a particular problem with respect to racial and ethnic differences, although in the nineteenth and early twentieth centuries, religious differences were also a significant source of workplace prejudice.

Should negatively held stereotypical assumptions about different people, and the distress deriving from discrimination in the workplace caused by these stereotypes, be characterized as a relational disorder? For example, a European American medical student who is pro-white and anti-black who has an African American supervisor who is pro-black but not anti-white will often disregard his supervisor's advice and direction because of his negatively held stereotypes of African Americans, and sooner or later both parties will be in a difficult relationship that will cause considerable distress for each. Furthermore, depending on the outcome of the medical student's rotation, administrative or legal intervention may be requested to resolve the conflict. As recognition that the world is a diverse multicultural environment becomes more widespread, society has become less tolerant of various forms of prejudice and discrimination. The result is that racism and sexism are less openly displayed, but they are still manifested in various forms (Bell 1996; Brantly 1983). Hostile work environments do exist, characterized by various levels of microinsults and microaggressions being made against minorities (Feagin and Sikes 1994; Pierce 1988). Examples of widely held racial and gender stereotypes would be a tall, stately, well-dressed African American judge waiting for his Mercedes-Benz in a parking garage being mistaken for a parking lot attendant by a hurried European American man, or a woman physician being automatically assumed to be a nurse by a male patient. (For a greater discussion on microaggressions and microinsults, see Chapter 6 in this volume.) These negative stereotypes may run quite deep in some people and exert a constant negative influence on workplace or personal relationships. The cumulative effect of such experiences may influence not only workplace and personal relationships, but also the presentation and treatment of serious mental illness. For example, it has been observed that one reason why African Americans with bipolar disorder are frequently misdiagnosed as having schizophrenia is that their "protective wariness" is frequently misattributed by clinicians to paranoid ideation (Jones and Gray 1986; Strakowski et al. 1993). Furthermore, negative stereotypes of African Americans held by European American clinicians may also contribute to the tendency to assign a diagnosis with a graver prognosis to the least valued African American patient (Bell and Mehta 1980, 1981).

Defining racism as a relational disorder, however, is fraught with potential for negative outcomes. By describing a dysfunctional relationship in terms of a diagnostic label, the holder of negative racial stereotypes may be relieved of personal responsibility for his or her attitudes, and the object of the negative racial stereotype may be inappropriately blamed for his or her supposedly contributory role when in fact he or she is actually just an unwitting victim (i.e., blaming the victim and excusing the perpetrator). More broadly, the concern exists that defining interactions outside the context of committed family relationships as disorders runs the risk of medicalizing a vast area of social behavior problems whose solutions are largely beyond the arena of psychiatry. In a related vein, patterns of discrimination are by no means confined to racism but also occur on the basis of religion, national origin, sexual orientation, gender, and age, among others (Sullaway and Dunbar 1996). These categories are comparable in terms of the factors that predispose to prejudicial attitudes and behavior and would also require attention in considering prejudice as a factor in relational disorders. Thus, it would be necessary to carefully consider the nature of an experimental program in this domain, in the context of defining the research agenda that is intended to provide a more adequate scientific basis for DSM-V. (For a greater discussion on the toxic influence of prejudicial attitudes and behaviors on mental health, symptom formation, diagnosis, and personality functioning, see Chapter 6, in this volume.)

Research Agenda for Clinical Classification and Validation of Relational Disorders

1. *Develop assessment modules for relationship disorders.* The next step in the practical assessment of clinical disorders is to develop a single, relatively brief assessment module that would include a brief clinical interview, selected questionnaires, and a sample of videotaped interaction evoked and coded in a standardized fashion. This module would have to be adapted for different types of relationships: parent-infant, parent-toddler, parent–older child, parent-adolescent, marriage, etc. A first order of business is to ensure that these modules show the same reliability and validity as do the measures from which they would be drawn. A second order of business is to begin studies of clinical validity. Can syndromes be defined using threshold or cutoff scores and clustering techniques, or do continuous dimensions of relational problems better cover the central clinical phenomena? Two crucial steps would follow.
2. *Determine clinical utility of relational diagnoses.* This task is critical in determining whether or not relational disorders deserve to be included in a future edition of the DSM. A prerequisite in ascertaining the clinical

utility of relational diagnosis is the establishment that the diagnoses can be made reliably (i.e., different clinicians classify the same pairs of patients in the same categories, and the categories are stable at least over the short term). In the absence of adequate reliability, further research to determine the clinical utility and validity of these categories is not possible.

The central aspect of clinical utility is that by classifying patient dyads according to whether criteria are met for a particular relational disorder, important information is added about these patients beyond what was known about them before. This added information can address issues of etiology, natural history, or response to treatment. If it is found that the classification of relational disorders adds little useful information for clinicians about these patients, then inclusion of relational disorders in the DSM would probably not be warranted. There are two components to this task: establishing the ability to adequately discriminate among relational problems, and discovering whether useful information is provided to the clinician by determining whether the inclusion of relational disorders will give the clinican useful information that is not available from the current assessments in the DSM system.

First, it is necessary to know how well standardized assessment modules discriminate among different relationship diagnoses and between relationship classifications and other psychiatric disorders. The distinction between marital conflict disorder and marital abuse disorder is not a very stringent test, because the defining characteristics of the latter is a pattern of physical aggression, which does not require an elaborate nosology or assessment battery to detect. However, the best-developed nosology for parent-child relational disorders requires, for example, a distinction between underinvolved and angry/hostile disorders. Can a practical clinical assessment module make this distinction reliably? In the former, the parent is unresponsive to the infant, and the affect in parent and child is constricted and flat. In the latter, the parent often teases or taunts the infant, and the affect of both parent and child is tense and angry.

For embedded disorders, it is important to demonstrate the utility of adding relational criteria. For example, in the case of feeding disorders, does adding relational information help distinguish among early appearing feeding disorders in ways that improve the effectiveness of treatment for each type? Desensitization procedures may be more appropriate for feeding disorders secondary to trauma, whereas intervention with parent-child relationships may be more appropriate for infantile anorexia. Correspondingly, the pervasive coercive parent-child relationships in most cases of conduct disorder should encourage a search for a subgroup, unresponsive to parent-child interventions, in which parent-child relationships are not a prominent feature. This subgroup may be more responsive to pharmacotherapeutic interventions.

3. *Conduct research on a broader range of relational disorders.* As noted, researchers have made promising starts in studying disorders of sibling relationships and gay relationships. Furthermore, relationships between adult children and their parents are increasingly important in the field of geriatric psychiatry. Research in this area is strongly encouraged. It should include the development of appropriate standardized assessment modules, assessments of their validity and clinical utility, and subsequent investigation of the roles of these relationships in the etiology and pathogenesis of individual psychiatric disorders.
4. *Determine the overlap of relational diagnoses with individual diagnoses.* With these new assessment tools available, it must be asked again, are relational diagnoses are just individual DSM diagnoses in disguise? For example, are all cases of marital abuse disorders just a reflection of the husband's antisocial personality disorder? Current evidence (O'Leary and Jacobson 1997) suggests this is not likely. It would be more useful to ask the following questions: If it is known that two people are involved in a relational disorder, how does such knowledge help to better fashion a prognosis, a treatment plan, and a program for prevention? What more is gained from a knowledge of the relational problem than from a detailed individual diagnosis of each partner? A closely related question is: How much can relational problems be predicted from knowledge of the individual attributes of each partner? There are correlations between measures on the five-factor model of personality (discussed elsewhere in this chapter) and relationship problems. However, because these dimensions are not specifically designed to predict behavior in marital and parent-child relationships, they are not stringent probes of this question. Dimensions of personality that are more specifically designed for these predictions may be a more stringent test (Benjamin 1996). In this work, it will be important to test whether these individual dimensions predict relational problems differently for men and for women. Finally, in assessments of individual attributes and relational problems, it is necessary to know what individual attributes of a *partner* are associated with conspicuous relational dysfunction in a target individual. For example, some of the relational processes of marital abuse disorder might be clarified if more data were available on victims' characteristics that predict her choosing an abusive partner or that anticipate her failing to protect herself from one. For example, data suggest that women who as children were themselves abused or witnessed interparental abuse are more likely to end up in abusive marriages (Stith

et al. 2000) and, even in the engagement phase, are more self-deprecatory during interaction with their partner (Halford et al. 2000).

5. *Determine the roles of relational disorders in the etiology and maintenance of individual diagnoses.* Once perfected, the new assessment module can also be put to work to clarify the etiology of major mental disorders of individuals. A critical need is for population-based epidemiologic studies that focus on relationships as the sampling unit. That is, representative samples would be composed of parent-child pairs or marital pairs. In conventional epidemiology, samples are developed of individuals with a known relationship to a specified population of individuals. We are proposing instead that dyads—marital or parent-child pairs—be sampled to be representative of a well-specified population of marital partners or parent-child pairs. Marital or parent-child units would be sampled and their relationships would be assessed systematically, including the use of direct observation. It is now quite feasible to collect and code videotaped records of large, epidemiologically sound samples of dyads and even larger family units (Reiss et al. 2001). Analyses would focus on the associations of these relationship measures with individual psychopathology on the one hand, and with risk and protective factors for relationships on the other.

   This research can address a fundamental question: Do relationship problems have to rise to the level of disorders to have a major impact on the course of individual mental disorders or on psychological adjustment? Data of this kind will help clarify the utility of a dimensional versus categorical approach to the definition and assessment of relational disorders.

   A matter of immediate importance is the significance of the comorbidity of relational diagnoses with other psychiatric diagnoses. For example, there is evidence from adoption studies that the genetic risk for schizophrenia, certain forms of alcoholism, depression, and antisocial behavior is enhanced in the presence of severe relational problems and may be suppressed altogether in the context of mentally healthy adoptive parents and positive family relationships (Cadoret and Cain 1981; Cadoret et al. 1983, 1995, 1996; Cloninger et al. 1981, 1996b; Tienari et al. 1985, 1994). However, these studies do not use widely established criteria for relational disorders nor standardized methods to assess them. Beyond these studies of the interplay of genetic and relationship factors, we recommend a full integration of social and biological studies in understanding the evolution of relational disorders and their impact on disorders of individuals.

6. *Consider the effect of individual differences (e.g., gender, culture) on relational disorders.* Researchers exploring the nature of relational disorders, in-

cluding those examining the overlap of relationship dysfunction with individual diagnoses, should consider aspects of these disorders that may be mediated or modulated by individual differences such as race, sex, age, culture, religion, and sexual preference. It will be important, in this regard, to take into account the nature of the relationships that are involved, for example, whether these involve relationships within a family unit (such as spousal/spouse-equivalent bonds or parent-child interactions) as opposed to those that occur in a workplace or other nonfamily social unit (e.g., a religious organization).

Implications of Proposals for DSM-V

Personality and relational disorders are commonly encountered in outpatient mental health practice. Yet the classification scheme offered by the DSM-IV for both of these domains is woefully inadequate in meeting the goals of facilitating communication among clinicians and researchers or in enhancing the clinical management of these conditions. This chapter presents a series of research agenda items that we hope will stimulate sufficient research into these areas. We hope that the future DSM-V work groups therefore have a large enough empirical data base to allow for the implementation of a significant overhaul in the classification of these conditions. Minor tweaking of the DSM-IV methodology is unlikely to correct the inadequacies that are identified here.

Regarding the domain of personality disorders, there is convincing evidence documenting their importance both as targets of treatment in their own right as well as their role as complicating factors in the management of other psychiatric and general medical conditions. The research agenda for personality disorder has two primary points of focus: 1) to reimplement the classification of personality disorders using a dimensional approach that avoids the artificiality of the current categorical approach and facilitates the identification and communication of the patient's clinically relevant personality traits; 2) to definitively address the confusion that has resulted from the current Axis I–Axis II delineation that has been an important (and irksome) feature of the classification system since 1980. We hope that over the next 10 years there will be a sufficient empirical base to allow for the identification of clinically useful and conceptually valid dimensions of personality and that they can be implemented in a way that clinicians will find acceptable. We also anticipate that the research agenda will allow for sufficient elucidation of the relationship between the possibly spectrum personality disorders and their Axis I counterparts to guide decisions regarding the fundamental organization of the DSM-V classification.

The current classification of relational problems is so nonspecific as to be a hindrance to both clinical practice and research. As discussed in this chapter, there is considerable evidence demonstrating the feasibility of the development of specific definitions for a number of relational disorders. With additional research along the lines of the research agenda outlined here, such categories could be defined in a way that is both reliable and clinically useful. A larger challenge facing the DSM-V work group considering these issues is how to implement the conceptual shifts and new forms of observation that would be entailed in including a classification of disorders in relationships among individuals, rather than disorders that are conceptualized to reside within an individual. The DSM-IV work groups were spared this dilemma because the empirical database available in the early 1990s was insufficient to even justify the development of specific relational disorders. Presumably, if the empirical database for DSM-V is sufficiently compelling, the mechanics of including disorders in both systems and individuals can be addressed.

References

Adebimpe VR, Gigandet J, Harris E: MMPI diagnosis of black psychiatric patients. Am J Psychiatry 136:85–87, 1979

Adler DA, Drake RE, Teague GB: Clinicians' practices in personality assessment: does gender influence the use of DSM-III Axis II? Compr Psychiatry 31:125–133, 1990

Ahadi SA, Rothbart MK: Temperament, development, and the Big Five, in The Developing Structure of Temperament and Personality From Infancy to Adulthood. Edited by Halverson CF, Kohnstamm GA, Martin RP. Hillsdale, NJ, Erlbaum, 1994, pp 189–207

Akiskal HS: The temperamental borders of affective disorders. Acta Psychiatr Scand Suppl 379:32–37, 1994

Akiskal HS, Yerevanian BI, Davis GC, et al: The nosologic status of borderline personality: clinical and polysomnographic study. Am J Psychiatry 142(2):192–198, 1985

American Psychiatric Association: Diagnostic and Statistical Manual of Mental Disorders, 3rd Edition. Washington, DC, American Psychiatric Association, 1980

American Psychiatric Association: Diagnostic and Statistical Manual of Mental Disorders, 3rd Edition, Revised. Washington, DC, American Psychiatric Association, 1987

American Psychiatric Association: Diagnostic and Statistical Manual of Mental Disorders, 4th Edition, Text Revision. Washington, DC, American Psychiatric Association, 2000

Angleitner A, Ostendorf F: Temperament and the Big Five factors of personality, in The Developing Structure of Temperament and Personality From Infancy to Adulthood. Edited by Halverson CF, Kohnstamm GA, Martin RP. Hillsdale, NJ, Erlbaum, 1994, pp 69–89

Angst J, Clayton P: Premorbid personality of depressive, bipolar and schizophrenic patients with special reference to suicidal issues. Compr Psychiatry 27:511–532, 1986

Angst J, Merikangas K: The depressive spectrum: diagnostic classification and course. J Affect Disord 45(1–2):31–39; discussion 39–40, 1997

Angst J, Sellaro R, Merikangas KR: Depressive spectrum diagnoses. Compr Psychiatry 41 (2 suppl 1):39–47, 2000

Babcock J, Waltz J, Jacobson NS, et al: Power and violence: the relationship between communication patterns, power discrepancies, and domestic violence. J Consult Clin Psychol 61(1):40–50, 1993

Bagby RM, Joffe RT, Parker JDA, et al: Major depression and the five-factor model of personality. J Personal Disord 9:224–234, 1995

Ball SA, Tennen H, Poling JC, et al: Personality, temperament, and character dimensions and the DSM-IV personality disorders in substance abusers. J Abnorm Psychol 106:545–553, 1997

Barnett PA, Gotlib IH: Psychosocial functioning and depression: distinguishing among antecedents, concomitants, and consequences. Psychol Bull 104:97–126, 1988

Beach SRH, Whisman MA, O'Leary KD: Marital therapy for depression: theoretical foundation, current status and future directions. Behavior Therapy 25:345–371, 1994

Bell CC: Treatment issues for African-American men. Psychiatric Annals 26(1):33–36, 1996

Bell CC, Mehta H: The misdiagnosis of black patients with manic depressive illness. J Natl Med Assoc 72(2):141–145, 1980

Bell CC, Mehta H: Misdiagnosis of black patients with manic depressive illness: second in a series. J Natl Med Assoc 73(2):101–107, 1981

Benjamin LS: Interpersonal Diagnosis and Treatment of Personality Disorders. New York, Guilford, 1993

Benjamin LS: Interpersonal Diagnosis and Treatment of Personality Disorders, 2nd Edition. New York, Guilford, 1996

Blashfield RK: The Classification of Psychopathology: Neo-Kraepelinian and Quantitative Approaches. New York, Plenum, 1984

Blashfield RK, Blum N, Pfohl B: The effects of changing Axis II diagnostic criteria. Compr Psychiatry 33:245–252, 1992

Bornstein RF: Reconceptualizing personality disorder diagnosis in the DSM-V: the discriminant validity challenge. Clinical Psychology: Science and Practice 5:333–343, 1998

Boyce P, Parker G, Barnett B, et al: Personality as a vulnerability factor to depression. Br J Psychiatry 159:106–114, 1991

Bradbury TN, Fincham FD: Attributions in marriage: review and critique. Psychol Bull 107(1):3–33, 1990

Brantly T: Racism and its impact on psychotherapy. Am J Psychiatry 140:1605–1608, 1983

Bray JH: Family assessment: current issues in evaluating families. Family Relations: Journal of Applied Family and Child Studies 44(4):469–477, 1995

Bray JH, Jouriles EN: Treatment of marital conflict and prevention of divorce. J Marital Fam Ther 21(4):461–473, 1995

Brooks R, Baltazar P, Munjack D: Co-occurrence of personality disorders with panic disorder, social phobia, and generalized anxiety disorder: a review of the literature. J Anxiety Disord 3:259–285, 1989

Burman B, Margolin G: Analysis of the association between marital relationships and health problems: an interactional perspective. Psychol Bull 112(1):39–63, 1992

Butzlaff RL, Hooley JM: Expressed emotion and psychiatric relapse: a meta-analysis. Arch Gen Psychiatry 55(6):549–562, 1998

Cadoret RJ, Cain CA: Genotype-environmental interaction in antisocial behavior. Psychol Med 12:235–239, 1981

Cadoret RJ, Cain CA, Crowe RR: Evidence for gene-environment interaction in the development of adolescent antisocial behavior. Behav Genet 13(3):301–310, 1983

Cadoret RJ, Yates WR, Troughton E, et al: Genetic-environmental interaction in the genesis of aggressivity and conduct disorders. Arch Gen Psychiatry 52(11):916–924, 1995

Cadoret RJ, Winokur G, Langbehn D, et al: Depression spectrum disease, I: the role of gene-environment interaction. Am J Psychiatry 153(7):892–899, 1996

Carey G, Goldman D: The genetics of antisocial behavior, in Handbook of Antisocial Behavior. Edited by Stoff DM, Breiling J, Maser JD. New York, Wiley, 1997, pp 243–254

Cascardi M, O'Leary KD, Lawrence EE, et al: Characteristics of women physically abused by their spouses and who seek treatment regarding marital conflict. J Consult Clin Psychol 63(4):616–623, 1995

Caspi A: Personality development across the life course, in Handbook of Child Psychology, Vol 3: Social, Emotional, and Personality Development. Edited by Damon W, Eisenberg N. New York, Wiley, 1998, pp 311–388

Cassano GB, Dell'Osso L, Frank E, et al: The bipolar spectrum: a clinical reality in search of diagnostic criteria and an assessment methodology. J Affect Disord 54(3):319–328, 1999

Chatoor I, Getson P, Menvielle E, et al: A feeding scale for research and clinical practice to assess mother-infant interactions in the first three years of life. Infant Mental Health Journal 18(1):76–91, 1997

Chatoor I, Ganiban J, Colin V, et al: Attachment and feeding problems: a reexamination of nonorganic failure to thrive and attachment insecurity. J Am Acad Child Adolesc Psychiatry 37(11):1217–1224, 1998a

Chatoor I, Hirsch R, Ganiban J, et al: Diagnosing infantile anorexia: the observation of mother-infant interactions. J Am Acad Child Adolesc Psychiatry 37(9):959–967, 1998b

Chatoor I, Ganiban J, Hirsch R, et al: Maternal characteristics and toddler temperament in infantile anorexia. J Am Acad Child Adolesc Psychiatry 39(6):743–751, 2000

Chatoor I, Ganiban J, Harrison J, et al: Observation of feeding in the diagnosis of posttraumatic feeding disorder in infancy. J Am Acad Child Adolesc Psychiatry 40(5):595–602, 2001

Cicirelli VG: Sibling influence throughout the lifespan, in Sibling Relationships: Their Nature and Significance Across the Lifespan. Edited by Lamb ME, Sutton-Smith B. Hillsdale, NJ, Erlbaum, 1982, pp 267–284

Clark LA: Resolving taxonomic issues in personality disorders. J Personal Disord 6:360–378, 1992

Clark LA: Manual for the Schedule for Nonadaptive and Adaptive Personality. Minneapolis, MN, University of Minnesota Press, 1993

Clark LA, Livesley WJ: Two approaches to identifying the dimensions of personality disorder: convergence on the five-factor model, in Personality Disorders and the Five-Factor Model of Personality. Edited by Costa PT, Widiger TA. Washington, DC, American Psychological Association, 1994, pp 261–278

Clark LA, Watson D: Temperament: a new paradigm for trait psychology, in Handbook of Personality: Theory and Research, 2nd Edition. Edited by Pervin LA, John OP. New York, Guilford, 1999, pp 399–423

Clark LA, Watson D, Mineka S: Temperament, personality, and the mood and anxiety disorders. J Abnorm Psychol 103:103–116, 1994

Clark LA, Watson D, Reynolds S: Diagnosis and classification of psychopathology: challenges to the current system and future directions. Annu Rev Psychol 46:121–153, 1995

Clark LA, Livesley WJ, Schroeder ML, et al: Convergence of two systems for assessing personality disorder. Psychol Assess 8:294–303, 1996

Clark LA, Livesley WJ, Morey L: Personality disorder assessment: the challenge of construct validity. J Personal Disord 11:205–231, 1997

Clarkin JF, Lenzenweger M (eds): Major Theories of Personality Disorder. New York, Guilford, 1996

Clarkin JF, Widiger TA, Frances A, et al: Prototypic typology and the borderline personality disorder. J Abnorm Psychol 92:263–275, 1983

Clarkin JF, Hull JW, Cantor J, et al: Borderline personality disorder and personality traits: a comparison of SCID-II BPD and NEO-PI. Psychol Assess 5:472–476, 1993

Clayton PJ, Ernst C, Angst J: Premorbid personality traits of men who develop unipolar and bipolar disorders. Eur Arch Psychiatry Clin Neurosci 243:340–346, 1994

Cloninger CR: The genetics and psychobiology of the seven-factor model of personality, in Biology of Personality Disorders. Edited by Silk KR. Washington, DC, American Psychiatric Press, 1998, pp 63–92

Cloninger CR: A practical way to diagnosis personality disorders: a proposal. J Personal Disord 14:99–108, 2000

Cloninger CR, Svrakic DM: Differentiating normal and deviant personality by the seven-factor personality model, in Differentiating Normal and Abnormal Personality. Edited by Strack S, Lorr M. New York, Springer, 1994, pp 40–64

Cloninger CR, Svrakic DM: Integrative psychobiological approach to psychiatric assessment and treatment. Psychiatry 60:120–141, 1997

Cloninger CR, Svrakic DM: Personality disorders, in Kaplan and Sadock's Comprehensive Textbook of Psychiatry, Vol 2. Edited by Sadock B, Sadock V. Philadelphia, PA, Lippincott Williams and Wilkins, 2000, p 1751

Cloninger CR, Bohman M, Sigvardsson S: Inheritance of alcohol abuse: cross-fostering analysis of adopted men. Arch Gen Psychiatry 38:861–868, 1981

Cloninger CR, Svrakic DM, Przybeck TR: A psychobiological model of temperament and character. Arch Gen Psychiatry 50:975–990, 1993

Cloninger CR, Przybeck TR, Svrakic DM, et al: The Temperament and Character Inventory: A Guide to Its Development and Use. St. Louis, MO, Center for Psychobiology of Personality, Washington University, 1994

Cloninger CR, Adolfsson R, Svrakic DM: Mapping genes for human personality. Nat Genet 12:3–4, 1996a

Cloninger CR, Sigvardsson S, Bohman M: Type I and type II alcoholism: an update. Alcohol Health and Research World 20(1):18–23, 1996b

Coccaro EF: Clinical outcome of psychopharmacologic treatment of borderline and schizotypal personality disordered subjects. J Clin Psychiatry 59:30–35, 1998a

Coccaro EF: Neurotransmitter function in personality disorders, in Biology of Personality Disorders. Edited by Silk KR. Washington, DC, American Psychiatric Press, 1998b, pp 1–25

Cole SW, Kemeny ME, Taylor SE: Social identity and physical health: accelerated HIV progression in rejection-sensitive gay men. J Pers Soc Psychol 72:320–335, 1997

Committee on the Family, Group for the Advancement of Psychiatry: A model for the classification and diagnosis of relational disorders. Psychiatr Serv 46(9): 926–931, 1995

Conger RD, Rueter MR: Siblings, parents and peers: a longitudinal study of social influences in adolescent risk for alcohol use and abuse, in Sibling Relationships: Their Causes and Consequences. Edited by Brody GH. Norwood, NJ, Ablex Publishing, 1996, pp 1–30

Contrada RJ, Cather C, O'Leary A: Personality and health: dispositions and processes in disease susceptibility and adaptation to illness, in Handbook of Personality: Theory and Research, 2nd Edition. Edited by Pervin LA, John OP. New York, Guilford, 1999, pp 576–604

Cordova JV, Jacobson NS, Gottman JM, et al: Negative reciprocity and communication in couples with a violent husband. J Abnorm Psychol 102(4):559–564, 1993

Costa PT, McCrae RR: Personality in adulthood: a six-year longitudinal study of self-reports and spouse ratings on the NEO Personality Inventory. J Pers Soc Psychol 54:853–863, 1985

Costa PT, McCrae RR: Revised NEO Personality Inventory (NEO-PI-R) and NEO Five-Factor Inventory (NEO-FFI) Professional Manual. Odessa, FL, Psychological Assessment Resources, 1992

Costa PT, McCrae RR: Set like plaster? evidence for the stability of adult personality, in Can Personality Change? Edited by Heatherton T, Weinberger JL. Washington, DC, American Psychological Association, 1994, pp 21–40

Costa PT, Widiger TA (eds): Personality Disorders and the Five-Factor Model of Personality. Washington, DC, American Psychological Association, 1994

Costa PT, Herbst JH, McCrae RR, et al: Personality at midlife: stability, intrinsic maturation, and response to life events. Assessment 7:365–378, 2000

Depue RA: A neurobiological framework for the structure of personality and emotion: implications for personality disorders, in Major Theories of Personality Disorder. Edited by Clarkin JF, Lenzenweger MF. New York, Guilford, 1996, pp 347–390

Depue RA, Lenzenweger MF: A neurobehavioral dimensional model, in Handbook of Personality Disorders. Edited by Livesley WJ. New York, Guilford, 2001, pp 136–176

Depue RA, Luciana M, Arbisi P, et al: Relationships of agonist-induced dopamine activity to personality. J Pers Soc Psychol 67:485–498, 1994

Digman JM: Child personality and temperament: does the five-factor model embrace both domains? in The Developing Structure of Temperament and Personality From Infancy to Adulthood. Edited by Halverson CF, Kohnstamm GA, Martin RP. Hillsdale, NJ, Erlbaum, 1994, pp 323–337

Dolan RT, Krueger RF, Shea MT: The relationship between personality disorders and syndrome disorders, in Handbook of Personality Disorders. Edited by Livesley WJ. New York, Guilford, 2001, pp 84–104

Dolz L, Cerezo MA, Milner JS: Mother-child interactional patterns in high- and low-risk mothers. Child Abuse and Neglect 21(12):1149–1158, 1997

Dunn J: Sibling influences on childhood development. J Child Psychol Psychiatry 29:119–127, 1988

Dunn J, Munn P: Siblings and the development of prosocial behavior. Int J Behav Dev 9:265–284, 1986

Ebstein RR, Novick O, Umansky R, et al: Dopamine D4 receptor (D4DR) exon III polymorphism associated with the human personality trait novelty seeking. Nat Genet 12:78–80, 1996

Ebstein RR, Nemanov L, Klotz I, et al: Additional evidence for an association between the dopamine (D4) receptor (D4DR) exon III repeat polymorphism and the human personality trait of novelty seeking. Mol Psychiatry 2:472–477, 1997

Egeland B, Sroufe LA: Attachment and early maltreatment. Child Dev 52(1):44–52, 1981

Fabrega H, Pilkonis P, Mezzich J, et al: Explaining diagnostic complexity in an intake setting. Compr Psychiatry 31:5–14, 1990

Fabrega H, Ulrich R, Pilkonis P, et al: On the homogeneity of personality disorder clusters. Compr Psychiatry 32:373–386, 1991

Feagin J, Sikes MP: Living With Racism: The Black Middle Class Experience. Boston, MA, Beacon Press, 1994

Floyd FJ, Weinand JW, Cimmarusti RA: Clinical family assessment: applying structured measurement procedures in treatment settings. J Marital Fam Ther 15(3):271–288, 1989

Frances AJ, Widiger TA: The classification of personality disorders: an overview of problems and solutions, in Psychiatry Update, Vol 5. Edited by Frances AJ, Hales RE. Washington, DC, American Psychiatric Press, 1986, pp 240–257

Frances AJ, Clarkin JF, Ross R: Introduction to Section V, family-relational problems, in DSM-IV Sourcebook, Vol 3. Edited by Widiger TA, Frances AJ, Pincus HA, et al. Washington, DC, American Psychiatric Association, 1996, pp 521–530

Friedman HS, Tucker JS, Tomlinson-Keasey C, et al: Does childhood personality predict longevity? J Pers Soc Psychol 65:176–185, 1993

Friedman HS, Tucker JS, Schwartz JE, et al: Childhood conscientiousness and longevity: health behaviors and cause of death. J Pers Soc Psychol 68:696–703, 1995

Gelernter J, Kranzler H, Coccaro E, et al: Serotonin transporter gene polymorphism and personality measures in African American and European American subjects. Am J Psychiatry 155:1332–1338, 1998

Glass MH, Bieber SL, Tkachuk MJ: Personality styles and dynamics of Alaskan Native and nonnative incarcerated men. J Pers Assess 66(3):583–603, 1996

Goldberg SC, Schulz SC, Schulz PM, et al: Borderline and schizotypal personality disorders treated with low-dose thiothixene vs placebo. Arch Gen Psychiatry 43(7):680–686, 1986

Goldman RG, Skodol AE, McGrath PJ, et al: Relationship between the Tridimensional Personality Questionnaire and DSM-III-R personality traits. Am J Psychiatry 151:274–276, 1994

Goldner V: The treatment of violence and victimization in intimate relationships. Fam Process 37(3):263–286, 1998

Gosling SD: From mice to men: what can we learn about personality from animal research? Psychol Bull 127:45–86, 2001

Gosling SD, John OP: Personality dimensions in nonhuman animals: a cross-species review. Current Directions in Psychological Science 8:69–75, 1999

Gottman JM: What Predicts Divorce? Hillsdale, NJ, Erlbaum, 1994

Gottman JM, Jacobson NS, Rushe RH, et al: The relationship between heart rate reactivity, emotionally aggressive behavior and general violence in batterers. J Fam Psychol 9(3):227–248, 1995

Gove WR, Hughes M, Style CB: Does marriage have positive effects on the psychological well-being of the individual? J Health Soc Behav 24(2):122–131, 1983

Greenberg BD, Li Q, Lucas FR, et al: Association between the serotonin transporter promoter polymorphism and personality traits in a primarily female population sample. Am J Med Genet 96:202–216, 2000

Grotevant HD, Carlson CI: Family Assessment: A Guide to Methods and Measures. New York, Guilford, 1989

Gunderson JG: Diagnostic controversies, in Review of Psychiatry, Vol 11. Edited by Tasman A, Riba MB. Washington, DC, American Psychiatric Press, 1992, pp 9–24

Gunderson JG, Sabo AN: The phenomenological and conceptual interface between borderline personality disorder and PTSD. Am J Psychiatry 150:19–27, 1993

Gunderson JG, Zanarini MC: Pathogenesis of borderline personality, in Review of Psychiatry, Vol 8. Edited by Tasman A, Hales RE, Frances AJ. Washington, DC, American Psychiatric Press, 1989, pp 25–48

Gunderson JG, Shea MT, Skodol AE, et al: The Collaborative Longitudinal Personality Disorders study, I: development, aims, design, and sample characteristics. J Personal Disord 14:300–315, 2000

Gynther MD, Fowler RD, Erdberg F: False positives galore: the application of standard MMPI criteria to a rural, isolated, Negro sample. J Clin Psychol 27:234–237, 1971

Halford WK, Sanders MR, Behrens BC: Repeating the errors of our parents? family-of-origin spouse violence and observed conflict management in engaged couples. Fam Process 39(2):219–235, 2000

Halverson CF, Kohnstamm GA, Martin RP (eds): The Developing Structure of Temperament and Personality From Infancy to Adulthood. Hillsdale, NJ, Erlbaum, 1994

Hamberger LK, Hastings JE: Racial differences on the MCMI in an outpatient clinical sample. J Pers Assess 58(1):90–95, 1992

Hamer DH, Greenberg BD, Sabol SZ, et al: Role of the serotonin transporter gene in temperament and character. J Personal Disord 13:312–328, 1999

Harkness AR, Lilienfeld SO: Individual differences science for treatment planning: personality traits. Psychol Assess 9:349–360, 1997

Hart SD, Hare RD: Psychopathy: assessment and association with criminal conduct, in Handbook of Antisocial Behaviour. Edited by Stoff DM, Maser J, Brieling J. New York, Wiley, 1997, pp 22–35

Hayden LC, Schiller M, Dickstein S, et al: Levels of family assessment, I: family, marital, and parent-child interaction. J Fam Psychol 12(1):7–22, 1998

Heath AC, Cloninger CR, Martin NG: Testing a model of the genetic structure of personality: a comparison of the personality systems of Cloninger and Eysenck. J Pers Soc Psychol 66:762–775, 1994

Helson R, Klohnen EC: Affective coloring of personality from young adulthood to midlife. Personality and Social Psychology Bulletin 24:241–252, 1998

Herbst JH, Zonderman AB, McCrae RR, et al: Do the dimensions of the Temperament and Character Inventory map a simple genetic architecture? evidence from molecular genetics and factor analysis. Am J Psychiatry 157(8):1285–1290, 2000

Herkov MJ, Blashfield RK: Clinicians' diagnoses of personality disorder: evidence of a hierarchical structure. J Pers Assess 65:313–321, 1995

Hetherington EM, Clingempeel WG: Coping with marital transitions: a family systems perspective. Monogr Soc Res Child Dev 57(2–3), 1992

Hirschfeld RMA, Klerman GL, Lavori P, et al: Premorbid personality assessments of first onset of major depression. Arch Gen Psychiatry 46:345–350, 1989

Holt C, Heimberg R, Hope D: Avoidant personality disorder and the generalized subtype of social phobia. J Abnorm Psychol 101:318–325, 1992

Holtzworth-Munroe A, Stuart GL: Typologies of male batterers: three subtypes and the differences among them. Psychol Bull 116(3):476–497, 1994

Holtzworth-Munroe A, Stuart GL, Hutchinson G: Violent versus nonviolent husbands: differences in attachment patterns, dependency, and jealousy. J Fam Psychol 11(3):314–331, 1997

Holtzworth-Munroe A, Smutzler N, Stuart GL: Demand and withdraw communication among couples experiencing husband violence. J Consult Clin Psychol 66(5):731–743, 1998

Huprich SK: Depressive personality disorder: theoretical issues, clinical findings, and future research questions. Clin Psychol Rev 18:477–500, 1998

Hyman SE: NIMH during the tenure of Director Steven E. Hyman, MD (1996–present): the now and future of NIMH. Am J Psychiatry 155 (suppl):36–40, 1998

Institute of Medicine: Exploring the Biological Contributions to Human Health: Does Sex Matter? Washington, DC, National Academy Press, 2001

Jackson JF: Multiple caregiving among African Americans and infant attachment: the need for an emic approach. Human Development 36(2):87–102, 1993

Jacobson NS, Gottman JM, Walz J, et al: Affect, verbal content and psychophysiology in the arguments of couples with a violent husband. J Consult Clin Psychol 62(5):982–988, 1994

Jacobson NS, Gottman JM, Berns S, et al: Psychological factors in the longitudinal course of battering: when do the couples split up? when does the abuse decrease? Violence Vict 11(4):371–392, 1996

Jang KL, Livesley WJ, Vernon PA: Heritability of the Big Five personality dimensions and their facets: a twin study. J Pers 64:577–591, 1996

Jang KL, McCrae RR, Angleitner A, et al: Heritability of facet-level traits in a cross-cultural twin sample: support for a hierarchical model of personality. J Pers Soc Psychol 74:1556–1565, 1998

Jansen M, Arntz A, Merckelbach H, et al: Personality disorders and features in social phobia and panic disorder. J Abnorm Psychol 103:391–395, 1994

John OP, Caspi A, Robins RW, et al: The "little five": exploring the nomological network of the five-factor model of personality in adolescent boys. Child Dev 65:160–178, 1994

Jones BE, Gray BA: Problems in diagnosing schizophrenia and affective disorders among blacks. Hosp Community Psychiatry 37:61–65, 1986

Kapfhammer H-P, Hippius H: Pharmacotherapy in personality disorders. J Personal Disord 12:277–288, 1998

Karney BR, Bradbury TN: The longitudinal course of marital quality and stability: a review of theory, method and research. Psychol Bull 118:3–34, 1995

Katigbak MS, Church AT, Akamine TX: Cross-cultural generalizability of personality dimensions: relating indigenous and imported dimensions in two cultures. J Pers Soc Psychol 70(1):99–114, 1996

Kass F, Skodol A, Charles E, et al: Scaled ratings of DSM-III personality disorders. Am J Psychiatry 142:627–630, 1985

Kazdin AE: Parent management training: evidence, outcomes, and issues. J Am Acad Child Adolesc Psychiatry 36(10):1349–1356, 1997

Kendell RE: The Role of Diagnosis in Psychiatry. London, Blackwell Scientific, 1975

Kendler KS: Diagnostic approaches to schizotypal personality disorder: a historical perspective. Schizophr Bull 11(4):538–553, 1985

Kendler KS: Parenting: a genetic-epidemiological perspective. Am J Psychiatry 153(1):11–20, 1996

Kendler KS, Neale MC, Kessler RC, et al: A longitudinal twin study of personality and major depression in women. Arch Gen Psychiatry 50:853–862, 1993

Kendler KS, Neale MC, Walsh D: Evaluating the spectrum concept of schizophrenia in the Roscommon Family Study. Am J Psychiatry 152(5):749–754, 1995

Kety SS: Mental illness in the biological and adoptive families of adopted individuals who have become schizophrenic, in On the Origin of Schizophrenic Psychoses. Edited by Van Praag HM. Amsterdam, De Erven Bohn BV, 1975, pp 19–26

Kety SS, Wender PH, Jacobsen B, et al: Mental illness in the biological and adoptive relatives of schizophrenic adoptees: replication of the Copenhagen Study in the rest of Denmark. Arch Gen Psychiatry 51(6):442–455, 1994

Kimmel PL, Peterson RA, Weihs KL, et al: Dyadic relationship conflict, gender, and mortality in urban hemodialysis patients. Journal of the American Society of Nephrology 11(8):1518–1525, 2000

Klein MH, Wonderlich S, Shea MT: Models of the relationship between personality and depression, in Personality and Depression: A Current View. Edited by Klein MH, Kupfer DJ, Shea MT. New York, Guilford, 1993, pp 1–54

Knutson B, Wolkowitz OM, Cole SW, et al: Selective alteration of personality and social behavior by serotonergic intervention. Am J Psychiatry 155:373–379, 1998

Knutson JF, Schartz HA: Physical abuse and neglect of children, in DSM-IV Sourcebook, Vol 3. Edited by Widiger TA, Frances AJ, Pincus HA, et al. Washington, DC, American Psychiatric Association, 1997, pp 713–804

Kochanska G: Socialization and temperament in the development of guilt and conscience. Child Dev 62:1379–1392, 1991

Koenigsberg HW, Kaplan RD, Gilmore MM, et al: The relationship between syndrome and personality disorder in DSM-III: experience with 2,462 patients. Am J Psychiatry 142:207–212, 1985

Kop WJ: Chronic and acute psychological risk factors for clinical manifestations of coronary heart disease. Psychosom Med 61:476–487, 1999

Lesch K, Bengel D, Heils A, et al: Association of anxiety-related traits with a polymorphism in the serotonin transporter gene regulatory region. Science 274:1527–1531, 1996

Lilienfeld SO, Waldman ID, Israel AC: A critical examination of the use of the term "comorbidity" in psychopathology research. Clinical Psychology: Science and Practice 1:71–83, 1994

Linehan MM: Cognitive-Behavioral Treatment of Borderline Personality Disorder. New York, Guilford, 1993

Liu D, Diorio J, Tannenbaum B, et al: Maternal care, hippocampal glucocorticoid receptors, and hypothalamic-pituitary-adrenal responses to stress. Science 277(5332):1659–1662, 1997

Livesley WJ: Suggestions for a framework for an empirically based classification of personality disorder. Can J Psychiatry 43:137–147, 1998

Livesley WJ (ed): Handbook of Personality Disorders. New York, Guilford, 2001

Livesley WJ, Jackson D: Manual for the Dimensional Assessment of Personality Pathology—Basic Questionnaire. Port Huron, MI, Sigma Press, in press

Livesley WJ, Jang KL: Toward an empirically based classification of personality disorder. J Personal Disord 14:137–151, 2000

Livesley WJ, Jackson DN, Schroeder ML: Factorial structure of traits delineating personality disorders in clinical and general population samples. J Abnorm Psychol 101:432–440, 1992

Livesley WJ, Jang KL, Vernon PA: Phenotypic and genetic structure of traits delineating personality disorder. Arch Gen Psychiatry 55:941–948, 1998

Loeber R, Stouthamer-Loeber M: Family factors as correlates and predictors of juvenile conduct problems and delinquency, in Crime and Justice. Edited by Morris N, Tonry M. Chicago, IL, University of Chicago Press, 1986, pp 29–149

Loehlin JC: Genes and Environment in Personality Development. Newbury Park, CA, Sage, 1992

Loranger AW: The impact of DSM-III on diagnostic practice in a university hospital. Arch Gen Psychiatry 47:672–675, 1990

Loranger AW, Satorius N, Andreoli A, et al: The International Personality Disorder Examination: the World Health Organization/Alcohol, Drug Abuse, and Mental Health Administration international pilot study of personality disorders. Arch Gen Psychiatry 51(3):215–224, 1994

Lynam DR: The early identification of chronic offenders: who is the fledgling psychopath? Psychol Bull 120:209–234, 1996

Lynam DR, Widiger TA: Using the five-factor model to represent the DSM-IV personality disorders: an expert consensus approach. J Abnorm Psychol 110:401–412, 2001

Lyons-Ruth K, Block D: The disturbed caregiving system: relations among childhood trauma, maternal caregiving, and infant affect and attachment. Infant Mental Health Journal 17(3):257–275, 1996

Lyons-Ruth K, Zoll D, Connell D, et al: Family deviance and family disruption in childhood: associations with maternal behavior and infant maltreatment during the first two years of life. Dev Psychopathol 1(3):219–236, 1989

Markman HJ, Renick MJ, Floyd FJ, et al: Preventing marital distress through communication and conflict management training: a 4- and 5-year follow-up. J Consult Clin Psychol 61(1):70–77, 1993

Maser JD, Kaelber C, Weise RF: International use and attitudes toward DSM-III and DSM-III-R: growing consensus in psychiatric classification. J Abnorm Psychol 100:271–279, 1991

McCord C: The cycle of crime and socialization practices. Journal of Criminality 82:211–228, 1991

McCrae RR, Costa PT Jr: Personality trait structure as a human universal. Am Psychol 52(5):509–516, 1997

McCrae RR, Yik MS, Trapnell PD, et al: Interpreting personality profiles across cultures: bilingual, acculturation, and peer rating studies of Chinese undergraduates. J Pers Soc Psychol 74(4):1041–1055, 1998

McCrae RR, Costa PT Jr, Pedroso deLima M, et al: Age differences in personality across the adult life span: parallels in five cultures. Dev Psychol 35(2):466–477, 1999

McDavid JD, Pilkonis PA: The stability of personality disorder diagnosis. J Personal Disord 10:1–15, 1996

McGlashan TH: Schizotypal personality disorder. Chestnut Lodge follow-up study, VI: long-term follow-up perspectives. Arch Gen Psychiatry 43(4):329–334, 1986

McGlashan TH, Grilo CM, Skodol AE, et al: The Collaborative Longitudinal Personality Disorders Study: baseline Axis I/II and II/II diagnostic co-occurrence. Acta Psychiatr Scand 102:256–264, 2000

McGue M, Lykken DT: Genetic influence on risk of divorce. Psychol Sci 3(6):368–373, 1992

McGuffin P, Thapar A: The genetics of personality disorder. Br J Psychiatry 160:12–23, 1992

Meehl P: The dynamics of "structured" personality tests. J Clin Psychol 1:296–303, 1945

Messer SC, Reiss D: Family and relational issues, in APA Handbook of Psychiatric Measures. Edited by Rush AJ, Pincus HA, First M, et al. Washington, DC, American Psychiatric Association, 1999, pp 239–260

Miller JD, Lynam DR, Widiger TA, et al: Personality disorders as extreme variants of common personality dimensions: can the five-factor model adequately represent psychopathy? J Pers 69:253–276, 2001

Millon T: Manual for the MCMI II, 2nd Edition. Minneapolis, MN, National Computer Systems, 1987

Millon T, Davis RD, Millon CM, et al: Disorders of Personality. DSM-IV and Beyond. New York, Wiley, 1996

Montgomery GT, Orozco S: Mexican Americans' performance on the MMPI as a function of level of acculturation. J Clin Psychol 41(2):203–212, 1985

Morey LC: Personality disorders under DSM-III and DSM-III-R: an examination of convergence, coverage, and internal consistency. Am J Psychiatry 145:573–577, 1988

Morey LC, Zanarini MC: Borderline personality: traits and disorder. J Abnorm Psychol 109:733–737, 2000

National Advisory Council on Violence Against Women: Ending Violence Against Women—An Agenda for the Nation. Washington, DC, Office of Justice Programs, U.S. Department of Justice, 2000

Nestadt G, Romanoski A, Chahal R, et al: An epidemiological study of histrionic personality disorder. Psychol Med 20:413–422, 1990

Newman JP: Conceptual models of the nervous system: implications for antisocial behavior, in Handbook of Antisocial Behavior. Edited by Stoff DM, Breiling J, Maser JD. New York, Wiley, 1997, pp 324–335

Nigg JT, Goldsmith HH: Genetics of personality disorders: perspectives from personality and psychopathology research. Psychol Bull 115:346–380, 1994

Nystrom S, Lindegard B: Predisposition for mental syndrome: a study comparing predispositions for depression, neurasthenia, and anxiety state. Acta Psychiatr Scand 51:69–76, 1975

O'Connor BP, Dyce JA: A test of models of personality disorder configuration. J Abnorm Psychol 107:3–16, 1998

O'Leary KD, Cascardi M: Physical aggression in marriage: a developmental analysis, in The Developmental Course of Marital Dysfunction. Edited by Bradbury TN. Cambridge, Cambridge University Press, 1998, pp 343–374

O'Leary KD, Jacobson NS: Partner relational problems with physical abuse, in DSM-IV Sourcebook, Vol 3. Edited by Widiger TA, Frances AJ, Pincus HA, et al. Washington, DC, American Psychiatric Association, 1997, pp 673–692

O'Leary KD, Curley A, Rosenbaum A, et al: Assertion training for abused wives: a potentially hazardous treatment. J Marital Fam Ther 11(3):319–322, 1985

O'Leary KD, Vivian D, Malone J: Assessment of physical aggression against women in marriage: the need for multimodal assessment. Behavioral Assessment 14(1):5–14, 1992

Oldham JM, Skodol AE: Charting the future of Axis II. J Personal Disord 14:17–29, 2000

Oldham JM, Skodol AE, Kellman HD, et al: Diagnosis of DSM-III-R personality disorders by two semistructured interviews: patterns of comorbidity. Am J Psychiatry 149:213–220, 1992

Olds DL, Henderson CR, Chamberlin R, et al: Preventing child abuse and neglect: a randomized trial of nurse home visitation. Pediatrics 78(1):65–78, 1986

Osher Y, Hamer D, Benjamin J: Association and linkage of anxiety-related traits with a functional polymorphism of the serotonin transporter gene regulatory region in Israeli sibling pairs. Mol Psychiatry 5:216–219, 2000

Paris J: Borderline personality disorder, in Oxford Textbook of Psychopathology. Edited by Millon T, Blaney PH, Davis RD. New York, Oxford University Press, 1999, pp 628–652

Patrick CJ: Emotion and psychopathy: startling new insights. Psychophysiology 31:415–428, 1994

Patrick CJ, Bradley MM, Lang PJ: Emotion in the criminal psychopath: startle reflex modulation. J Abnorm Psychol 102:82–92, 1993

Patterson CJ: Family relationships of lesbians and gay men. Journal of Marriage and the Family 62(4):1052–1069, 2000

Patterson G: Coercive Family Process: A Social Learning Approach. Eugene, OR, Castalia, 1982

Patterson GR, Forgatch MS: Predicting future clinical adjustment from treatment outcome and process variables. Psychol Assess 7(3):275–285, 1995

Patterson GR, Reid JB, Dishion TJ: Antisocial Boys: An Interactional Approach. Eugene, OR, Castalia, 1992

Peltonen L, McKusick VA: Genomics and medicine. Dissecting human disease in the postgenomic era. Science 291:1224–1229, 2001

Perry JC, Banon E, Ianni F: Effectiveness of psychotherapy for personality disorders. Am J Psychiatry 156:1312–1321, 1999

Phillips KA, Hirschfeld RMA, Shea MT, et al: Depressive personality disorder, in The DSM-IV Personality Disorders. Edited by Livesley WJ. New York, Guilford, 1995, pp 287–302

Piedmont RL: The Revised NEO Personality Inventory. Clinical and Research Applications. New York, Plenum, 1998

Pierce CM: Stress in the workplace, in Black Families in Crisis. Edited by Conner-Edwards AF, Spurlock J. New York, Brunner/Mazel, 1988, pp 27–33

Pincus HA, Frances AJ, Davis WW, et al: DSM-IV and new diagnostic categories: holding the line on proliferation. Am J Psychiatry 149:112–117, 1992

Pinshof WM, Wynne LC: The efficacy of marital and family therapy: an empirical overview, conclusions and recommendations. J Marital Fam Ther 21(4):585–613, 1995

Pinto OC, Akiskal HS: Lamotrigine as a promising approach to borderline personality: an open case series without concurrent DSM-IV major mood disorder. J Affect Disord 51(3):333–343, 1998

Plomin R, Caspi A: Behavioral genetics and personality, in Handbook of Personality, 2nd Edition. New York, Guilford, 1999, pp 251–276

Reich J, Noyes R, Yates W: Alprazolam Treatment of Avoidant Personality Traits in Social Phobic Patients. J Clin Psychiatry 50:91–95, 1989

Reiss D: The Suicide Six: Observations on Suicidal Behavior and Group Function. Int J Soc Psychiatry 14:201–212, 1968

Reiss D: The Family's Construction of Reality. Cambridge, MA, Harvard University Press, 1981

Reiss D, Neiderhiser J, Hetherington EM, et al: The Relationship Code: Deciphering Genetic and Social Patterns in Adolescent Development. Cambridge, MA, Harvard University Press, 2000

Reiss D, Cederblad M, Pedersen NL, et al: Genetic probes of three theories of maternal adjustment: genetic and environmental influences. Fam Process 40(3):261–272, 2001

Robins E, Guze SB: Establishment of diagnostic validity in psychiatric illness: its application in schizophrenia. Am J Psychiatry 126:983–987, 1970

Robins LN, Tipp J, Przybeck T: Antisocial personality, in Psychiatric Disorders in America. Edited by Robins LN, Regier DA. New York, Free Press, 1991, pp 258–290

Robins RW, John OP, Caspi A: Major dimensions of personality in early adolescence: the Big Five and beyond, in The Developing Structure of Temperament and Personality From Infancy to Adulthood. Edited by Halverson CF, Kohnstamm GA, Martin RP. Hillsdale, NJ, Erlbaum, 1994, pp 267–291

Rothbart MK, Ahadi SA: Temperament and the development of personality. J Abnorm Psychology 103:55–66, 1994

Rozanski A, Blumenthal JA, Kaplan J: Impact of psychological factors on the pathogenesis of cardiovascular disease and implications for therapy. Circulation 99:2192–2217, 1999

Rutter M, Giller H, Hagell A: Antisocial Behavior by Young People. New York, Cambridge University Press, 1998

Ryder AG, Bagby RM: Diagnostic viability of depressive personality disorder: theoretical and conceptual issues. J Personal Disord 13:99–117, 1999

Sampson RJ, Laub JH: Crime in the Making: Pathways and Turning Points Through Life. Cambridge, MA, Harvard University Press, 1993

Sanderson C, Clarkin JF: Use of the NEO-PI personality dimensions in differential treatment planning, in Personality Disorders and the Five-Factor Model of Personality. Edited by Costa PT, Widiger TA. Washington, DC, American Psychological Association, 1994, pp 219–235

Sanderson WC, Wetzler S, Beck AT, et al: Prevalence of personality disorders among patients with anxiety disorders. Psychiatry Res 51:167–174, 1994

Sanislow CA, McGlashan TH: Treatment outcome of personality disorders. Can J Psychiatry 43:237–250, 1998

Schneier FR, Spitzer RL, Gibbon M, et al: The relationship of social phobia subtypes and avoidant personality disorder. Compr Psychiatry 32:496–502, 1991

Schneier FR, Johnson J, Hornig CD, et al: Social phobia: comorbidity and morbidity in an epidemiological sample. Arch Gen Psychiatry 49:282–288, 1992

Schroeder ML, Wormworth JA, Livesley WJ: Dimensions of personality disorder and their relationship to the Big Five dimensions of personality. Psychol Assess 4:47–53, 1992

Segerstrom SC: Personality and the immune system: models, methods, and mechanisms. Ann Behav Med 22:180–190, 2000

Segraves RT: Marriage and mental health. Journal of Sex and Marital Therapy 6(3):187–198, 1980

Serban G, Siegel S: Response of borderline and schizotypal patients to small doses of thiothixene and haloperidol. Am J Psychiatry 141(11):1455–1458, 1984

Shaffer D, Gould MS, Rutter M, et al: Reliability and validity of a psychosocial axis in patients with child psychiatric disorder. J Am Acad Child Adolesc Psychiatry 30(1):109–115, 1991

Shea MT: Some characteristics of the Axis II criteria sets and their implications for assessment of personality disorders. J Personal Disord 6:377–381, 1992

Shea MT, Widiger TA, Klein MH: Comorbidity of personality disorders and depression: implications for treatment. J Consult Clin Psychol 60:857–868, 1992

Sher KJ, Trull TJ: Methodological issues in psychopathology research. Annu Rev Psychol 47:371–400, 1996

Shiner RL: How shall we speak of children's personalities in middle childhood? a preliminary taxonomy. Psychol Bull 124:308–332, 1998

Siever LJ: Schizophrenia spectrum personality disorders, in Review of Psychiatry, Vol 11. Edited by Tasman A, Riba MB. Washington, DC, American Psychiatric Press, 1992, pp 25–42

Siever LJ: Biologic factors in schizotypal personal disorders. Acta Psychiatr Scand Suppl 384:45–50, 1994

Siever LJ, Davis KL: A psychobiological perspective on the personality disorders. Am J Psychiatry 148:1647–1658, 1991

Siever LJ, Kalus OF, Keefe RS: The boundaries of schizophrenia. Psychiatr Clin North Am 16(2):217–244, 1993

Siever LJ, New AS, Kirrane R, et al: New biological research strategies for personality disorders, in Biology of Personality Disorders. Edited by Silk KR. Washington, DC, American Psychiatric Press, 1998, pp 27–61

Silverman JM, Pinkham L, Horvath TB, et al: Affective and impulsive personality disorder traits in the relatives of patients with borderline personality disorder. Am J Psychiatry 148:1378–1385, 1991

Skodol A, Oldham JM, Hyler SE, et al: Patterns of anxiety and personality disorder comorbidity. J Psychiatr Res 29:361–374, 1995

Smith BM: The measure of narcissism in Asian, Caucasian, and Hispanic American women. Psychol Rep 63:779–785, 1990

Snyder D, Smith GT: Classification of marital relationships. Journal of Marriage and the Family 48:137–146, 1986

Soldz S, Budman S, Demby A, et al: Representation of personality disorders in circumplex and five-factor space: explorations with a clinical sample. Psychol Assess 5:41–52, 1993

Spitzer RL, Williams JBW: Revising DSM-III: the process and major issues, in Diagnosis and Classification in Psychiatry. Edited by Tischler G. New York, Cambridge University Press, 1987, pp 425–434

Spitzer RL, Endicott J, Gibbon M: Crossing the border into borderline personality and borderline schizophrenia. Arch Gen Psychiatry 36:17–24, 1979

Stallings MC, Hewitt JK, Cloninger CR, et al: Genetic and environmental structure of the Tridimensional Personality Questionnaire: three or four temperament dimensions? J Pers Soc Psychol 70:127–140, 1996

Stein G: Drug treatment of the personality disorders. Br J Psychiatry 161:167–184, 1992

Steinglass P, Wolin S, Bennett L, et al: The Alcoholic Family. New York, Basic Books, 1987

Stith SM, Rosen KH, Middleton KA, et al: The intergenerational transmission of spouse abuse: a meta-analysis. Journal of Marriage and Family 62(3), 2000

Stocker C, Dunn J, Plomin R: Sibling relationships: links with child temperament, maternal behavior, and family structure. Child Development 60:715–727, 1989

Stoff D, Breiling J, Maser JD (eds): Handbook of Antisocial Behavior. New York, Wiley, 1997

Stoolmiller M, Patterson GR, Snyder J: Parental discipline and child antisocial behavior: a contingency-based theory and some methodological refinements. Psychological Inquiry 8(3):223–229, 1997

Strack S, Lorr M (eds): Differentiating Normal and Abnormal Personality. New York, Springer, 1994

Strakowski SM, Shelton RC, Kolbrener ML: The effects of race and comorbidity on clinical diagnosis in patients with psychosis. J Clin Psychiatry 54:96–102, 1993

Straus MA: Measuring intrafamily violence and conflict: the Conflict Tactics (CT) Scale. Journal of Marriage and the Family 41:75–85, 1979

Sullaway M, Dunbar E: Clinical manifestations of prejudice in psychotherapy: toward a strategy of assessment and treatment. Clinical Psychology: Science and Practice 3(4):296–309, 1996

Suomi SJ: A biobehavioral perspective on developmental psychopathology: excessive aggression and serotonergic dysfunction in monkeys, in Handbook of Developmental Psychopathology. Edited by Sameroff AJ, Lewis M, Miller SM. New York, Kluwer Academic/Plenum, 2000, pp 237–256

Svrakic DM, Whitehead C, Przybeck TR, et al: Differential diagnosis of personality disorders by the seven-factor model of temperament and character. Arch Gen Psychiatry 50:991–999, 1993

Szapocznik J, Hervis O, Rio AT, et al: Assessing change in family functioning as a result of treatment: the Structural Family Systems Rating scale (SFSR). J Marital Fam Ther 17(3):295–310, 1991

Taylor RJ, Chatters LM: Religious life, in Life in Black America. Edited by Jackson JS. Newbury Park, CA, Sage, 1991, pp 105–123

Tellegen A: Structures of mood and personality and their relevance to assessing anxiety, with an emphasis on self-report, in Anxiety and the Anxiety Disorders. Edited by Tuma AH, Maser JD. Hillsdale NJ, Erlbaum, 1985, pp 681–706

Tienari P, Sorri A, Lahti I: Interaction of genetic and psychosocial factors in schizophrenia. Acta Psychiatr Scand 71:19–30, 1985

Tienari P, Wynne LC, Moring J, et al: The Finnish Adoption Family Study of Schizophrenia: implications for family research. Br J Psychiatry 164:20–26, 1994

Tillfors M, Furmark T, Ekselius L, et al: Social phobia and avoidant personality disorder as related to parental history of social anxiety: a general population study. Behav Res Ther 29:289–298, 2001

Torgersen S: Genetics in borderline conditions. Acta Psychiatr Scand Suppl 379: 19–25, 1994

Trull TJ: DSM-III-R personality disorders and the five-factor model of personality: an empirical comparison. J Abnorm Psychol 101:553–560, 1992

Trull TJ: Dimensional models of personality disorder. Current Opinion in Psychiatry 13:179–184, 2000

Trull TJ, Geary DC: Comparison of the big-five factor structure across samples of Chinese and American adults. J Pers Assess 69(2):324–341, 1997

Trull TJ, Widiger TA, Useda JD, et al: A structured interview for the assessment of the five-factor model of personality: facet level relations to the Axis II personality disorders. J Pers 69(2):175–198, 2001

Turner SM, Beidel DC, Borden JW, et al: Social phobia: Axis I and II correlates. J Abnorm Psychol 100:102–106, 1991

Tyrer P, Alexander J: Classification of personality disorder. Br J Psychiatry 135:163–167, 1979

Tyrer P, Johnson T: Establishing the severity of personality disorder. Am J Psychiatry 153:1593–1597, 1996

Waldner-Haugrud LK: Sexual coercion in lesbian and gay relationships: a review and critique. Aggression and Violent Behavior 4(2):139–149, 1999

Wasserman GA, Green A, Rhianon A: Going beyond abuse: maladaptive patterns in abusing mother-infant pairs. J Am Acad Child Psychiatry 22:245–252, 1983

Watson D, Clark LA, Harkness AR: Structures of personality and their relevance to psychopathology. J Abnorm Psychol 103:18–31, 1994

Westen D: Divergences between clinical and research methods for assessing personality disorders: implications for research and the evolution of Axis II. Am J Psychiatry 154:895–903, 1997

Westen D, Arkowitz-Westen L: Limitations of Axis II in diagnosing personality pathology in clinical practice. Am J Psychiatry 155:1767–1771, 1998

Westen D, Shedler J: Revising and assessing Axis II, I: developing a clinically and empirically valid assessment method. Am J Psychiatry 156:258–272, 1999a

Westen D, Shedler J: Revising and assessing Axis II, II: toward an empirically based and clinically useful classification of personality disorders. Am J Psychiatry 156:273–285, 1999b

Westen D, Shedler J: A prototype matching approach to personality disorders. Journal of Personality Disorders 14:109–126, 2000

Wetzler S, Morey LC: Passive-aggressive personality disorder: the demise of a syndrome. Psychiatry 62:49–59, 1999

Widiger T: Categorical versus dimensional classification: implications from and for research. J Personal Disord 6:287–300, 1992

Widiger TA: The DSM-III-R categorical personality disorder diagnoses: a critique and an alternative. Psychological Inquiry 4:75–90, 1993

Widiger TA: Deletion of the self-defeating and sadistic personality disorder diagnoses, in The DSM-IV Personality Disorders. Edited by Livesley WJ. New York, Guilford, 1995, pp 359–373

Widiger TA: Personality disorder dimensional models, in DSM-IV Sourcebook, Vol 2. Edited by Widiger TA, Frances AJ, Pincus HA, et al. Washington, DC, American Psychiatric Association, 1996, pp 789–798

Widiger TA: Four out of five ain't bad. Arch Gen Psychiatry 55:865–866, 1998

Widiger TA: Personality disorder dimensional models, in DSM-IV Sourcebook, Vol 2. Edited by Widiger TA, Frances AJ, Pincus HA, et al. Washington, DC, American Psychiatric Association, 1996, pp 789–798

Widiger TA: Personality disorders in the 21st century. J Personal Disord 14:3–16, 2000

Widiger TA: Official classification systems, in Handbook of Personality Disorders. Theory, Research, and Treatment. Edited by Livesley WJ. New York, Guilford, 2001, pp 60–83

Widiger TA, Clark LA: Toward DSM-V and the classification of psychopathology. Psychol Bull 126:946–963, 2000

Widiger TA, Corbitt E: Normal versus abnormal personality from the perspective of the DSM, in Differentiating Normal and Abnormal Personality. Edited by Strack S, Lorr M. New York, Springer, 1994, pp 158–175

Widiger TA, Costa PT: Personality and personality disorders. J Abnorm Psychol 103:78–91, 1994

Widiger TA, Lynam DR: Psychopathy from the perspective of the five-factor model of personality, in Psychopathy: Antisocial, Criminal, and Violent Behaviors. Edited by Millon T, Simonsen E, Birket-Smith M, et al. New York, Guilford, 1998, pp 171–187

Widiger TA, Sanderson CJ: Towards a dimensional model of personality disorders in DSM-IV and DSM-V, in The DSM-IV Personality Disorders. Edited by Livesley WJ. New York, Guilford, 1995, pp 433–458

Widiger TA, Sankis L: Adult psychopathology: issues and controversies. Annu Rev Psychol 51:377–404, 2000

Widiger TA, Trull TJ: Performance characteristics of the DSM-III-R personality disorder criteria sets, in DSM-IV Sourcebook, Vol 4. Edited by Widiger TA, Frances AJ, Pincus HA, et al. Washington, DC, American Psychiatric Association, 1998, pp 357–373

Widiger TA, Frances A, Spitzer RL, et al: The DSM-III-R personality disorders: an overview. Am J Psychiatry 145:786–795, 1988

Widiger T, Frances A, Harris M, et al: Comorbidity among Axis II disorders, in Axis II: New Perspectives on Validity. Edited by Oldham J. Washington, DC, American Psychiatric Press, 1991, pp 163–194

Widiger TA, Trull TJ, Clarkin JF, et al: A description of the DSM-III-R and DSM-IV personality disorders with the five-factor model of personality, in Personality Disorders and the Five-Factor Model of Personality. Edited by Costa PT, Widiger TA. Washington, DC, American Psychological Association, 1994, pp 41–56

Widiger TA, Verheul R, van den Brink W: Personality and psychopathology, in Handbook of Personality, 2nd Edition. Edited by Pervin L, John O. New York, Guilford, 1999, pp 347–366

Widiger TA, Costa PT, McCrae RR: Diagnosis of personality disorders using the five-factor model, in Personality Disorders and the Five-Factor Model, 2nd Edition. Edited by Costa PT, Widiger TA. Washington, DC, American Psychological Association, 2002, pp 431–456

Wiebe DJ, Smith TW: Personality and health: progress and problems in psychosomatics, in Handbook of Personality Psychology. Edited by Hogan R, Johnson J, Briggs S. New York, Academic Press, 1997, pp 892–918

Wiggins JS, Pincus AL: Personality: structure and assessment. Annu Rev Psychol 43:473–504, 1992

Wilberg T, Urnes O, Friis S, et al: Borderline and avoidant personality disorders and the five-factor model of personality: a comparison between DSM-IV diagnoses and NEO-PI-R. J Personal Disord 13:226–240, 1999

Wilson M, Daly M, Wright C: Uxoricide in Canada: demographic risk patterns. Canadian Journal of Criminology 35(3):263–291, 1993

Wolfe DA: Child-abusive parents: an empirical review and analysis. Psychol Bull 97(3):462–482, 1985

Yehuda R: Psychoneuroendocrinology of post-traumatic stress disorder. Psychiatr Clin North Am 21:359–379, 1998

Zanarini MC: Childhood experiences associated with the development of borderline personality disorder. Psychiatr Clin North Am 23:89–101, 2000

Zimmerman M: Diagnosing personality disorders. A review of issues and research methods. Arch Gen Psychiatry 51:225–245, 1994

Zimmerman M, Coryell W: Diagnosing personality disorders in the community. A comparison of self-report and interview measures. Arch Gen Psychiatry 47:527–531, 1990

Zimmerman M, Mattia JI: Psychiatric diagnosis in clinical practice: is comorbidity being missed? Compr Psychiatry 40:182–191, 1999

CHAPTER 5

Mental Disorders and Disability

Time to Reevaluate the Relationship?

Anthony F. Lehman, M.D., M.S.P.H.,
George S. Alexopoulos, M.D., Howard Goldman, M.D., Ph.D.,
Dilip Jeste, M.D., Bedirhan Üstün, M.D.

Impairment and Disability in DSM-IV

A primary purpose of the current DSM-IV diagnostic system is to facilitate the reliable communication of clinically important descriptive information regarding individuals' psychiatric presentations. This diagnostic information can conceptually be separated into two components: *psychiatric symptoms* experienced by the patient that are produced by dysfunctions in biological or psychological processes, and the effects of these symptoms on the patient's ability to perform important functions, called *functional impairment.* Although they are certainly related and intercorrelated, these two domains are not equivalent. A patient can experience relatively pronounced symptoms that result in little or no functional impairment; conversely, a patient can have rather severe functional impairment with relatively few psychiatric symptoms. In recognition of the fact that symptoms and functioning represent two distinct components of an individual's psychiatric presentation, the DSM multiaxial system encourages the rating of functional impairment on a separate axis (i.e., Axis V) from those devoted to the reporting of specific disorders (i.e., Axes I, II, and III) to facilitate the reporting of these two independent contributions.

Despite the acknowledgment of this conceptual separation between symptoms and functioning, in practice the DSM combines symptoms and functioning in a way that makes them difficult to disentangle. When the multiaxial system was first introduced as part of DSM-III in 1980 (American Psychiatric Association 1980), Axis V was intended to allow for the independent reporting of the highest level of adaptive functioning (independent of symptoms) in the past year on a scale that ranged from 1 (superior) to 7 (grossly impaired). In DSM-III "adaptive functioning" was conceptualized as a composite of three major areas: social relations, occupational functioning, and use of leisure time. In DSM-III-R, Axis V was replaced with the Global Assessment of Functioning (GAF) scale, which asks the clinician to consider not only social and occupational functioning but also "psychological functioning," which includes current symptoms. This change was motivated by evidence that "clinical ratings of overall severity of disturbance are reliable and related to treatment utilization" (American Psychiatric Association 1987, p. 410). Thus, rather than measuring functional impairment or disability, Axis V actually measures a conglomeration of the two factors, with the expressed goal of facilitating prediction of treatment utilization.

Functional impairment and symptoms are also inextricably bound up in terms of the definition of the various disorders in the DSM. One significant advance of DSM-III over prior editions of the DSM was its provision of operationalized diagnostic criteria that defined the various mental disorders in terms of their symptomatic presentations, rather than in terms of unproven theoretically based assumptions about their etiology. The presence or absence of a particular mental disorder is thus determined by whether or not an individual's symptomatic presentation meets the diagnostic criteria. Because the symptoms that make up the definitions (e.g., depression, anxiety, fear, or poor concentration) commonly occur in individuals without a mental disorder, diagnostic thresholds must be set at a high enough level to avoid excessive false-positive results. A number of potential factors make up the particular diagnostic thresholds for each disorder, including symptom counts, modifiers indicating the severity of a particular item (e.g., "grossly disorganized behavior"), duration, distress, and functional impairment. From DSM-III onward, functional impairment was an important component of the definition of many disorders, reflecting its inclusion as part of the definition of mental disorder. Some disorders specifically required evidence of functional impairment, including dementia and schizophrenia. Functional impairment was also used to help set the diagnostic boundary for many disorders that are especially likely to blur with normality (e.g., simple phobia, obsessive-compulsive disorder, hypochondriasis). During the DSM-IV revision process, concerns about potential false-positive results led to the addition of a "clinical significance criterion" to more than 70% of the disorders (e.g., "the disturbance causes clinically significant distress or impairment in social, occupational, or other important areas of functioning"). This criterion has been criticized on several grounds (Spitzer and Wakefield 1999): 1) it is redundant with the thresholds already in the criteria sets; 2) it is tautological and in fact is not particularly helpful in setting the threshold because the concept of "clinically significant" remains undefined; 3) although it was added based on the supposed requirement for distress or impairment in the 1987 definition of mental disorder, it may in fact be too restrictive because the actual definition of mental disorder also allows for a disturbance that is associated with a "significantly increased risk of suffering death, pain, disability, or an important loss of freedom" (American Psychiatric Association 2000, p. xxxi).

There are several disadvantages of having impairment and disability so intertwined with symptoms. Combining both symptoms and functional impairment in one scale, as the GAF does, makes it impossible to measure functional impairment apart from symptoms. Including functional impairment in the definition of disorder brings psychiatric disorders further away from other medical conditions, such as diabetes, tuberculosis, and cancer, which are defined based on the presence or absence of a particular pathophysiological disturbance or infectious agent. Requiring functional impairment may impede early diagnosis and provision of care before a disorder is severe enough to actually produce distress or disability in the individual. It also may have a negative impact on research by potentially interjecting bias into studies of underlying disease processes by excluding subjects who have not developed impairment. Finally, it may inhibit research into the understanding of the interaction between the symptoms and the various individual factors that may ameliorate or exacerbate them, leading to variable levels of disability or impairment The need to better understand the relationships between mental disorders and disability is further bolstered by recent international research that that revealed mental disorders to be among the leading causes of disability worldwide (Murray and Lopez 1997).

The thesis of this chapter is that research into disability and impairment requires that the diagnosis of mental disorders be uncoupled from disability in order to foster a more vigorous research agenda on the etiologies, courses, and treatments of mental disorders *as well as* disabilities and to avert unintended consequences of delayed diagnosis and treatment. The independent assessment and classification of disability carries two important implications. First, disabilities warrant interventions and research efforts that may differ from those needed for the clinical symptoms of mental disorders. Uncoupling the two concepts will facilitate research on treatments for disabilities. Second, we anticipate that the diagnosis of mental disorders will be increasingly driven by knowledge about etiology and risk factors rather than by phenomenology. Ideally, the presence or absence of distress or disability should not govern the determination of the presence of a mental disorder or the need for treatment; removing the requirement for impairment from diagnostic criteria will encourage early intervention for those at risk for future morbidity and death rather than delaying intervention until after significant morbidity has occurred.

Defining and Assessing Disability

Conceptual Framework and Terminology

An attempt to uncouple diagnosis and disability underlies the model used in the World Health Organization's Family of International Classifications. The *International Statistical Classification of Diseases and Related Problems*, 10th Revision (ICD-10) (World Health Organization 1992) provides diagnostic definitions that, for the most part, do not require any level of functional impairment. Associated functioning and disability are classified in the International Classification of Functioning, Disability and Health (ICF) (World Health Organization 2001). The terminology of the ICD-10 and ICF are instructive for this discussion.

ICF defines *functioning* as general aspects of a person's body functions, activities, and social participation. *Disability* indicates problems in any one of these dimensions. The system can be summarized in more detail as shown in Table 5–1.

TABLE 5–1. International Classification of Functioning, Disability and Health classification of functioning and disability

Level	Functioning	Disability
Body	Functions	Impairments
Person	Activities	Activity limitations
Society	Participation	Participation restrictions

Body functions are the physiological or psychological processes of body systems. *Body structures* are anatomical parts of the body such as organs, limbs, and their components. *Impairments* are problems in body processes or structures, mainly significant deviations or losses. Mental or psychological functions are subsumed under body functions. Impairments related to mental disorders can involve anomalies, defects, losses, or other significant deviations in the processes or structure of the central nervous system. Impairments can be temporary or permanent; progressive, regressive, or static; intermittent or continuous. Deviations from the norm may be slight or severe and may fluctuate over time.

These characteristics are captured in further qualifier codes in ICF, labeled *activity* (person-level functioning) and *participation* (society-level functioning). *Activity limitations* and *participation restrictions* are difficulties an individual may have at these levels of functioning. Activities and participation are qualified further by the concepts *performance* and *capacity*. The former describes what an individual does in his or her current environment, and the latter describes an individual's capability to execute a task or an action described in the classification in a uniform environment. The domains assessed are learning and applying knowledge; general tasks and demands; communication; mobility; self-care; domestic life; interpersonal interactions and relationships; major life areas; and community, social, and civic life. Using these concepts of disability, the intent of ICF is to provide an operational framework to describe a person's functioning and disability in a manner unconnected from the description of the disease.

When considering disability, one also needs to characterize an individual's background and life situation. These are called *contextual factors* in ICF and include *environmental* and *personal* factors that may have an impact on the individual's health state. *Environmental factors* include the physical, social and attitudinal environments in which people live. *Personal factors* encompass a range of individual characteristics and include age, race, gender, educational background, experiences, personality and character style, aptitudes, other health conditions, fitness, lifestyle, habits, upbringing, coping styles, social background, profession, and past and current experience.

Functioning and disability are complex concepts with multiple dimensions. International research (Üstün et al. 2001; World Health Organization 2000) suggests that activities of a person can be grouped according to the following categories:

- Understanding and communicating with the world (cognition)
- Moving and getting around (mobility)
- Self-care (attending to one's hygiene, dressing, eating, and staying alone)
- Getting along with people (interpersonal interactions)
- Life activities (domestic responsibilities, leisure, and work)
- Participation in society (joining in community activities)

This formulation is grounded in a model of disablement originally presented by Nagi (1976). Figure 5–1 includes a modification of Nagi's model suggested by Jette (1997) that the model include both intraindividual and extraindividual influences on the disablement process.

This conceptual model of disablement may be readily applied to mental disorders. For example, in the case of schizophrenia, the neurobiology manifests in a variety of physical abnormalities (e.g., enlarged ventricles

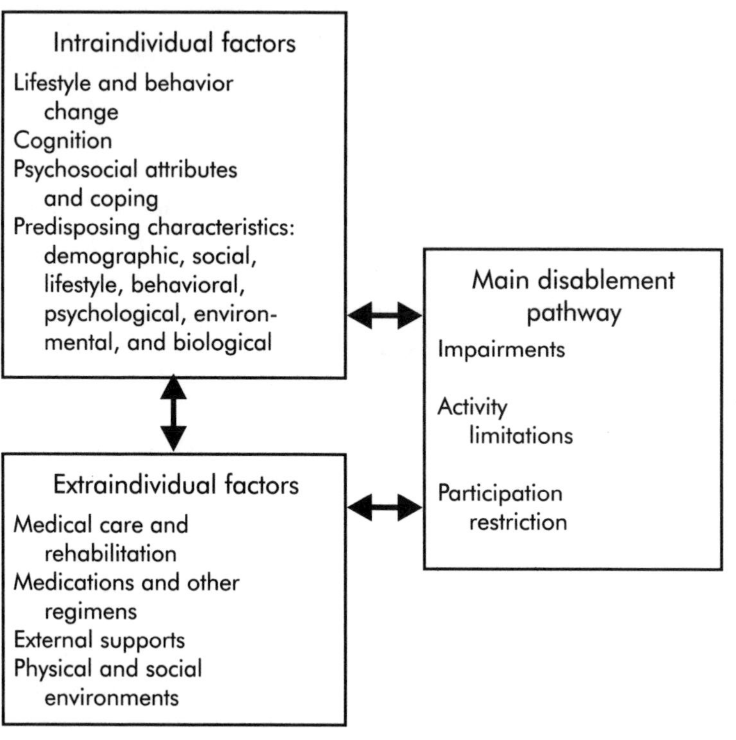

FIGURE 5–1. Conceptual model of disablement.

and sulci, neuronal disarray, excess of dopamine, and reduced frontal lobe blood flow) and psychological abnormalities (e.g., hallucinations, delusions, disorganized cognition, and basic cognitive disturbances, including input, memory, and abstraction). These abnormalities (i.e., impairments) may lead to various difficulties (i.e., activity limitations) for persons with schizophrenia, including the inability to speak in coherent sentences, to concentrate, and to remember and organize details. Without some or all of these abilities, an individual with schizophrenia will have great difficulty meeting certain expectations such as being able to manage finances, establish social relationships, or use public services. Thus he or she may experience participation restriction. Such contextual issues as stigma and impaired social support networks can exacerbate participation restrictions by limiting access to resources and opportunities.

Measuring Disability

There are several different approaches to assessing disability and functioning: self-reports; proxy (e.g., confidant, caregiver) reports; clinician ratings; direct observations of behavior in settings where patients live; and performance-based measures that use tasks in clinical settings. A wide variety of self-report measures of functioning have been extensively used in the field (e.g., regarding social and occupational adjustment) (Loew and Rapin 1994; Rohland and Langbehn 1997; Schooler et al. 1979; Weissman 1975; Weissman et al. 1981). Performance-based measures present a number of attractive features, including less dependence on patient insight and a potential for focusing on real-life skills that may be targets for interventions. These advantages should be tempered with potential pitfalls, including the use of contrived environments, which may bring their validity into question. Although a number of performance-based measures have been developed for use with cognitively impaired individuals (e.g., Structured Assessment of Independent Living Skills [Mahurin et al. 1991]; Performance Test of Activities of Daily Living [ADL] [Kuriansky and Gurland 1976]; Refined ADL Assessment [Tappen 1994]; the ADL Situational Test [Skurla et al. 1988]; Dressing Performance Scale [Beck 1988]; Kitchen Task Assessment [Baum and Edwards 1993]; Medicine Management Test [Gurland et al. 1994]; UCSD Performance-Based Skills Assessment [Patterson et al. 2001a]; Medication Management Ability Assessment [Patterson et al. 2002]; and Social Skills Performance Assessment [Patterson et al. 2001b]), little work has been conducted with the severely mentally ill.

Although direct measures of social functioning (Bellack et al. 1990) and other functional dimensions have been developed for psychiatric patients, available measures have been narrow in their focus, require extensive time commitments for both participants and researchers, and may be impractical for use in large-scale clinical trials. Moreover, the reasons for poor performance may or may not be related to psychopathology. Social performance can be extensively influenced by other health problems, level of motivation, and a wide range of environmental opportunities and incentives not directly related to mental illness. More research is needed on how to identify the impacts of psychopathology on functional status and to differentiate these from effects from other influences on functional status. Some measures of disability ask about whether a person "does" a certain task (*performance*), whereas others ask about whether he or she "can do" the task (*capacity*). It is important to evaluate reasons for a discrepancy between actual behavior and perceived ability (Glass 1998; Sherman and Reuben 1998). As emphasized by Bruce (2001), part of the challenge is determining the extent to which social roles, environmental options, or decisions to forgo an activity are actually independent of disability.

The Context of DSM-IV

Under the ICD-10 concept of mental disorder, a disorder is necessary but not sufficient to produce the functional limitations that result in disability. Individuals may experience the signs and symptoms of mental disorders without having "clinically significant" conditions as defined by DSM-IV, that is, without significant distress or dysfunction. Thus, under these ICD-10 guidelines, an individual living in New York City who has a snake phobia but who never has any occasion to encounter a snake would be diagnosed as having a mental disorder. In contrast, DSM-IV would make this diagnosis only if the individual either had some functional impairment associated with the phobia or was distressed about having the phobia.

The major problem for mental disorders as currently defined is that their causes and pathophysiological mechanisms remain largely unknown. It is expected that, at some point in the future (perhaps decades from now), the pathophysiological states predisposing or contributing to major mental disorders will be identified. These might take the form of an anatomical or cellular defect, a physiochemical laboratory abnormality, or even a genetic defect. Once it is possible to define a mental disorder based on the identification of its underlying pathology, then it would surely make sense to follow the course of other medical conditions and have the presence of disorder be based solely on pathology and not on the effect this pathology exerts on the individual's functioning. Medicine recognizes conditions that do not produce either distress or dysfunction but that indicate an increased risk for illness and later impaired functioning, disability, or death. These include conditions in which the abnormality is in a laboratory value rather than in a function, such as hypertension or hyperlipidemia. They include genetic abnormalities and certain "silent" structural defects. In each case, some aspect of human functioning is expected to result in an abnormality of the phenotype now or in the future. In these cases a lesion is implied but not yet identified. Absent definable lesions, however, it is extremely difficult to predict future morbidity or mortality from nondisabling and nondistressing mental signs and symptoms.

Research on disabilities among elderly persons with mental disorders illustrates the complex relationships between mental disorder (specifically depression in this example), medical comorbidity, and disability. The reasons for the association between late-onset depressive disorder and disability are unclear. Depression with onset in late life is a heterogeneous condition and includes a large group of patients in whom medical and neurologic disorders play an important role (Alexopoulos 1990). This position is supported by 1) reports of greater medical morbidity and death in patients with late-onset depression than in patients with early onset depression of similar age (Jacoby et al. 1981; Roth and Kay 1956); 2) studies suggesting higher frequency of neuropsychological (Alexopoulos et al. 1993a, 1993b) and neuroradiological abnormalities (Alexopoulos et al. 1992; Coffee et al. 1988; Jacoby and Levy 1980) in late-onset than in early onset geriatric depression; and 3) family studies showing lower familial prevalence of affective disorders in patients with late-onset depression than in those with early-onset depression (Baron et al. 1981). However, some studies failed to confirm the association between late depression onset and high medical and neurologic morbidity (Conwell et al. 1989; Greenwald and Kramer-Ginsberg 1988; Herrmann et al. 1989). These discrepancies may be explained by biased mortality estimates, difficulties in ascertaining age at onset, and the biological heterogeneity of late-life depressive disorders. The biological contributors to early life depression (usually genetic) may or may not be the causes of depression occurring in late life (usually brain lesions), although they may have an additive or synergistic effect; patients may experience episodes with different etiologies at various points in their lives. Therefore, age at onset alone may be a critical clue to etiology. The association of late-onset depression with disability may be due to underlying subclinical medical or neurologic disorders or to present cognitive dysfunction and thus cannot be rated by the instruments of medical burden or cognitive impairment used by a specific study. In that event, both late onset and presence of disability may be proxies for subclinical medical and neurologic diseases in elderly depressed persons.

The absence of identifiable lesions and abnormal laboratory findings for most mental disorders creates a problem for proper diagnosis. The problem was partly solved by the introduction of explicit diagnostic criteria for each disorder. This was the hallmark advance of DSM-III. Unfortunately, the lack of identifiable lesions or laboratory abnormalities makes reliance on somewhat arbitrary criteria necessary and creates a special problem for establishing a threshold for the number and severity of sign and symptom criteria for determining a "case" of mental disorder. This is particularly problematic because of the ubiquitous nature of abnormal mental phenomena, such as manifestations of anxiety or depression, which do not necessarily indicate the presence of mental disorder.

Achieving the status of a case requires that several signs and symptoms occur together for some period of time—to meet the criteria for any mental disorder, more than a single transient symptom is required. Even then, such conditions are common and may not impose any real burden on the individual or society. If not, then the condition is not viewed to be clinically significant and does not require identification or treatment. Such individuals and their families may not wish to be stigmatized by such a diagnosis. Society may see no reason to allocate scarce resources for treatment or services. This dilemma was the reason for establishing an additional criterion for defining a mental disorder: that the syndrome of co-occurring signs and symptoms also causes distress or dysfunction. At times, the threshold is set at a severity sufficient to lead to help-seeking behavior. For those concerned about allocating scarce resources, however, this threshold is tautological as a measure of the need for treatment or services. Establishing a definition of clinical significance as the point at which an individual seeks help or is brought for clinical attention does not add much information. At other times, the threshold is established on some measure of severity of psychopathology, such as a symptom severity scale (e.g., Hamilton Rating Scale for Depression) or a functioning measure (such as the GAF scale). In all circumstances, the threshold for defining a case is arbitrary, even if it is reliable. The threshold is established by convention according to the need for setting boundaries.

The DSM-IV approach leads to a reification of the syndromes it defines without actual lesions. The inclusion of a threshold of distress and dysfunction in defining a case has two problems. First, distress and disability are behavioral domains that are conceptually and clinically distinct from each other and are influenced by different factors. Therefore, diagnostic categories assigned on the basis of distress may be different from the same diagnostic categories assigned because of disability. Second, despite these shortcomings of such a threshold, the lack of a severity threshold would allow almost everyone to qualify for the diagnosis of a mental disorder (e.g., a mood or anxiety disorder not otherwise specified). Were there lesions, there would be less doubt about there being a disease, but the question of treatability and clinical significance would remain. If resources were unlimited and there was no stigma associated with having a mental disorder, there would not be the debate about "caseness" for the mental disorders. But resource limits and stigma abound, and so the debate has importance.

Under the current diagnostic system the threshold for a case is determined by a level of distress and/or dysfunction. This has become an apparent necessity in an era of scarce resources and continued stigma for the mental disorders. Intellectually it is important not to confuse the potential significance of conditions below the current threshold for severity and caseness with the current need to limit the boundaries of mental illness. Some conditions, such as subsyndromal depression, appear to impose as much disability as cases above the current threshold for DSM-IV disorders, such as major depressive disorder. Other conditions, such as specific genetic abnormalities that cause no current distress or dysfunction, may turn out to be markers for significant risk for future mental illness. Effective preventive interventions may make them clinically significant in the future—like abnormal blood pressure measurements in asymptomatic individuals today. Just as it is intellectually critical to remain open to the idea that there may be clinically significant conditions (e.g., genotypes) that impose no current distress or disability, it is equally critical to accept that a threshold for distress and disability may be required by the current realities of scarcity and restrictions on services and treatments. Perhaps most important is an awareness of the difference between symptoms and disability as targets for treatment and rehabilitation.

As attention turns toward defining clinical significance as a means to establish priorities for who receives treatment, it is important to recognize that it may be used as a key criterion for determining who gains access to mental health care and what services they will receive. Although the intent of establishing clinical significance criteria is to maximize the use of scarce resources, there is the potential that inequities may be created regarding who gets access to valued services. It is clear that careful monitoring of the consequences of using different criteria for clinical significance is needed to assess whether those criteria discriminate against certain groups.

A Research Agenda on Defining, Preventing, and Treating Disability

Going forward, a national research agenda must provide substantial new knowledge on the etiology, course, and treatment of disabilities to make the transition to a diagnostic system that allows for separate but coordinated consideration of disease and disability. An important task is to develop a classification of disability states associated with psychiatric disorders for which effective treatments exist or can be developed. The conceptual model of disablement in Figure 5–1 provides a guide to the research needed.

First, more research is needed on methods to define and assess disability for both clinical and research applications. Second, a multifaceted research program is needed that examines the intraindividual factors at the biological and psychological levels that contribute to disability. Third, a multifaceted program of research is also needed to examine the extraindividual factors that contribute to disability, including influences from family, social networks, the community, and the cultural context in which patients live. Fourth, considering these intraindividual and extraindividual factors, research must examine the pathways to and from disability, including natural course and the impacts of interventions to alter the course. Finally, health services research needs to examine the role of the health care system and government policy in promoting recovery and addressing barriers to overcoming disabilities.

Measuring Disability

To proceed with any research agenda on functional impairment and disability, it is first essential to define and measure these concepts. A variety of measurement issues need to be tackled. Measures that purport to assess disease symptoms and signs on the one hand and disability on the other must be free of confounding effects. The GAF is a prime example of a measure that combines the ratings of symptoms and functioning in such as way as to obscure their relationship. For example, a patient with a GAF of 20 may have been given this rating because of severe delusions (the symptom contribution to the GAF) or because of an inability to function in almost all areas; there is no way to know which. Furthermore, two patients with severe delusions may function at completely different levels but will still receive the same GAF score of 20 because of the symptoms. Also, patient-reported disability may be altered by symptoms, as exemplified by the tendency for depressed patients to underestimate their functional status and manic patients to overestimate their functioning. Therefore, interpretation of the relationships of disability to psychopathology may be limited by the potential misperceptions of disability by the patients. Corroboration by informants and use of objective measures of disability may be helpful in identifying the impact of symptoms on self-ratings of disability.

However, even objective measures of disability cannot clarify if a patient does not perform a function because of mental disorder, because of another condition, or because of environmental expectations. Instruments using combinations of assessment approaches need to be developed. As there is agreement that psychopathology is linked with medical morbidity and disability, treatment studies need to introduce measures not only of psychiatric symptoms and signs but also of specific medical conditions, overall medical burden, and broad and specific aspects of disability. Measures must incorporate contextual, environmental, life span, and cultural considerations. Researchers also must ask whether there are universal dimensions of disability and to what extent measures must be culturally specific.

Intraindividual Factors in Disability

Biological Factors

As illustrated in Figure 5–1, disability is a final common pathway on which multiple influences converge, and any research agenda on disability must include a focus on the biological substrates of impaired functioning. Research is needed that clarifies the mechanisms through which brain pathology produces disability and the degree to which disability affects the course of psychiatric illnesses and even their underlying brain pathophysiology. Do patients with different courses of disability have different disorders? What are the natural course trajectories for the development of disabilities in relation to the development of the signs and symptoms of illness? How do neuropsychological, neuroanatomical, and neurophysiological processes relate to the development of disability? An extremely intriguing issue is how to account for apparent resilience against disability among some individuals with mental disorders.

Individual Psychopathology

Studies conducted so far have not identified whether and to what extent psychopathology increases disability, how much disability contributes to psychopathology, or whether the relationship is bidirectional. Cognitive impairment is one factor that may affect treatment outcome. There is evidence that cognitive impairment is associated with poor adherence to medication regimens (Marder 1998) and is one of the best predictors of social adaptive functioning and outcome in psychosocial interventions (Bowen et al. 1994; Green 1993, 1996; Lysaker et al. 1995; McKee et al. 1997; Penn et al. 1995).

Comorbidity

Substance abuse is similarly associated with poor outcome, including occurrence of new psychotic episodes and high rehospitalization rates (Ayuso-Gutierrez and del Rio Vega 1997). Other comorbid disorders can influence the rehabilitation process in two ways: 1) by preventing, delaying, or interrupting services because of new symptoms (e.g., drug-induced delirium in patients taking anticholinergic medications), or 2) by requiring adaptations to rehabilitation services (e.g., comorbid hypertension in psychiatric patients) (Studenski et al. 1999). A major challenge in the assessment of disability is attribution of the disability. To what extent is disablement attributable to a mental disorder and to what extent is it attributable to other comorbid conditions? One approach for studying this attribution problem is to compare disablement across groups who have single versus multiple potential causes of impaired function in order to estimate the unique and combined contributions of sources of disability. For example, patients with only one diagnosis could be compared with those with the same diagnosis but an additional complicating comorbidity or adverse social circumstance. Answers to this question are highly relevant to the design and evaluation of treatments for disabilities.

Extraindividual Factors in Disability

It is important to recognize the importance of the social environment that influences the development of disability and the effects of treatment. Even if an individual improves in strength and balance, the individual may remain dependent if his or her social world of family and friends continue to do everything for the person (Studenski et al. 1999). Similarly, living in areas that restrict opportunities (areas with high unemployment, poverty, or racism) can be equally disabling for a person (Hohmann 1999). Research on contextual factors in disability need to address such issues as the role of stigma and social supports.

Disability Pathways

The natural course of disabilities remains unclear and requires examination in order to understand the relationship of disabilities to underlying individual and contextual factors and to provide a meaningful baseline against which to assess the efficacy and effectiveness of interventions. Although the primary goal of treatment studies is to improve outcomes, such studies can be useful for learning about the mechanisms underlying the disabilities associated with a disorder. Intervention studies may solely target treatment of a psychopathological impairment, or may focus on reduction of disability, or may be specially designed for people with both psychopathology and disability (Bruce 2001). For example, changes in disability might be observed in depressed patients receiving antidepressant treatment, or changes in depression might be observed in persons with disabilities undergoing physical rehabilitation. Conversely, a therapy traditionally used in one domain may be substituted for use in the other. Thus, one could test the effect of physical rehabilitation on changing the course of depression in depressed persons (Singh et al. 1997), or could test the effect of antidepressants in improving the function of persons with disabilities.

Health Services and Government Policy

Finally, health services research can address issues related to the interplay between approaches to nosology and health service utilization. This is especially relevant to assessing the impacts of changes in the "clinical significance" criteria on resource allocation. The Surgeon General's Report on Mental Health (U.S. Department of Health and Human Services 1999) mentions three types of barriers to psychiatric patients having adequate access to necessary health care. These include patient barriers (e.g., preference for primary care, tendency to emphasize physical problems, denial of psychological symptoms), provider barriers (e.g., lack of awareness of the manifestations of mental disorders among primary care clinicians, complexity of treatment, and reluctance to inform patients of a diagnosis), and mental health delivery system barriers (e.g., time pressures, reimbursement policies). Through health service intervention research, different systems of care may be compared with respect to their effects on patient disability. Some of the barriers to care may be difficult to remove in short order, whereas others may be more easily amenable to change. Thus, inadequate social support as well as adverse psychosocial and economic factors are harder to correct, whereas physical obstacles (e.g., location or layout of health care facilities) would be easier to modify, thereby allowing a comparative study of the effects of such changes on patient disability. Longstanding problems with reimbursement of mental health care are a significant barrier to care for psychiatric patients. These include discriminatory copayments, limits on inpatient care, and discouragement of specialized services even when warranted. Well-designed interregional or even international studies comparing the levels of disability among similar patient groups exposed to different systems of health care delivery would be useful.

Conclusion

As the field of psychiatric nosology moves forward in the era of genomics and more precise neuroscience, considerable opportunities exist to develop a much better understanding of the etiology and course of disability. This will best be accomplished by uncoupling disability and diagnosis. Disabilities warrant interventions that may differ from those needed for the relief of disease symptoms. Uncoupling the two concepts will facilitate research on the development of treatment for disabilities, especially as the diagnosis of mental disorders is increasingly driven by knowledge about etiology rather than phenomenology. Public health implications of investigations such as the ones mentioned here may go beyond their impact on the patient groups studied. It is conceivable that a focus on reducing disability and improving everyday function and independence may result in a greater acceptance of psychiatric treatment by patients and their families. Possible long-term impact of such a shift in emphasis in treatment and research can be examined over a period of time.

References

Alexopoulos GS: Clinical and biological findings in late-onset depression, in Review of Psychiatry, Vol 9. Edited by Tasman A, Goldfinger SM, Kaufmann CA. Washington, DC, American Psychiatric Press, 1990, pp 249–262

Alexopoulos GS, Young RC, Shindledecker R: Brain computed tomography in geriatric depression and primary degenerative dementia. Biol Psychiatry 31:591–599, 1992

Alexopoulos GS, Meyers BS, Young RC, et al: The course of geriatric depression with reversible dementia. Am J Psychiatry 150:1693–1699, 1993a

Alexopoulos GS, Young RC, Meyers BS: Geriatric depression: age of onset and dementia. Biol Psychiatry 34:141–145, 1993b

American Psychiatric Association: Diagnostic and Statistical Manual of Mental Disorders, 3rd Edition. Washington, DC, American Psychiatric Association, 1980

American Psychiatric Association: Diagnostic and Statistical Manual of Mental Disorders, 3rd Edition, Revised. Washington, DC, American Psychiatric Association, 1987

American Psychiatric Association: Diagnostic and Statistical Manual of Mental Disorders, 4th Edition, Text Revision. Washington, DC, American Psychiatric Association, 2000

Ayuso-Gutierrez JL, del Rio Vega JM: Factors influencing relapse in the long-term course of schizophrenia. Schizophr Res 28:199–206, 1997

Baron M, Mendlewicz J, Klotz J: Age-of-onset and genetic transmission in affective disorders. Acta Psychiatr Scand 64:373–380, 1981

Baum C, Edwards DF: Cognitive performance in senile dementia of the Alzheimer's type: the kitchen task assessment. Am J Occup Ther 47:431–436, 1993

Beck C: Measurement of dressing performance in persons with dementia. American Journal of Alzheimer Care Related Disorder Research 3:21–25, 1988

Bellack A, Morrison R, Wixted J, et al: An analysis of social competence in schizophrenia. Br J Psychiatry 156:809–818, 1990

Bowen L, Wallace CJ, Glynn SM, et al: Schizophrenic individual's cognitive functioning and performance in interpersonal interactions and skills training procedures. J Psychiatr Res 28:289–301, 1994

Bruce JL: Depression and disability in late-life: directions for future research. Am J Geriatr Psychiatry 9(2):102–112, 2001

Coffee CE, Figiel GS, Djang WT, et al: Leukoencephalopathy in elderly depressed patients referred for ECT. Biol Psychiatry 24:143–161, 1988

Conwell Y, Nelson JC, Kim KM, et al: Depression in late life: age of onset as marker of a subtype. J Affect Disord 17:189–195, 1989

Glass TA: Conjugating the "tenses" of function: discordance among hypothetical, experimental, and enacted function in older adults. Gerontologist 38:101–112, 1998

Green MF: Cognitive remediation in schizophrenia: is it time yet? Am J Psychiatry 150:178–187, 1993

Green MF: What are the functional consequences of neurocognitive deficits in schizophrenia? Am J Psychiatry 153:321–330, 1996

Greenwald BS, Kramer-Ginsberg E: Age of onset in geriatric depression: relationship to clinical variables. J Affect Disord 15:61–68, 1988

Gurland BJ, Cross P, Chen J, et al: A new performance test of adaptive cognitive functioning: the Medication Management (MM) Test. International Journal of Geriatric Psychiatry 9:875–885, 1994

Herrmann N, Lieff S, Silberfeld M: The effect of age of onset on depression in the elderly. J Geriatr Psychiatry Neurol 2:182–187, 1989

Hohmann A: A contextual model for clinical mental health effectiveness research. Mental Health Services Research 1:83–91, 1999

Jacoby RJ, Levy R: Computed tomography in the elderly, 3: affective disorder. Br J Psychiatry 136:270–275, 1980

Jacoby RJ, Levy R, Bird JM: Computed tomography and the outcome of affective disorder: a follow-up study of elderly subjects. Br J Psychiatry 139:288–292, 1981

Jette AM: Disablement outcomes in geriatric rehabilitation. Med Care 35:JS28–JS37, 1997

Kuriansky JB, Gurland B: Performance test of activities of daily living. International Journal of Aging and Human Development 7:343–352, 1976

Loew F, Rapin H: The paradoxes of quality of life and its phenomenological approach. J Palliat Care 10:37–41, 1994

Lysaker PH, Bell MD, Zito WS, et al: Social skills at work: deficits and predictors of improvement in schizophrenia. J Nerv Ment Dis 183:688–692, 1995

Mahurin RK, DeBettignies BH, Pirozzolo FJ: Structured assessment of independent living skills: preliminary report of a performance measure of functional abilities in dementia. J Gerontol 46:58–66, 1991

Marder SR: Facilitating compliance with antipsychotic medication. J Clin Psychiatry 59:21–25, 1998

McKee MB, Hull JW, Smith TE: Cognitive and symptom correlates of participation in social skills training groups. Schizophr Res 23:223–229, 1997

Murray JL, Lopez AD: Global mortality, disability, and the contribution of risk factors: global burden of disease study. Lancet 349:1436–1442, 1997

Nagi SZ: An epidemiology of disability among adults in the United States. Milbank Memorial Fund Quarterly. Health and Society 54:439–467, 1976

Patterson TL, Goldman S, McKibbin CL, et al: UCSD Performance-Based Skills Assessment: development of a new measure of everyday functioning for severely mentally ill adults. Schizophr Bull 27(2):235–245, 2001a

Patterson TL, Moscona S, Davidson K, et al: Social skills assessment among older patients with schizophrenia. Schizophr Res 48:351–360, 2001b

Patterson TL, Lacro J, McKibbin CL, et al: Medication management ability assessment: results from a performance-based measure in older outpatients with schizophrenia. J Clin Psychopharmacol 22(1):11–19, 2002

Penn DL, Mueser KT, Spaulding W, et al: Information processing and social competence in chronic schizophrenia. Schizophr Bull 21:269–281, 1995

Rohland BM, Langbehn DR: Self-reported life satisfaction. Am J Psychiatry 154:1478–1479, 1997

Roth M, Kay DWK: Affective disorders arising in the senium, ii: physical disability as an etiological factor. Journal of Mental Science 102:141–150, 1956

Schooler N, Hogarty G, Weisman MM: Social Adjustment Scale II (SAS II), in Resource Materials for Community Mental Health Program Evaluators. Edited by Hargreaves WA, Attkisson CC, Sorenson JE. Washington, DC, Superintendent of Documents, Government Printing Office, 1979, pp 290–303

Sherman SE, Reuben D: Measures of functional status in community-dwelling elders. J Gen Intern Med 13:817–823, 1998

Singh NA, Clements KM, Fiatrarone MA: A randomized controlled trial of progressive resistance training in depressed elders. J Gerontol A Biol Sci Med Sci 52:M27–M35, 1997

Skurla E, Rogers JC, Sunderland T: Direct assessment of activities of daily living in Alzheimer's Disease. J Am Geriatr Soc 36:97–103, 1988

Spitzer RL, Wakefield JC: DSM-IV Diagnostic criterion for clinical significance: does it help solve the false positives problem? Am J Psychiatry 156:1856–1864, 1999

Studenski SA, Duncan P, Maino JH: Principles of rehabilitation in older patients, in Principles of Geriatric Medicine and Gerontology. Edited by Hazzard WR, Blass JP, Ettinger WH, et al. New York, McGraw-Hill, 1999, pp 435–455

Tappen RM: Development of the refined ADL assessment scale for patients with Alzheimer's and related disorders. Journal of Gerontology Nursing 20:36–42, 1994

U.S. Department of Health and Human Services: Mental Health: A Report of the Surgeon General. Rockville, MD, U.S. Department of Health and Human Services, Substance Abuse and Mental Health Services Administration, Center for Mental Health Services, National Institute of Mental Health, 1999

Üstün TB, Chatterji S, Bickenbach J, et al: Disability and Culture: Universalism and Diversity. Seattle, WA, Hogrefe and Huber, 2001

Weissman MM: The assessment of social adjustment: a review of techniques. Arch Gen Psychiatry 32:357–365, 1975

Weissman MM, Sholomskas D, John K: The assessment of social adjustment: an update. Arch Gen Psychiatry 38:1250–1258, 1981

World Health Organization: International Statistical Classification of Diseases and Related Health Problems, 10th Revision. Geneva, World Health Organization, 1992

World Health Organization: World Health Organization Disability Assessment Schedule (WHODAS II). Geneva, World Health Organization, 2000

World Health Organization: International Classification of Functioning, Disability and Health—ICF. Geneva, World Health Organization, 2001

CHAPTER 6

Beyond the Funhouse Mirrors

Research Agenda on Culture and Psychiatric Diagnosis

Renato D. Alarcón, M.D., M.P.H., Carl C. Bell, M.D., Laurence J. Kirmayer, M.D., Keh-Ming Lin, M.D., M.P.H., Bedirhan Üstün, M.D., Katherine L. Wisner, M.D., M.S.

> There is increasing recognition that we have failed to see others clearly but have instead treated their cultural worlds like funhouse mirrors that hold up distorted reflections of our own cultural preoccupations.
>
> Kirmayer and Minas (2000), p. 434

Sociodemographic and political changes, and the technological and scientific advances of recent decades, have contributed to a growing consideration of culture and cultural factors as essential in all aspects of health care (Brody 1990; Duff and Hollingshead 1968; Harwood 1981). Assessment and management of psychiatric conditions are not an exception, given that culture permeates every facet of human behavior (Kleinman et al. 1978; Littlewood and Lipsedge 1987). The coming of age of cultural psychiatry—not so much a clinical subspecialty as a systematic body of knowledge that addresses the multidimensional relationship between culture and psychopathology (Favazza and Oman 1984; Mezzich et al. 2001)—has undoubtedly contributed to these developments.

The relevance of culture for contemporary psychiatry stems from the fundamental value of social context and meaning in the human experience. Context can be conceived of as the multilayered matrix in which interper-

---

Thanks to those who served as chapter consultants: Margarita Alegria, Ph.D.; Cheryl Boyce, Ph.D.; James S. Jackson, Ph.D.; Steven Lopez, Ph.D.; Maritza Rubio-Stipek, Ph.D.; and David Takeuchi, PhD.

sonal transactions take place. Meaning reflects both the intimate, uniquely personal nature of such events and their wider social consequences (Geertz 1973; Hannerz 1992). Together, context and meaning define the distinctiveness of the individual vis-à-vis his or her own cultural background and that of others, and the comprehensiveness indispensable in the correct assessment of clinical information.

Historically, the association between culture and psychiatric diagnosis shows three strands. The earliest entailed a comparative psychiatry seen from the vantage point of asylums and colonialist psychiatrists. This work led to the description of so-called culture-bound syndromes (CBSs). A second strand fostered the study of cultural diversity within multicultural populations, with a particular focus on the illness behavior and psychiatric diagnoses of immigrants, refugees, and established ethnocultural communities or ethnoracial blocs. This type of research has examined the stress of migration and acculturation, as well as ethnocultural aspects of trauma-related disorders. The third and most recently developed strand includes the comprehensive analysis of psychiatric knowledge and practice as the outcome of social, cultural, economic, political, and historical factors. This analysis serves as a useful basis for rethinking the applicability of current nosologic and diagnostic practices to diverse populations, both in the United States and internationally.

The progress made in recent decades does not preclude the need to continue fostering the integration of cultural factors as strong features in the internal consistency and the external presentation of psychiatric diagnoses. Culture introduces a complicating but essential element of heterogeneity in a task that nevertheless entails ecumenical aspirations. In this chapter we examine the importance of culture in psychopathology, and the main cultural variables at play in the diagnostic process. We also review the current status of research and formulate specific suggestions for an agenda aimed at making culture an integral part of the scientific foundation of DSM-V. In the final section we elaborate on the agenda's priorities and on the scope and limits of research on culture and psychiatric diagnosis.

Cultural Variables and Psychiatric Diagnosis

Mental disorders are multifactorial in nature. It follows that for any psychiatric diagnosis to be truly comprehensive, it has to take into account a multitude of variables that contribute not only to the etiology and pathogenesis of the disorder but also to a thorough understanding of its treatment and outcomes (Group for the Advancement of Psychiatry 2001). A critically important debate centers on whether race and ethnicity should be considered cultural variables or broader theoretical constructs (Schermerhorn 1970). In fact, many authors characterize *race* as a social construct created from prevailing social perceptions about physiognomic features, an "arbitrary biological fiction" (Witzig 1996) that nevertheless has an undeniable emotional impact on individuals and groups and on patients, practitioners, and researchers.

Ethnicity, on the other hand, is understood as the subjective and objective belonging to a specific group whose members share geographic and historical origins, beliefs, traditions, housing and employment patterns, dietary preferences, migratory status, and even genetic ancestry (Harwood 1981; E. Pinderhughes 1989). It crystallizes in what is known as personal or group identity. Identity relies on cultural influences as strongly as personality may be based on psychodynamics or genetics. Ethnicity provides an important interpretive, explanatory, and measurement perspective of behaviors and symptoms, particularly in the case of those who confront acculturative and socioeconomic stresses while handling the behavioral and interpersonal dysfunctions of mental illness.

Language is another cultural variable that conveys a wealth of information about the speaker and his or her culture, allowing clinically relevant insights into the patient's education, social class, intelligence, and other aspects of interpersonal and cognitive development (Westermeyer and Janca 1997). The internalization of language reflects life experiences, notions of self, and emotional and interpersonal styles. Although it is unlikely that any one language possesses the full range of terms for describing psychological experiences, it assists in shaping their context, severity, and specificity through denotative and connotative equivalences (Molesky 1988).

Education articulates the reporting and modes of clinical presentations and perceptions of severity (Eccles 1983). *Religion* and its spiritual component influence mental status, the experiencing of illness and disease, coping styles, and even clinical outcomes (Lukoff et al. 1995). *Gender and sexual orientation* and the roles they generate are significant variables in risk assessment, perception, and impact of potentially stereotyping descriptions (Almeida 1994; Cabaj and Stein 1996). Cultural *values* influence age group and family dynamics; beliefs about health and health care; social networks; and perspectives on migration, acculturation patterns, socioeconomic status, and occupational hierarchies that have also a definite impact on psychiatric diagnosis (Geertz 1973).

Culture and Psychopathology: General Issues

There is clear evidence that cultural processes can 1) define and create specific sources of stress and distress; 2) shape the form and quality of illness experience; 3) influence the symptomatology of generalized distress and of specific syndromes; 4) determine the interpretation of symptoms and hence their subsequent cognitive and social impact; 5) provide specific modes of coping with distress; 6) guide help-seeking and the response to treatment; and 7) govern social responses to distress and disability (Alarcón et al. 1999; Kirmayer and Young 1999). As a result of these pervasive and ubiquitous effects, there is no "natural history" of disease but rather a social course that must be described relative to specific contexts.

One of the main points of contention in this area is the commission of a "category fallacy" (Kleinman 1988b; Littlewood and Lipsedge 1987), the tendency of conventional clinicians to pigeonhole behaviors inherent to some cultures or societies within the diagnostic terms of Western taxonomic systems. The diagnostic construct then becomes a culturally determined belief and a value judgment. Moreover, in influencing the expressions of discomfort underlying the symptomatology of a given condition, culture delineates the so-called idioms of distress, the patient's unique styles of expressing uncomfortable illness-related experiences (Nichter 1981). The same occurs with the explanatory models offered by the patient in his or her efforts to make sense out of disturbing clinical phenomena and to assess their level of severity (Kleinman 1988b; Lopez 1994). The latter is also closely related to the creation, translation, adaptation, and cultural validity of qualitative and quantitative assessment tools. Clearly, no diagnostic approach would be complete without all these strong cultural components.

Most of the developments in cultural psychopathology research have been largely unnoticed by mainstream investigators and policy makers in the United States and around the world. The attitudes of researchers and clinicians—and the extent to which they assess and report on culture in the diagnostic process—have shown divergent and at times ambiguous results. For instance, more attention was paid to cultural issues in DSM-IV (American Psychiatric Assocation 1994) than in its predecessors, but DSM-IV still did not acknowledge the dynamic role of culture, intricately tied to the social world of the patient. It also tended to "exoticize" the cultural approach by ascribing it only to ethnic minorities (Lopez and Guarnaccia 2000). The normality-psychopathology boundaries entail cultural thresholds for all clinical populations (i.e., culture seems to influence perceptions of levels of severity, causation, or even identification and labeling of syndromes and clinical entities) compared with the "normal problems of living" (Kirmayer 1989). Comorbidity may be determined by as-yet unidentified cultural factors that contribute, for instance, to the internalization of personality features or the externalization of clinical symptoms (Lilienfield et al. 1994). The clarification of terminological distinctions (distress, dysfunction, impairment, disability, and handicap) has not been exhausted from the perspective of culture and must also be considered a worthy research topic (Widiger and Sankis 2000).

The social desirability factor in diagnosis-making processes (Kirmayer and Young 1999) and the ethnocultural and linguistic biases in mental health evaluations also deserve serious investigation (Malgady et al. 1987). Standards of research and evidence need to give increased credence to qualitative and ethnographic data. There is consensus in that a rigid or universalistic diagnostic frame subverts the essential scope of the cultural perspective. The actual diagnostic and assessment process needs to address cultural differences, language barriers, and the implications of nosologic labeling in clinical reasoning and as determinants of the patient's behaviors.

An Agenda for Research on Culture and Psychiatric Diagnosis[1]

Research on cultural psychiatry and psychiatric diagnosis can be examined from different perspectives. Methodologically, it has evolved within clinical, epidemiologic, ethnographic, and experimental contexts. Thematically, it includes universalistic and relativistic areas of inquiry, acculturation-related issues, or cultural critiques of biomedicine and conventional psychiatry. From an ideological vantage point, it has used a purely culturalistic, quasi-dogmatic, essentially anthropological approach, as well as being the recipient of multiple theoretical influences (i.e., psychoanalysis), sociopolitical phenomena (i.e., colonialism, racism, refugee issues), intellectual propositions such as decontextualization, and technological advances such as those from the cybernetic-electronic era. In short, research in cultural psychiatry requires a truly integrative approach aimed at the elimination of false dichotomies (Kirmayer and Minas 2000). Likewise, there are five interrelated questions (Bibeau 1997; Kirmayer and Young 1999) that can guide cultural research on diagnosis:

1. *Has the right nosologic system been conceptualized?* A nosologic system is constructed for multiple purposes, and the one that works best for one purpose may not be ideal for another. It is broader than its purely taxonomic component (see below). In contemporary psychiatry, existing nosologies represent a compromise among different goals from many

---

[1] A preliminary list of areas, items, and specific topics of suggested research is included in Appendix 6–1.

different interest groups with distinct agendas. Internationally, compromises have been made among different traditions of nosology. Social science research on the development of psychiatric nosology is helpful to identify deforming or distorting factors that privilege one interest or agenda over another. Finally, attempts to define the overall boundaries of psychiatric disorders in terms of some universal notion of dysfunction may obscure important cultural dimensions.

The overall architecture of a diagnostic system is therefore more than a matter of editorial convenience. The placing of diagnoses in larger groups conveys implicit information about which conditions are thought to be related and which are distinct in their manifestations, putative causes, treatment, or prognosis. Thus, it is important whether affective, anxiety, somatoform, or dissociative disorders are classified as discrete, interrelated, or comorbid clinical occurrences.

2. *Are the right diagnostic categories and criteria being used?* Diagnoses are made by applying sets of criteria that define discrete entities. If an epidemiologic instrument is used to diagnose depression based on an application of universally defined (and accepted) criteria sets, it can never be known whether vast regions of related forms of distress (not captured by the criteria built into the diagnostic instrument) have been left out. With such standardized, cookie-cutter methodology, what lies outside the preexisting definitions of disorder cannot be captured. Therefore, research is needed that extends beyond standard symptom checklists, diagnostic interviews, and algorithms to consider alternative symptoms, syndromes, and corresponding criteria.

   Single key symptoms or skip-outs also need to be avoided in collecting data because they preclude post hoc comparisons of alternative criteria sets. For example, if an interview instrument skips the somatic symptoms of depression in the absence of typical depressive mood or loss of interest, not only will it be impossible to determine the prevalence of somatic symptoms (which may be the most important indicators of depression in an alternative criteria set), but it will also be impossible to ascertain the prevalence of depression in the population thus studied. Similarly, surveys conducted in the clinical and cultural contexts of other countries are needed, because Western-style health care systems select for similar patients. Ethnographic and longitudinal studies can address issues such as false-positive results or the delineation of better outcome predictors and treatment response.

3. *Has the diagnostic threshold been set at the right level?* Points of rarity or discontinuity may suggest a natural cutoff point, but for many psychiatric conditions, distress varies continuously along a dimension, and setting the threshold for pathology (whether in terms of epidemiologic

caseness or clinical impairment) is arbitrary. Measures of functioning, adaptation, and disability need to be included to validate pathology (Widiger and Clark 2000). Most importantly, longitudinal research, with culturally or ecologically valid indicators, is needed to establish that a particular threshold or configuration of symptoms predicts course and treatment response in ways that validate it as a diagnostic entity.

4. *Have the course and characteristics of disorders been correctly typified?* DSM-IV includes accompanying descriptive material that creates prototypes in the clinician's mind and sets broad, overgeneralizing parameters for common variations related to gender, age, and sociocultural correlates, based on limited information. Studies are needed that address the full range of populations commonly seen in clinical settings. Where information is not available, the text must remain agnostic and carefully indicate the boundaries of existing knowledge.
5. *Are existing diagnostic criteria being employed in an unbiased and culturally appropriate way?* There is evidence for systematic biases in diagnosis and for unequal distribution of treatment interventions. These issues can be addressed at the level of cautions or caveats in the application of existing nosology, in terms of changes in criteria and hierarchical exclusion rules, and in refinements of clinical practice such as the use of the cultural formulation. It is also necessary to give careful consideration to the potentially harmful impact of labeling as psychotic conditions that are transitory, culturally sanctioned, and nonstigmatized by members of non-Western communities, such as reporting hearing the voice of a deceased relative in the midst of the grief process.

In the following sections we describe research done so far on these issues, and also outline a research agenda for the future, grouping the research topics into five main areas: methodological issues; epidemiology; clinical and health services/outcomes; culture and neurobiology; and special topics such as gender, violence, religion, and spirituality (Figure 6–1).

Methodological Issues

Rogler (1997, 1999b) has consistently identified areas of methodological concern in diagnosis research. Of particular value are his critiques about cultural biases (or "insensitivity") of assessment and epidemiologic instruments, his proposal of using help-seeking pathways as a unifying concept of research in mental health diagnosis and care of different ethnic groups, the difficulties in clarifying the culture–socioeconomic status dilemma, and the nuances of the categorical-dimensional debate. Arguing against what

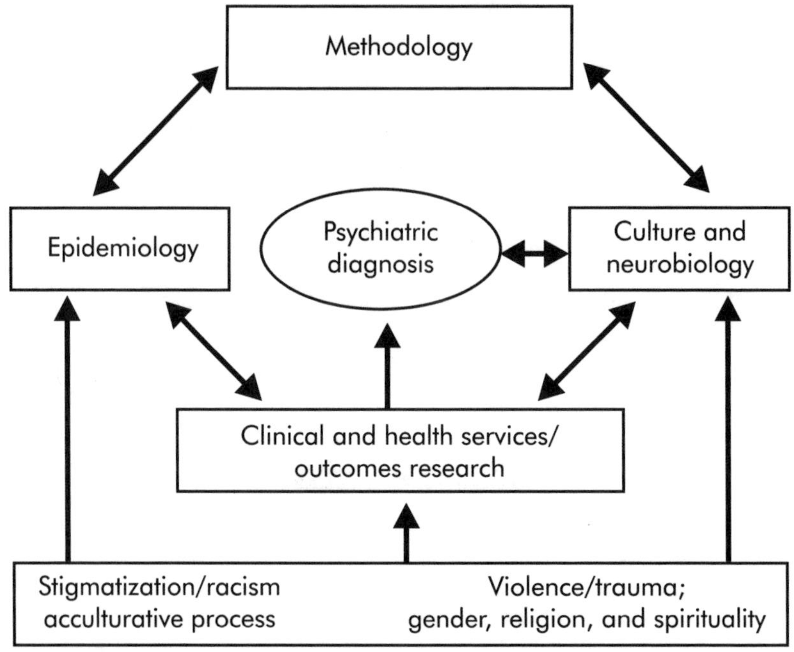

FIGURE 6–1. Research areas in cultural psychiatry and psychiatric diagnosis.

he sees as a purely descriptive, strong, research-oriented approach in the structure of the diagnostic categories in DSM-III, DSM-III-R, and DSM-IV, Rogler decries this type of "contextualization" implicit in the multiaxial system: he calls it a by-product of social and ideological forces bent on the "remedicalization of psychiatry" (Rogler and Cortes 1993).

Canino et al. (1997) point out the problems derived from the emic (from within) versus the etic (externally validated) method: that is, obtaining clinical information from the sources of study themselves (patients, communities, ethnic groups) framed in their own words versus generating clinical information through instruments devised and administered by the clinician or researcher. These writers also question the tendency of clinical epidemiologists to sanction a dubious generalizability of findings, as if their instruments captured *all* relevant information. Anthropologically oriented researchers, in turn, demand that nosologic criteria be significantly recast or even derived anew on the basis of culture-specific information. The problem with this approach is that it makes case ascertainment, epidemiologic testing of causal hypotheses, and comparability across cultures very difficult indeed, given the inherent heterogeneity of the subjects under study. In short, the main methodological problem—in itself an appallingly complex research item—is "to incorporate cultural flexibility...while retaining cross-cultural generalizability of the findings" (Canino et al. 1997, p. 169).

The statistical methods that have been most frequently used in the study of ethnic psychopathology are regression models that compare rates of subgroups to assess differences in prevalence or symptomatology. Several steps are taken to control for a variety of other factors (variables), and if differences persist, then cultural factors are implicated (Lopez and Hernandez 1986). Likewise, when cultural factors are not directly measured, the findings can only speculatively be assigned to cultural sources (Draguns 1990). Similar considerations apply to studies of observer bias (Lopez 1989).

A reasonable program of research on culture and psychiatric diagnosis would combine the following methods:

1. Clinical descriptions should be formulated in such a way that they can identify salient symptoms and syndromes through systematic case studies and detailed phenomenology. The DSM system was built on phenomenological descriptions of cases drawn from a relatively limited range of clinical contexts in the United States. Cultural variations in the clinical populations must be studied to assess the relevance of existing prototypes, establish the range of variation, and potentially identify new syndromes. These objectives can also be reached, according to Kirmayer (1989), by keeping a clear distinction between psychology (behavioral mechanisms) and metapsychology (theories of the self) in ethnopsychological studies.
2. Ethnographic research that uses participant observation, as well as social, cultural, historical, and political analyses of local worlds can be significantly helpful. The study of discursive practices, including the clinical narratives of patients and clinicians, as well as everyday talk about symptoms and affliction, assists in the identification of cultural models that influence symptom reporting, help-seeking, and response to treatment. Ethnography sacrifices generalizability for an in-depth exploration of a specific community or group. It allows study of symptoms and syndromes in community contexts to discover how individuals understand and describe their problems and to establish thresholds of pathology and clinical impairment.
3. Epidemiologic methods, applied to both clinical and community samples, characterize the prevalence, stability, and correlates of diagnostic entities. Epidemiology offers the best tool to explore the generalizability of categories and their distribution across populations. This area is examined below.

4. Experimental methods that involve intervention studies of clinical and nonclinical samples under controlled conditions with standardized measures should be used. For example, the work on ethnoracial differences in drug metabolism described elsewhere in this chapter documents clinically relevant cultural variations. Experimental work can establish the links between symptom experience and the underlying pathophysiological, psychological, and social/interactional bases of psychiatric disorders.

An overall cultural framework for programmatic and longitudinal research on psychiatric diagnosis and care is mandatory (Rogler 1992). It should cover the diagnostic process itself; the predictive power of alternative categories, criteria, and axes; and help-seeking pathways (Rogler 1997, 1999a, 1999b). Case definition is an eminently cultural process, and that makes clinical outcomes a cultural product as well. The issue of *conceptual equivalence* of symptoms and syndromes across different cultures is critical in this arena.

Two other methodological propositions with potential cultural implications linger on the flanks of the current version of DSM. One is the challenge posed by the demand to consider psychiatric entities as relational rather than individual events (Group for the Advancement of Psychiatry 1989). To these critics, the V codes of DSM-IV represent an "inadequate miscellany" full of vague labels and illegitimate categories that clearly need to be major diagnostic concerns. From a cultural perspective, relational issues clearly entail an interaction of views, styles, attitudes, and behaviors that vary according to the individuals and/or groups so involved.

Fabrega (2001) and Fabrega et al. (1990) suggest the study of "intracultural variations" among psychiatrists as a research strategy that could assist in conducting better initial patient evaluations and reaching more reliable diagnoses. Psychiatrists are informants of the culture of their profession (which is shown in their use of the knowledge pool linked to the disorders they study) and are makers of what these authors call diagnostic signatures. This feature is characterized by the psychiatrist's use of the lexical/semantic inventory of DSM that, due to the psychiatrists' different cultural backgrounds, results in discrepancies with regard to number, patterning, and redundancy of diagnostic formulations. The clarification of these discrepancies through protocols in different settings, and with psychiatrists and other mental health professionals of different theoretical orientations, could be a valuable research objective.

The assumption that European American categories are universally acceptable or valid requires, in turn, additional methodological approaches. Ethnographic tools would identify alternative symptoms and emic categories, novel methods of interviewing would tap knowledge structures and symptom experience, ecological validators would help ascertain appropriate thresholds, and keeping anchor points in current nosology would allow for comparison and cumulative knowledge. The result may very well be the emergence of new criteria and categories, or the regrouping of existing ones.

Assessment Instruments

Progress in the field of assessment instruments has been uneven. A number of scales and questionnaires have been validated throughout the past three decades in clinical and nonclinical populations, particularly for the assessment of depression. The only one intended from the outset to ensure validity across gender, age, and ethnic groups is the Center for Epidemiological Studies–Depression (CES-D) Scale (Roberts and Vernon 1983). Structured instruments such as the Diagnostic Interview Schedule (DIS; Robins et al. 1981) have been used for case ascertainment by the National Institute of Mental Health–sponsored Epidemiologic Catchment Area (ECA) Survey, and the Taiwan Psychiatric Epidemiological Project (Compton et al. 1991; Regier et al. 1998). The DIS was a precursor of the Composite International Diagnostic Interview (CIDI), currently considered the instrument of choice for cross-cultural surveys (Wittchen et al. 1991). In the field of personality assessment, applying various instruments, such as the Minnesota Multiphasic Personality Inventory (Hathaway and McKinley 1967) and the Millon Clinical Multiaxial Inventory (Millon 1977) results in different scores for different ethnic groups, making it necessary to search for scientifically adequate explanations (Pritchard and Rosenblatt 1980). Not surprisingly, Kinzie and Manson's (1987) review of the use of self-rating scales in cross-cultural psychiatry concluded that no truly etic self-reporting measures exist because all of these tests are ultimately based on the respondent's subjective sense of distress, which is a function of culture and language and therefore requires an emic perspective.

The reliance of both clinical and research practices on purely subjective and idiosyncratic interviewing styles fosters false assumptions, attributional errors, and misleading expectations, mostly due to the absence of a solid cultural anchor (Rogler 1999a). Guarnaccia et al. (1993) have dealt with the issue of "normative uncertainty" of assessment tools, that is, the possibility of instruments distinguishing between psychiatric illnesses and culturally determined responses to questions. As a result, these investigators assert that "cross-cultural validity can occur only when indigenous categories of experience are incorporated into assessment schedules" (p. 160).

Thus, culturally standardized assessment instruments (epidemiologic and clinical) are mandatory. Although methodology and the tools that configure it are also, in and of themselves, cultural creations, their most important features are reliability and validity. Cross-cultural research requires both, and psychiatric diagnoses must be reliable and valid regardless of which approach (categorical or dimensional), or set of criteria (idiographic or nomothetic), is used. Ultimately, the quest is not to find a single correct instrument but to apply instruments that reflect multiple perspectives or cultural "lenses" (Lopez and Guarnaccia 2000).

Psychological tests must be considered to be as relevant for the diagnosis of some psychiatric conditions as are laboratory tests (e.g., neuroendocrine or neurocognitive tests) (Westermeyer 1987). For example, assessment of personal identity, personality disorders , quality of life, and other culture-influenced areas requires proven instruments. In the case of quality of life, research offers a chance to dissect the various sources of expectations nurtured by the microcultural family world, work expectations, social status, locus of control, self-perception, and perception (judgment) (Lopez 2000). The validity and reliability of translated instruments should be continually assessed (Malgady 1996).

Flaherty et al. (1988) more than a decade ago postulated a stepwise validation of selected instruments with five measured dimensions of cross-cultural equivalence: content (relevant to the phenomena of each culture), semantic (similarities in meaning of individual items), technical (comparable assessment in each culture), criterion (interpretation remains the same when compared with the norm), and conceptual (measuring the same theoretical construct in each culture). These proposals are still valid today.

Context, Meaning, and Interpretation

Over- and under-pathologization of individual and group behaviors have resulted from not considering the cultural context and the unique meaning of such behaviors (Alarcón 1983; Hannerz 1992). A number of researchers have assumed a straightforward relationship between symptoms and disease, whereas others have incompletely and inconsistently considered culture and context. As a result, stereotypes rather than prototypes may have been described, with obvious negative consequences for diagnosis and treatment.

Kirmayer and Young (1999) find fault in Wakefield's (1992, 1999) exclusive emphasis on a "harmful dysfunction" approach to psychiatric diagnosis because it is not grounded in social norms and practices among clinicians. Even if most psychiatric disorders would qualify as diseases (i.e., having a biological substrate), this would not cover the whole purpose or nature of the diagnostic process, that is, the social embedding of clinical constructs attempting to capture complex human experiences. Biological reductionism (of which the modular design of brain and other central nervous system structures is a good example)—as much as the "inappropriateness" or incompleteness of the assessment process outlined above (Greenfield and Cocking 1996; Patcher and Harwood 1996)—fails to recognize that making a diagnosis implies using social standards as the measure of dysfunction, and not simply of harm.

Although context is configured by most or all of the cultural variables enumerated at the beginning of the chapter, research conducted so far has not covered them systematically and comprehensively; therefore, the potential protective or risk-inducing nature of such context has not been accurately evaluated. Clinicians and researchers can make errors of omission or of commission regarding the interpretation of child-rearing practices, social context, or more specific parameters such as neighborhood, political climate, or migratory status. All these areas are still subjects of great controversy.

Studies of immigrant and refugee groups may be ideal to delineate context, meaning, and interpretation of anamnestic data leading to diagnosis (Westermeyer 1989). The stresses of migration, flight, and resettlement provide a variety of contextual scenarios and interpretive perspectives. Similarly, studies on individuals victimized by torture and human rights violations highlight the context and meaning of internal (intrapersonal) constructs such as attachment, identity, and existential impact, or of external systems such as safety, justice, and social roles (Herman 1992; Silove 1999). Widening the focus from individual to family and community would also serve the purpose of enriching the diagnostic context.

The risk of overdiagnosing can be addressed by avoiding the use of idioms of distress as subclinical "entities" (Kirmayer and Minas 2000; Littlewood and Lipsedge 1987). Preventing underdiagnosing would require studies on culture-specific symptoms, illness behavior, or evidence of reluctance to seek help. These objectives can also be accomplished if the diagnostician pays attention to larger, pluralistic health care and other healing systems, rather than following a purely individualized perspective. Essentially, this area of inquiry implies an anthropological-cultural critique of the theory, epistemology, political and economical features, and actual practice of psychiatry (Kleinman 1980, 1988b) and of nosology as a cultural construction at the levels of scientific research, clinical work, and popular understanding.

Epidemiology

Psychiatric epidemiology is based on the general assumption that answers to survey questionnaires more or less accurately reflect bodily and personal experiences and events. However, it must be recognized that errors are possible due to perceptual imprecision or strategic self-representations. Symptom reports are based on a search and reconstruction of memories guided by tacit cultural knowledge or templates. Memory is state dependent, context sensitive, and organized in terms of salient events and conceptual modules, which change with subsequent experience. The resultant reports therefore reflect not simply the occurrence of natural events but also the occurrence of social constructions.

On the other hand, epidemiologic surveys provide a useful source of prevalence and incidence data from different communities, allowing for comparisons between diverse ethnic, demographic, and socioeconomic groups. Such comparisons, however, may not be as inclusive as the diversity of the populations under study would require. Furthermore, the methodology may be insufficient to delineate diagnostically useful information, and the results may not be generalizable due to the limitations of the study settings. These problems may result in underestimation of levels of distress or prevalence data in minority groups, and missing information on, for example, dual diagnoses or the impact of medical complications on psychiatric conditions among the same groups.

In much epidemiologic research in the United Sates, culture has been defined in terms of categories derived from the national census (African American, American Indian and Alaska Native, Asian and Pacific Islander, Caucasian, and Hispanic). These categories are not equivalent, as they represent groupings based on the history of ethnoracial blocs and their language, geographic or national origin, and experience of racism. Furthermore, there is great ethnocultural diversity within each group. Research based on these categories reflects important political realities but cannot give clear answers to scientific questions. Clearer definitions of the ethnocultural composition of samples and of the distribution of specific culture-related behaviors within a group are needed. This is likely to show that the degree of variation is greater within than between cultural groups. Because most groups will have high levels of variation among their subgroups, it may be more useful to measure specific social and cultural parameters in such subgroups (e.g., the level of conviction about explanatory models of illness, or the willingness to seek professional help) and determine their correlation with specific outcomes.

Estimates of disease burden and a framework for the study of its determinants are also important contributions of epidemiologic research. They have been useful in pointing out, for instance, the overdiagnosis of psychoses among African Americans and of violent behavior among Hispanics (Blue and Griffith 1995); the resilience and reduced prevalence of mental illness among Mexican immigrants compared with U.S.-born Mexican

Americans (Vega et al. 1998); the higher risk in minority women and adolescents for alcohol and drug abuse and suicide (Roberts et al. 1997); the preferred use of injectable medications among Caribbean Islanders (Lin et al. 1995); or the sociocentric (i.e., group-oriented) approach to mental illness by Asians and Asian Americans (Lin 1996). Yet most researchers agree that the data are insufficient and superficial at best. In short, conventional epidemiologic approaches lack the essential cultural ingredients to cover a variety of areas of inquiry.

Cultural Epidemiology

Epidemiologists can use standardized measures and random samples of clinical and community populations and enhance them with ethnographically informed, culture-specific measures to establish the distribution and correlates of clinical syndromes. Provided the right variables are measured in a valid manner, multivariate statistics can be used to determine the effects of specific social and cultural variables and thereby develop interactional models of the role of cultural factors in psychiatric disorders (Weiss 2001) (Figure 6–2).

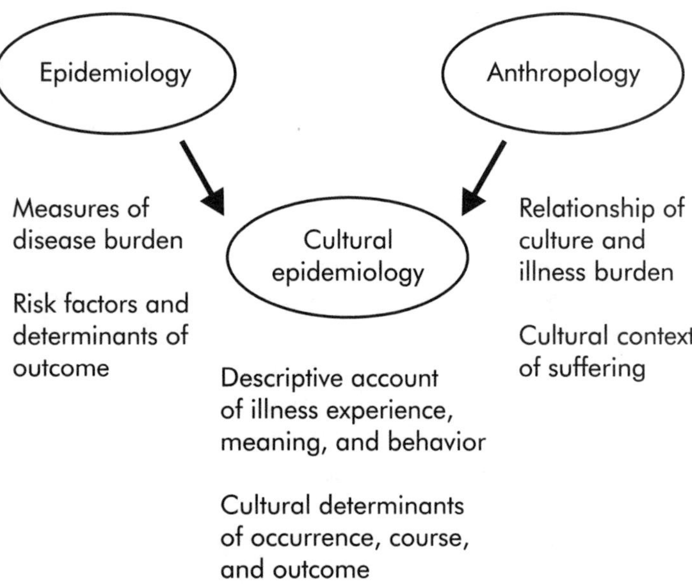

FIGURE 6–2. Integrative framework for cultural epidemiology.

Source. Reprinted from Weiss MG, Cohen A, Eisenberg L: "Mental Health," in *Introduction to International Health.* Edited by Merson M, Black B, Mills A. Gaithersburg, MD, Aspen, 2001, p. 356. Used with permission.

Cultural epidemiology focuses on the study of locally valid representations of illness and their distribution. These representations are specified by variables, descriptions, and narratives accounting for the experience of illness, its meaning, and associated illness behavior (risk-related or help-seeking). Qualitative and quantitative research methods provide a descriptive account; facilitate comparisons; and clarify the cultural basis of risk, course, and outcomes of practical significance to clinical practice and public health (Heggenhougen and Shore 1986; Lopez and Nunez 1987). Although it focuses on locally identified problems, it also considers a range of issues encompassing emotional and social distress, disordered behavior (for example, deliberate self-harm in clinical and community settings), intervention studies, and conventional clinical categories in specialty and health service settings (Weiss 2001).

A crucial feature of the cultural epidemiologic context in relation to diagnosis is who decides on the values and priorities that transform findings into authoritative evidence. The cultural representation of mental illness requires a categorical identification but also a narrative account and a full assessment of the social context in which illness occurs. An excellent example of this approach is the work of Weiss and his collaborators on the Explanatory Model Interview Catalogue (EMIC) (Weiss 1997; Weiss and Kleinman 1988), a semistructured instrument that elicits information needed for coding and comparing responses from large numbers of respondents. It also provides a framework for eliciting narratives required for interpreting the meaning of categories and dynamic relationships. These data components are then cross-referenced for analysis to clarify key diagnostic and explanatory features and to answer important questions about patterns of distress, perceived causes, and help-seeking behaviors (Jadhav et al. 2001). It also makes possible the collection of qualitative data to be maintained in appropriate databases (Figure 6–3).

Epidemiologic research should therefore encompass not only community-based surveys but also special age, gender, occupational, and geodemographic populations as well as groups such as refugees, legal and illegal immigrants, displaced and emerging communities, homeless, and so-called fringe groups. Each one contains a wealth of culturally determined features that would broaden the diagnostic coverage (Neff 1984; Westermeyer 1989). Cultural risk and protective factors and quality-of-life issues, when assessed by appropriate instruments, will sharpen the cultural facets of psychiatric diagnosis (Lefley 1990; Susser 1990). Joint work of clinical researchers, social scientists, and linguists leads to the comprehensiveness demanded by the diagnostic task. Linguists, for instance, can assist in diluting biases regarding language, translation, communication barriers, and the patient's world perspective in the diagnostic process (Brislin 1970; Rubio-Stipec et al. 1990; Schumman 1986).

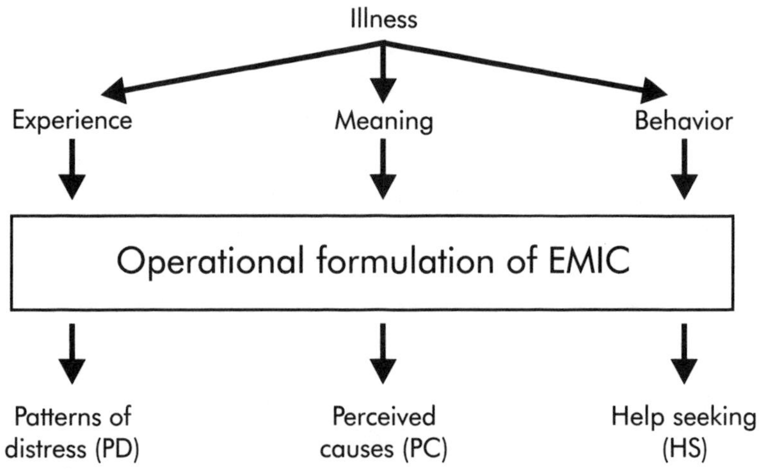

FIGURE 6–3. Cultural epidemiology of illness representations.
Note. EMIC=Explanatory Model Interview Catalogue.
Source. Reprinted from Weiss MG: "Cultural Epidemiology: An Introduction and Overview." *Anthropology and Medicine* 8:5–29, 2001. Used with permission from Taylor & Francis, Ltd. (Web, http://www.tandf.co.uk/journals).

International Studies

At the international level, the two most important developments in the diagnostic/nosologic area during the past decade are the varying levels of acceptance and use of the tenth edition of the International Classification of Diseases (ICD-10) by member countries of the World Health Organization (1992) (WHO), and the extraordinary diffusion of DSM-IV. Many studies have pointed out similarities and differences between the two systems (Alarcón 1995; Jablensky 1993; Mezzich et al. 2001). Work has taken place on both sides to make most diagnostic categories more compatible for both clinical and research uses. Local efforts in different parts of the world, aimed at making both systems more user friendly by reflecting sociocultural realities, have focused mostly on adding glossaries, dissecting culture-related syndromes, or adapting axes and instruments (Berganza et al. 2001; S. Lee 2001; Lu et al. 1995; Mezzich 1984; Olatawura 2001; Weiss et al. 2001b).

Collaborative studies among different countries are scarce. The most prominent was certainly the International Pilot Study of Schizophrenia (IPSS) (World Health Organization 1973, 1979), conducted during the 1970s in nine sites. The main finding, from the diagnostic perspective, was the demonstration of cross-national agreement based on a well-structured set of diagnostic criteria. Nevertheless, some critics of this study still point out the percentages of disagreement as a possible reflection of culturally based, instrument-based, or interviewer-based deficiencies (Kleinman 1988b).

The WHO is perhaps the most significant player in this field. The impact of the WHO's World Mental Health Report (Desjarlais et al. 1995) and disease burden studies (Murray and Lopez 1999) has been notable, and new initiatives on primary and secondary prevention open the way to epidemiologic research studies on cultural and culture-related factors, including vulnerability, resilience, and social networks (Aguilar-Gaxiola 1999). In addition, the WHO has developed a number of assessment tools, which are widely used but are still subject to improvement in relation to culture, gender, age, and population needs. Moreover, the WHO is paying attention to health care–seeking behaviors and the links between psychosocial and biological factors and treatment strategies. These assessment tools could gain in feasibility by being more client and symptom oriented, eventually providing rapid evaluations suitable for use in direct care.

Operationalization of diagnostic concepts and terminology is a prominent item in the WHO's research agenda. In 2001 the WHO published the *International Classification of Functioning, Disability and Health* (World Health Organization 2001), which includes descriptions and assessment guidelines as well as assessment criteria for research on disabilities, distress, and handicaps. In trying to operationalize and measure disability in a multicultural world, one confronts the same universalism versus diversity dilemma encountered in the assessment of other diagnostic constructs (Üstün et al. 2000), with the concomitant need to study conceptual equivalencies, translatability, usability, and cross-population comparability. A series of collaborative cultural applicability studies of classification systems, survey instruments, and assessment tools across the world would assist in identifying assessment domains, patterns, scales, and other parameters in order to evaluate current practices and identify potential level of use. Metric, conceptual, and functional-operational equivalencies need to be instrumentalized. International studies such as WHO disability assessment surveys have explored issues of understanding communication, self-care, and social interaction within and between societies throughout the world (Üstün and Sartorius 1995).

The WHO's agenda also includes focus on the mind-body interaction and its context; the stability of classification across cultures; and specific topics such as bereavement, social phobias, personality disorders, *ataque de nervios,* and schizotaxia. Differences between urban and rural areas, the hidden burden of stigmatization and human rights violations, technology transfer and dissemination, primary mental health care intervention protocols, and promotion of the social capital of all countries also figure prominently. All these areas do have, of course, a notable impact on the diagnosis of mental disorders.

International mental health research confronts the same tensions generated by the perceived Eurocentrism or Western-centrism denounced by ethnic minority groups within the United States. The overriding objective is, like in the United States, the development of culturally sensitive models, methods, and instruments for understanding psychopathology and for the formulation of a truly comprehensive diagnosis.

Clinical, Health Services, and Outcomes Research

DSM-IV represented a modest advancement in the study of culture as part of the diagnostic process (Mezzich et al. 1999; Rogler 1997). On the positive side, DSM-IV made cultural considerations a regular part of the description of each diagnostic category. These considerations summarized information on cultural variations in the description, patterns, course, sociodemographic correlates, and level of dysfunction of most disorders. However, the cultural perspective was read only as a mere addendum to the manual's introduction. Furthermore, any mention of ethnocentric bias was deleted, and suggested cultural annotations for the multiaxial assessment section were not included. Obviously clinical, health services, and outcomes research can be better only if the diagnostic bases of such endeavors are sound, valid, and reliable. Psychiatric diagnosis, in turn, would be enhanced by solid research in many clinical areas.

Cultural Formulation

Many authors point out that the most relevant cultural addition to DSM-IV was the inclusion of the cultural formulation (CF) guidelines that "supplement the nomothetic or standardized diagnostic ratings with an idiographic statement, emphasizing the patient's personal experience and the corresponding cultural reference group" (Mezzich et al. 1999, p. 459). Composed of five elements (cultural features of identity, explanatory models, psychosocial environment and functioning, patient-clinician relationship, and overall formulation), the CF filled a gap in the preceding DSMs and made clinicians explicitly aware, for the first time, of the cultural dimension in the patient's clinical presentation. The CF was complemented by a collation of the so-called culture-bound syndromes and terms (or "idioms of distress") likely to be encountered in cross-cultural psychiatric work. These were included in recognition of the difficulties of locating culturally based conditions in the conventional nosology and in assessing their true clinical nature as well as the validity of their local explanations (Group for the Advancement of Psychiatry 2001).

On the other hand, critics of the CF argue that the clinician may "lose the story" within the frame the CF provides (Rousseau 2000). They point out the risks of fragmentation of the information, dichotomization of the sources, simplification of the documented parameters, and impersonalization of the clinical description thus obtained. Purporting to offer an emic perspective, the CF nevertheless ends up making the clinician the ultimate judge of the overall relevance of the patient's clinical and human experience. This "hierarchy of power," to use Foucault's term, may be unavoidable and makes clear that the value of the CF as an integrating (hybridizing) tool deserves heuristic exploration.

The first research work using the CF was the pilot project designed to appraise its feasibility, before its inclusion in DSM-IV (Mezzich et al. 1996). As of this writing, no valid assessment of the systematic use, usefulness, and relevance of the CF has been published. It remains a promising instrument in cultural psychiatric diagnosis, as proven by its use in a variety of clinical case reports (Group for the Advancement of Psychiatry 2001; Yilmaz and Weiss 2000). In fact, it can make possible the creation of an enlarged database for diagnostic complementation and multiaxial diagnostic rating.

The next few years offer perhaps the last opportunity to explore the value of the CF. Proposals have been made for the refinement of its content, organization, and actual administration to patients. The impact of different cultural variables should also be addressed. Research on cultural explanations of illness and idioms of distress has already been outlined. The role of support systems and of the patient's socioenvironmental world in the diagnostic process offers a dynamic field of inquiry on notions with a heavy cultural component such as privacy and confidentiality (Littlewood 1990; Lopez and Guarnaccia 2000; Wohlfarth et al. 1993). Transference—as attribution and expectation of cultural assumptions—is as relevant in psychotherapy research (Comas-Díaz and Jacobsen 1991) as it is for the study of culture and psychiatric diagnosis. Social differences and the notion of cultural identity, akin to those of self or ego from other theoretical orientations, require additional research (Alarcón 1990; Kleinman et al. 1997).

The standardization of all or selected components of the CF (and an inherent need to quantify them) to be used in culturally based measures of clinical severity, quality of life, or personal or group identity is a desirable development. The value of the CF in assessing naturalistic clinical contexts, treatment effectiveness, and outcome prediction must also be studied (Lewis-Fernandez 1996). These issues are more relevant considering the role and impact of managed care and cost-effectiveness precepts in medical and psychiatric practice (Kleinman 1980).

Specific Clinical Entities

It is reasonable to assume that the psychiatric nomenclature of the near future will retain at least an element of the categorical approach. Clinical research, therefore, will focus on these categories or sets of symptoms and syndromes to complement expected progress in the understanding of the etiopathogenesis of mental illnesses. This approach appears even more justified if clinicians do not lose sight of the cultural components of the patient's diagnosis, as the patient's cultural background colors every facet of his or her illness experience—from the linguistic structure and the form and content of delusions in psychotic patients of different ethnicities, to the unique meaning of expressed emotions such as grief or terror, and to the cultural nuances and variants of depression, somatization, panic, dissociation, or anxiety. On the other hand, doubts remain about pervasive Western views that may cause false assessment of behaviors, adscription of symptom clusters, and determination of severity (Sartorius et al. 1993; Westermeyer 1987).

The anthropological basis of all the types of research described above is self-evident and thereby presents a solid critique of the artificiality of a professed atheoreticism of the diagnostic and nosologic task. It also provides further validation of the usefulness of ethnographic narratives and the strength of a pluralistic perspective in the assessment of mental disorders (Kleinman 1988a).

Psychotic disorders. Misdiagnosis due to a different cultural perspective of bizarreness is rather frequent. Individual emotions vary as a function of previous experience, and this results in difficulties in the assessment of symptoms such as flat affect, paranoia, alogia, and avolition (Grier and Cobbs 1968; Lin and Kleinman 1988; Ndetei and Vadher 1984; Sartorius et al. 1986). This finding is more evident in comparison studies between different ethnic groups (Trierweiler et al. 2000). In schizophrenia, the review by Karno and Jenkins (1993) corroborates the cross-cultural validity of the criteria included in DSM-III and ICD-9 and of the Schneider's first-rank symptoms. It also substantiates the better course and outcome of schizophrenic patients in developing countries than in developed nations (World Health Organization 1973, 1979). However, research on expressed emotions (Jenkins and Karno 1992; Lefley 1992) appears to be only beginning and needs methodological improvement in terms of cultural validity of the protocols, that is, normative baselines, rules for family display of affect, and culturally specific meanings.

Depression and other mood disorders. Conventional epidemiology has shown the relevance of cultural factors for mood disorders in populations as different as the Amish of Pennsylvania (Egeland 1986) and the Chinese Americans in Los Angeles (Takeuchi et al. 1998). Among contemporary Chinese, for instance, the tendency to either deny depression or express it somatically may be changing as a result of growing Western influences (Parker et al. 2001). Golding et al. (1992) also demonstrated culturally determined risk factors for depression secondary to other medical, psychiatric, or interpersonal conditions among Mexican Americans (e.g., "drinking to forget"). An association between stigma and both depression and somatization was observed in studies conducted in India (Raguram et al. 1996, 2001).

Delineating depression as a normal mood state, symptom, or disorder is a complicated task because such experiences are not unidimensional, linear, or additive; not only might the scales of measurement differ (minimally in some cases), but the significant categories of aggregation may not correspond either (Mezzich et al. 1999). Furthermore, how the duration of symptoms (an important criterion in most DSM categories) is perceived requires a strong level of cultural awareness of mood states that, like all other parameters, generates differences in narrative and diagnostic contexts.

One of the greatest difficulties for research on dysphoria lies in determining its true clinical presence, largely because of the attendant cultural assumptions by both patient and clinician (Manson 1997). Jenkins et al. (1990) point out that key elements in understanding these variations involve definitions of selfhood, indigenous categories of emotion, emphasis on particular aspects of emotional life, emotion-based patterning of relationships, precipitating social situations, and ethnophysiologic accounts of emotionality. The latter element has a close link with the different magnitude of somatic symptoms among several ethnic groups (Alarcón and Ruiz 1995; Escobar et al. 1983; Marsella et al. 1985).

Anxiety disorders. D.M. Clark (1991) conceives these conditions not simply as biological perturbations but as a reflection of vicious cycles of bodily arousal, cognitive interpretations, and ineffective coping in a runaway feedback loop. Cultural beliefs and practices influence coping styles, context, interpretations and responses to threats, and concomitant fears. These disorders show perhaps the most convincing prevalence rate differences along ethnic lines (Eaton et al. 1991). The exact reasons for these differences are still unknown, although explanations based on mislabeling, help-seeking practices, socioeconomic status, religious beliefs, and instrumental limitations have been advanced and require additional research (Brown et al. 1990).

Cross-cultural studies have also revealed substantial differences among ethnic groups in the prominence and type of specific fears, phobic and obsessive-compulsive disorders, and associated somatic, dissociative, and affective symptoms and syndromes (Eaton et al. 1991; Gothe et al. 1995; Okasha et al. 1994). Outcomes of severe anxiety in psychotic-like or dissociative syndromes also vary as a function of ethnicity (Kirmayer et al. 1995).

Posttraumatic stress disorder. Although it is classified as an anxiety disorder, posttraumatic stress disorder (PTSD) in fact appears to be a clinically more complex condition than others in the same category. It also offers significant challenges to a cultural diagnostic approach, particularly because charges of Western-centrism have been more intense for it than for other clinical entities (Boehnlein and Kinzie 1992; Marsella et al. 1996). From the characterization of stressors to the peculiar memory distortions created by the traumatic event and its sequelae; from its close links to violence in its different expressions to the production of symptoms as opposite as numbness and emotional arousal; from a varied "typology of forms of uncertainty" (Young 1995) as a cardinal clinical and behavioral feature to the role of shame, guilt, anger, and resentment; and from a presumed diathesis to the existential debacle it may lead to, PTSD is an extraordinarily rich area of research in cultural psychiatry and cultural diagnosis (Boehnlein and Alarcón 2000). Ideal settings and groups in which diagnostic and other clinical comparisons can take place include survivors of massive collective traumas, refugees and other displaced groups, military populations, and victims of natural and technological disasters or of political persecution (Fullerton et al. 2001; Kleinman et al. 1997; Root 1996). Environmental and family culture-related factors are extremely relevant in diagnosing PTSD. Eisenbruch (1992) suggests that posttraumatic behavior presents a clear example of what he calls "cultural grief" in the sense that it mainly manifests itself in clinical presentations that are highly influenced by cultural precepts in the patient or the patient's community of origin. Eisenbruch therefore questions the efficacy of Western-based treatment modalities.

Cognitive disorders. There are culturally based problems in the assessment and conceptualization of space and time; fund of knowledge; family, community and societal tolerance of pathology; level of isolation of the affected individual; and familiarity with diagnostic and testing methods (de la Monte et al. 1989; Group for the Advancement of Psychiatry 2001; Williams 1987). The very definition of cognitive pathology in different cultures, and the clinical recognition of Alzheimer's disease and related dementias present significant obstacles that feed (or are fed by) denial, underlying hostility, depression, and personal devastation among family members. Epidemiologically relevant items are age groups, educational level, language familiarity, and skills. Checking out of other sources provides information to test the validity and usefulness of the instruments used. Sample selection, bias analyses, and the search for a gold standard of cross-cultural cognitive comparability are research subjects as well (Lopez and Taussig 1991). On the clinician's side, stereotype, stigma, or deeper personal factors such as religiosity or lifestyle may affect the thoroughness of the diagnostic approach. In addition, issues such as clinical progression and biological correlates of the disorder must be the subject of correlational cultural and medico-anthropological research.

Substance use disorders and alcoholism. In DSM-IV there seems to be a greater emphasis on the neurophysiologic nature of substance dependence, expanding this notion to features such as maladaptive motivation, interest, desire, and craving (Kosten 1998). However, social learning and cultural or environmental contingencies cannot be simply set aside, particularly in the area of diagnosis. The clinician should keep in mind cultural prescriptions for and proscriptions against substance use; pathogenic patterns, including culturally determined risk factors (i.e., leaving one's culture of origin, poor acculturation); and even the metabolic pathways in specific ethnic groups (Westermeyer 1995; Westermeyer and Canino 1997). The cultural assessment should also involve patterns of use throughout the life cycle, family response, and idiosyncratic aspects of sanctions, social tolerance, and religious and spiritual interactions (Vaillant 1986).

Eating disorders. The diagnosis, nosology, and cultural context of eating disorders is a matter of intense debate. Weiss (1995) analyzed in detail the terminological variations in the description of the disorders in DSM-III, DSM-III-R, and DSM-IV. Cross-cultural studies raise questions about how to interpret low rates and distinctive clinical features of eating disorders in non-Western cultures. On the other hand, the effects of rapid acculturation and/or industrialization on the frequency and symptomatology of eating disorders, age-related vulnerabilities (Gordon 1990; Ritenbaugh et al. 1997), and clinical and diagnostic differences in core features of anorexia nervosa by clinicians from different countries require validation (Habermas 1991; Iancu et al. 1994). Weiss (1995) proposes comparative studies of current criteria, and S. Lee (1993) suggests that inquiries of a culture-free nature should be conducted along with a systematic use of the CF parameters, cultural assessment instruments, and field studies in communities at risk.

Personality disorders. Personality disorders represent perhaps the most challenging field of research on cultural issues. Beyond the question of boundaries between normality and abnormality in personality functions, an examination of cultural factors can contribute to the debate on whether personality disorders should or should not be considered autonomous mental disorders, or whether some of them are best considered as variants of Axis I disorders (e.g., schizotypal personality disorder as a variant of schizophrenia) (Alarcón et al. 1998). There is growing evidence that culture can help refine clinical descriptors in different groups, thus contributing to a more realistic assessment of a current requirement in the definition of personality disorder: that the behavior deviates from the expectations of the individual's subculture. In this area more than any other, the main issue is whether a new classification system will maintain the current categorical and axial implementation of personality disorders or move on to an entirely different perspective (Widiger and Clark 2000). (See also Chapter 4, this volume, for a more detailed discussion of this issue.) Clinicians tend to use a combination of categorical and dimensional approaches to diagnose personality disorders, whereas researchers, especially psychologists, appear to be more inclined to use dimensional approaches. In recent times, the purely dimensional approach seems to be gaining recognition as a focus of research, due to its broad, more thoroughly encompassing scope (Livesley 1998). Riso et al. (1994) conclude that patient-informant concordance for personality disorders is poor for categorical diagnoses but somewhat better for dimensional scores. Similarly, culture has a relevant role in the structure, performance, evaluation, and usefulness of specific diagnostic instruments and in the study of eventual interrelationships between Axis I and Axis II conditions.

From a strictly clinical research perspective, there is a need to assess the homogeneity (or lack of it) of personality disorder diagnostic criteria within and across the existing clusters, and within and across different cultural groups (Fabrega et al. 1991). The diagnostician's stands on gender as related to personality disorders; the utility of personality traits in tests of adaptability to environmental changes; and the presence, perception of, and interpretation or explanation of physical symptoms by individuals with personality disorders are urgent research issues (Alarcón et al. 1998; Oldham 1994; Siever and Davis 1991). Suggestions related to measurement of cultural distance between the patient and the clinician, assignment of a cultural profile, and assignment of complementary roles to specific personality disorder categories have been advanced (Abroms 1981; Alarcón and Foulks 1995; Benjamin 1999).

Family and Support Systems

Child-rearing practices and family-based experiences are potent pathogenic and pathoplastic sources in clinical psychiatry. Both respond to particular elements of the individual's family microculture and, in the diagnostic arena, shape the form and expression of behaviors that the clinician must catalog either as symptoms or as unique forms of culturally determined thoughts, feelings, or actions (Kaslow et al. 1995).

Although family members are valuable providers of information leading to diagnosis, their role is even more important as vehicles of cultural messages regarding the interpretation and explanation of events that cause behavioral disturbances, their actual presentation, and the strategies patients choose to handle them. Research in this area should be oriented to recognize the family's (and the surrounding community's) role in the generation of symptoms, the explanatory models, the behavior-labeling practices, and their attitudes vis-à-vis the helping professions. Cultural and environmental family-based factors must be investigated vis-à-vis risk-taking, novelty-seeking, or reward-dependent behaviors, and even verbal and cognitive skills (Svrakic et al. 1999). Research on the relationship of a number of these variables with the family's microcultural features (belief systems, social expressiveness, group-connectedness, acceptance of authority) along developmental phases may produce significant findings.

The severity of symptoms may be either exacerbated or attenuated by the nature and strength of family and social support systems. It is important to study this relationship to separate neurobiological from psychosociocultural factors and to pave the way for the development and application of better diagnostic measures. Finally, the role of family and social factors in the differential diagnosis of several entities, and in the assembling of treatment options, must be investigated (Alarcón et al. 1999; Lewis-Fernandez and Kleinman 1993).

Culture-Bound Syndromes

Appendix I in DSM-IV-TR (American Psychiatric Association 2000), devoted to culture-bound syndromes (CBSs), was originally intended as a glossary to clarify terms that would appear elsewhere in the volume in association with specific disorders. The editors cut much of the suggested material and, as a consequence, the glossary may give some the impression that these CBSs are candidate disorders with status comparable to those listed in the main text but awaiting further research. Although the introduction of this glossary states that it contains "some of the best-studied culture-bound syndromes and idioms of distress that may be encountered in clinical practice in North America and includes relevant DSM-IV categories when data suggest that they should be considered in a diagnostic formulation" (American Psychiatric Association 2000, p. 899), the fact is that most of the entities listed are not CBSs. Many are not restricted or "bound" to one culture, because they appear in closely analogous forms in many different settings (e.g., *taijin kyofusho* in Japan and Korea) and are best termed "culture-related." Many are not syndromes (co-occurring sets of symptoms with a characteristic course), but are instead causal explanations that can be applied to a wide range of conditions (e.g., *susto* or fright illness) or can be considered only as cultural idioms of distress that help to understand the patient's social world. In these cases, the cultural labels cut across other DSM categories and represent an axis of cultural meanings that is orthogonal to conventional psychiatric nosology. This does not mean, however, that the local labels are irrelevant to proper diagnosis. They may affect symptom experience, help-seeking, disability, stigmatization, and response to treatment.

The crucial question is whether CBSs are superficially atypical variants of conventional psychiatric diagnoses or, on the contrary, examples of mutually incompatible nosologies (Lewis-Fernandez et al. 2000). A current definition of CBSs (Prince and Tcheng-Laroche 1987) excludes a notion of causality and limits them to the medical meaning of the term *syndrome*—a thorough, stable, and verifiable picture. Simons and Hughes (1985) use a well-defined taxonomic principle to group the CBSs on the basis of phenomenological similarities and across diverse cultural settings. Another approach classifies the syndromes according to the most dominant symptom(s) and considers them as culturally modeled versions of traditional diagnostic categories (Levine and Gaw 1995). Some CBSs, however, escape this attempt and are defined in "attributional," etio-pathogenic (e.g., *dhat*, described in some Far Eastern cultures as being due to semen loss and attributed to a heterogeneous range of ailments), or powerful clinically expressive terms (e.g., *ataque de nervios*).

The somewhat arbitrary nature of these conceptualizations demands serious research. The technical difficulties related to the assignment of popular expressions of psychopathology to conventional categories are enormous and require careful methodological approaches. A possible compromise is postulated by Carr and Vitaliano (1985), who maintain that CBSs represent final common pathways of culturally sanctioned behaviors. These pathways, although molded by culture, are mediated by universal mechanisms of learning and cognition. Such alternative expressions of suffering are therefore cultural variants of responses not to universal forms of psychopathology but to universal stress factors. Idiosyncratic responses to stress must be understood as a function of a complex interaction of experiences that trigger specific physiologic reactions, personality functions, cognitive processes, and problem-solving skills. Responses to stress also reflect perceptual styles, self-concept parameters, and the individual's expectations of effectiveness and adaptability. These concepts, quite close to Jilek and

Jilek-Aall's (1985) model of "feelings of powerlessness caused by perceived threats to ethnic survival" generate hypotheses that call for potent multidisciplinary research.

From the medico-anthropological vantage point, Good and Delvecchio-Good (1982) propose the analysis of "semantic networks"—groups of experiences, words, and interpretations that, occurring together within a specific cultural context, end up producing uniquely labeled ailments. Indeed, the CBSs test the claims of ecumenical validity made by existing professional nosologies. Kirmayer (1989) suggests research on the gap between experience and expression, the voluntary or accidental labeling of deviant behavior and distress, and the interpretation of symptoms as symbols or as meaningless events. Regardless of current uncertainties about the viability of the CBS notion, new or revived old names and categories continue to pour into the literature in search of validation (Hatta 1996; Lin 1983; Paradis et al. 1995; Zheng et al. 1997).

Guarnaccia and Rogler (1999) have recently suggested a broad research program centered on four key topics related to each CBS: 1) defining characteristics of the phenomenon; 2) its position in the social and personal context of the sufferer; 3) its relationship with existing psychiatric disorders, and 4) the clinical sequence as related to the experiencing of traumatic events. The proposal entails a hybrid methodology that, although essential for the generation of a truly global psychopathological catalogue, should also be able to include categorizations at different levels: descriptive, comparative, and etio-pathogenic (neurobiological and psychosocial).

Special Populations

Most of the research areas discussed so far apply to the so-called special populations within the United States, which include, in addition to ethnic minorities, age-related (children, adolescents, and the elderly), gender-related, and sexual orientation subgroups. These populations possess singular characteristics in demographic, clinical, health-related, socioeconomic, and even political terms and receive varying levels of attention from government and legislative agencies, insurance companies, and health professionals. Not surprisingly, health services and outcomes researchers have focused with growing interest on these groups. Epidemiologic, methodological, clinical, and diagnostic matters are relevant research areas if for no other reason than that the existing literature is still considered small and rather tentative.

By 2030, 70 million people will be 65 or over in the United States, making up 20% of the American population. Poverty rates, however, may remain high for elderly persons, women, and minorities. Indeed, the health and economic status of the next generations of special populations is threatened by current realities such as the number of young black men in prison and the higher rates of acquired immunodeficiency syndrome and drug abuse in minority communities. The increase of physical and biological vulnerabilities among the elderly makes them more likely candidates for diagnoses of cognitive and affective disorders, as well as for central nervous system–related complications of medical disorders (Federal Interagency Forum 2000).

Fabrega et al. (1994) deplore the fact that the role of ethnicity in the psychiatric problems of older patients is virtually unexplored. In their own study, they found that the diagnosis of psychoses was significantly higher in African American than among European American elderly persons, thus weakening the claim that such an association stems from the confounding effects of social class. Similar trends were observed by Leo et al. (1997) regarding rates of consultations: significantly more consultations were made for Caucasian than for African American elderly persons, the latter being mostly referred for evaluation of psychosis, and significantly less for assessment of suicide potential. The issue of Alzheimer's disease prevalence among African Americans (with concomitant questions about higher predisposition and different metabolic processes for Alzheimer's disease medications) remains extremely pertinent. On the other hand, African Americans appear to have less of an alcohol problem than do white Americans but appear to engage in more illicit drug use (Howard University Symposium 2000).

Culturally sensitive assessment is extremely important for an accurate diagnosis among elderly minority persons. This is even more important in non-English-speaking, nonimpaired elderly persons, who are prime candidates for misdiagnosis, as demonstrated by Lopez and Taussig (1991) using the Wechsler Adult Intelligence Scale—Revised in a group of Spanish-speaking individuals.

Even more dramatic findings among members of aboriginal groups in the United States and Canada make the case for serious diagnostic and clinical research in these communities, where cultural discontinuity and oppression have been linked to high rates of depression, alcoholism, suicide, and violence (Kirmayer et al. 2000; Thompson 2000). Suicide is the second leading cause of death for 15- to 24-year-olds in these ethnic groups. The alcoholism mortality rates are nearly 1,000% greater than the national average, and an estimated 95% of American Indians and Alaskan natives are affected directly or indirectly by alcohol abuse (Walker et al. 1994). Comorbid diagnoses of personality disorders, depression, and PTSD are also more prevalent among American Indians (Eaton et al. 1991).

The mental health and adjustment of immigrant and refugee children offer an extraordinary source of diagnostic and service-related research from a cultural perspective. The story of children's migration has unique features in its context, stress experiences, and the impact of the human and social capital of migrants (Guarnaccia and Lopez 1998). Acculturative stress in these groups also has special characteristics related to language problems, perceived discrimination, perceived cultural incompatibilities, and intergenerational conflicts. The contexts of receptiveness by and concomitant support from the host culture appear to be particularly powerful (McKelvey and Webb 1996). Family and developmental issues in children are also relevant and different from those affecting adult migrants and refugees (Aronowitz 1984). The instruments used and the reliability of informants are critical research topics for this population. Guarnaccia and Lopez (1998) remark on the need for special attention by researchers to areas such as assessment of second-language acquisition and school performance processes, family contexts, academic motivation, multilingual and multicultural service programs, and adjustment facilitation policies.

Care Disparities

There is overwhelming systematic documentation showing that ethnic minorities experience disparities in the availability of mental health care services and in the access, provision, and use of those services (Alegría et al. 2000a; Pescosolido 1992; Rogler 1999b; Rogler et al. 1989, Satcher 1999; U.S. Department of Health and Human Services 2000). From a cultural perspective, areas such as expressed emotions, explanatory models of illness, cultural competence, and therapist-client matching provide abundant but still inconclusive findings (Leff and Vaughn 1985; S. Sue 1998). Disparities result from a complex set of factors and pertain to individual, interpersonal, and organizational sources (Kessler et al. 1999; Solís et al. 1993).

What is the diagnostic relevance of research on mental health care disparities? Once the significant sociocultural basis of this phenomenon is demonstrated, the answer has to do primarily with its sequence: care cannot be appropriately provided if a correct diagnosis is not made (Bird et al. 1988). Thus, first, disparities may be the result of misdiagnosis or nondiagnosis due to unfamiliarity with the culturally determined pathoplastic components of any clinical entity (Alarcón et al. 1999). Second, differences in measures employed to assess psychiatric disorders can generate response biases (Alegría et al. 2000a). Third, factors such as discrimination, racism, social position, and even expectations about services and treatment may cloud the diagnostic process and be the "omitted factor" in clinical assessment (Alegría et al. 2000b). Fourth, linguistic limitations on the patient's and the clinician's sides produce a formidable (and obvious) communication obstacle (Lopez 1988; Malgady et al. 1987). Fifth, diagnosis in psychiatry is meant to reflect individual coping styles on the one hand, and customary treatment options on the other; both factors are culturally charged, and both are also parcels of the disparities field.

Vega (2000) lists research topics in the disparities area that apply to all minority groups and that have cogent connections with psychiatric diagnosis. These topics include effective screening and referral of patients by primary care physicians; profiling of successful case managers; assessment of clinical and community factors in dual diagnoses; determinants of relapse; roles of the juvenile justice system; identification of effective treatment modalities; issues of substance abuse, trauma, and violence; health policies; quality of care and cultural competence; and performance differences on standardized instruments for clinical evaluation and research.

Along these lines, Vega (2000) advocates, for instance, comparative studies among U.S. Latino groups, and with other ethnic and nonethnic groups in the United States and populations in Latin America, to "gauge the shortfall of services utilization among those with diagnosed disorders" (p. 8). High levels of demand on support networks are more likely to generate higher levels of symptoms, and vice versa (Vega and Kolody 1985). The variance of cultural factors such as poor interpersonal relations and awareness of the medical model–based interpretation of diagnoses has been investigated by Guarnaccia et al. (1992). Steps of translational action research as outlined by Aguilar-Gaxiola et al. (2000) include delineation of philosophies and strategies; dialogues with community members and leaders, administrators, and providers; consensus building; actual data translation for the understanding of multiple stakeholders; and implementation and evaluation of best-practice models. In the realm of idioms of distress, it is good to remember that they often reflect the sufferer's little power and disrupted social relations, another cultural connection of psychiatric diagnosis (Littlewood 1990).

As for clinical competence research, factors that advance it—such as a true acceptance of a scientific/empirical mentality by the system, clinicians' awareness of their own assumptions about the patient's culture and cognition, and cultural proficiency in the care-providing system—await methodical studies (Cross et al. 1989; Rogler 1992). Cultural competence narrows the distance between patient and clinician, thereby creating a common cultural zone and reducing the likelihood of diagnostic errors, inappropriate treatment, and poor outcomes. Clearly, the study of disparities also places the researcher and the clinician much closer to the role of a true advocate, which many consider essential if the problem is ever going to be solved (S. Sue 1998).

Culture and Neurobiology

Contemporary cognitive neuroscience underscores the importance of a nonreductionistic analysis of the interactions between person and environment (Henningsen and Kirmayer 2000; Kendler 2001). Recent neurobiological advances recognize the significance of sociocultural contexts and of different levels of explanation in models of both normal and pathological behavior. Arriving at this understanding has not been a smooth process, however. The notion that bodies and brains are engaged in an interaction with the social world, interaction that ultimately guides thought and action (Hutchins 1995), still lacks a totally coherent theoretical framework. Mind has been redefined—far from the metaphorical and abstract perspective of psychodynamics—as a control system of cognitive processes involving the interplay between intrinsic mechanisms and productions of the body-brain system (from neuronal plasticity to neuroendocrine changes, for instance) and external structures in the environment—from social contexts to cultural meanings (A. Clark 1995; Henningsen and Kirmayer 2000; Hinton 1999; Hutchins 1995). A purely neuronal (functionalist or connectivist) account cannot analyze the interactions between organism and environment. Its subproduct, the "localization fallacy" or "intracranial phrenology" is a considerable oversimplification (George 1996).

On the other hand, a systems approach fails to conceptually include the subject's internal representations of prior interactions and makes no reference to the actual structure of the mechanism(s) whose behavior it is explaining. Even the notion of *convergence zones,* neural circuits onto which multiple feedforward and feedback loops concur, expands control functions into distribution, activation, retrieval, and coordination representations but still omits crucial interactions with the actual human agent and his or her internalized representations, which are a product of cultural influences. Symptoms of a mental disorder, therefore, only manifest themselves in a person who is interacting with others in one way or another, and explanations of these interactions have to be set at a level higher than the subpersonal, brain-centered accounts of cognitive functions and neural components.

One of the fundamental aspects of these explanations is the phase of the process of diagnosis that covers predisposition, onset, form, and course of the disorder. A multilevel, coherent description and explanation of behaviors encompasses neurobiological bases but also individual expectations, narrative style, social context, and other cultural factors (Kirmayer 1996). On the other hand, the meaning of behaviors and experiences being diagnosed is viewed as a sequential pattern codetermined by the patient's internal representations and by the significant others with whom he or she has interacted (Oyama 2000). The interactions that shape the structure and function of the brain are culturally meaningful actions. A cultural neurobiology thus would provide a rather dynamic, multilevel, multidimensional perspective to diagnostic endeavors, rather than accepting diagnostic dictates based on physiopathologic a prioris.

Complex diseases, including many medical problems (e.g., asthma, hypertension, diabetes, and malignancies) and most psychiatric conditions, are determined by the presence of, and interactions between, multiple genetic and environmental factors. Similarly, genetic variations of numerous biological traits are extremely common throughout the genome, and their distribution often varies substantially across ethnic groups, modulated by environmental (including cultural) inputs (Kandel 1998, 1999). Paralleling these examples, there is now substantial evidence supporting the heritability and varied distribution of different types of temperaments (Heath et al. 1999).

These considerations, and the unequivocal influence of culture in areas such as cognitive appraisals of distress or coping styles, make ethnicity and culture crucial variables in attempts to delineate the biological processes associated with psychiatric morbidities and their diagnosis, that is, the search of neurobiological markers. Unfortunately, the overwhelming majority of studies have not included subjects with multiethnic or multicultural backgrounds, and very few examine the potential effects of ethnicity (Lawson 1986), despite suggestive findings in areas such as abnormal sleep electroencephalographic patterns, or dysfunction of the hypothalamic-pituitary-adrenal (HPA) axis associated with depression (Cowen and Wood 1991; Mendlewicz and Kerkhofs 1991; Rush et al. 1982). Further research demands that ethnicity and culture vis-à-vis psychiatric diagnosis be examined at and across the genetic-molecular-cellular (genotype), neurobiological (endophenotype), clinical (phenotype), and epidemiologic levels.

Biocultural Linkages in Psychopathology

Depression and anxiety are, for a variety of reasons, the main areas of current research in biocultural connections (Alarcón 2000). Kendler et al. (1992) demonstrated in a long-term study of a large cohort of female twins that the genetic factors responsible for the vulnerability or predisposition to major depression and generalized anxiety disorder were essentially the same, which would help explain the high levels of comorbidity of the two disorders. On the other hand, the question of why some patients who have the same genetic load develop anxiety and others develop depression was answered with the hypothesis that environmental risk factors (i.e., well-defined stressors or sociocultural challenges) were different for each disorder. This clearly would move the focus of research from the genetic-molecular to the socioenvironmental level. Diagnosis would be more comprehensive with a clearer delineation of the impact of each component beyond the view that a lower level of description and explanation is the causally decisive factor (Henningsen and Kirmayer 2000).

Cultural factors may trigger, perpetuate, or prevent psychopathological phenomena (mostly depression or anxiety) through two main sets of mechanisms: individual, microsocial learning or modeling, and macrosocial (or societal) influences. The former, more operative in the family microcosm, includes coping styles, idioms of distress, explanatory models of illness, or the psychodynamic concept of repetition compulsion. Macrosocial influences comprise processes of social contagion, stressful events of the most diverse nature, adaptive and social survival mechanisms, and ethical standards transmitted throughout generations (Alarcón 2000; Eisenberg and Kleinman 1981; Wierzbick 1986). It is clear that all of these processes have both harmful and pathogenic, or beneficial and even therapeutic potential. As such, all deserve systematic research.

Some of the most productive and promising areas of inquiry in the study of biocultural links in psychopathology are as follows:

- The genetic-epidemiologic perspective (Kendler et al. 1992, 1997)
- The ethnophysiologic approach (which includes contributions from the fields of psycho-neuroendocrinology, neuroimaging, and neuropsychology) (Grigsby and Stevens 2000; Manson 1995)
- The cognitive-interpretive view (which includes topics ranging from hypnotic suggestibility to psychotherapy-induced changes in genetic expressiveness) (Kandel 1998, 1999; Paulesu et al. 2000; Wilson 1998)
- The psychopathology-creativity model, based on the findings of significantly high rates of psychiatric diagnoses in groups of artists, writers, and intellectuals (Alarcón 2000; Andreasen 1987; Schildkraut and Otero 1996)

Ethnic and Cultural Factors in Psychopharmacology

Ethnic variations in the response to different psychotropic medications have been clearly documented. The mechanisms responsible for these interindividual variations are of a pharmacokinetic, pharmacodynamic, and behavioral nature (Lin et al. 1993). Practically all the genes encoding drug-metabolizing enzymes and proteins involved in drug transport are highly polymorphic, and the frequency of most of the functional alleles varies widely across ethnic groups, often leading to substantial differences in their activity (Leathart et al. 1998; Weber 1997).

There is also evidence of ethnic variations in pharmacodynamics. Substantial ethnic differences in the therapeutic levels of lithium, clozapine, and antidepressants, and a differential prolactin response to haloperidol between Asians and Caucasians, have been reported (Hu et al. 1983; Lin and Smith 2000; Matsuda et al. 1996). Mechanisms that might be responsible for such variations have not been elucidated. Significant ethnic variations also exist in transporter-controlling genes, receptors, and other proteins (e.g., catechol-*O*-methyl-transferase) regarded as putative therapeutic targets of psychotropics.

Nonbiological processes—including therapeutic alliance, adherence, and the so-called placebo effect—may exert even more powerful influences on diagnosis and treatment outcome than the biological variables discussed above. However, these nonbiological processes remain largely elusive and have not been systematically investigated (Smith et al. 1993). Limited data indicate that difficulties in medication adherence are aggravated in cross-cultural clinical encounters (Kinzie et al. 1987; Sclar et al. 1999) and that the interpretation of both therapeutic and adverse effects is strongly influenced by culturally shaped beliefs and expectations (S. Lee et al. 1992). Even less is known about how sociocultural factors affect clinicians' prescription patterns.

The diagnostic implications of ethno-psychopharmacologic research are manifold. The study of a possible subjection of neurobiological markers to ethnic variations will enhance the clinician's ability to identify symptoms and syndromes with greater precision and to establish more reliable correlations. Understanding the connection between culture and biology (as demonstrated by pharmacokinetic and pharmacodynamic variations) will also improve the level of diagnostic sensitivity among mental health professionals. Ethno-psychopharmacologic research may also exert an influence in potential diagnostic revisions on the basis of clinical response, clinical course, and collateral effects.

Behavioral Traits and Emotional Processes

A number of authors opine that the current nosologic characterizations of clinical entities exhibit limits that may force a reformulation of research efforts, with a greater emphasis on normal behaviors or temperamental traits. This reformulation would have the added effect of making the evaluation of environmental (sociocultural) factors more reachable and more accurate. Studies in this new wave focus on both animal and human models of resilience, happiness, fear, shyness, altruism, or love (Alarcón 2000). On the topic of resilience, for instance, Schissel (1993) elegantly examines the ability of adult children of problem drinkers to resist the negative effects of their parents' pathology, and the disposition of schizophrenic patients to develop depression. Through the use of regression models, he shows that individuals have varying degrees of susceptibility to adversity and that these variations are based, to a large degree, on psychosocial concerns. The concept of resilience exists, of course, across many or all cultures and phenomenologically entails notions such as courage, energy, altruism, resourcefulness, intellectual mastery, compassion ("learned helpfulness"), and vision. It is conceivable that specific research initiatives could be formulated that are aimed at dissecting the sociocultural and biological elements of these attributes.

At the other side of the spectrum, the mostly (or purely) biological basis of heavily culturally charged behaviors such as social attachment is described as the result of hormonal variations in adult species of laboratory animals (Insel 1997). Obviously, the integrative approach advocated throughout this chapter would lead one to expect the active consideration of sociocultural (environmental) ingredients in this equation. A multidimensional interactive systemic strategy (aided by the tremendous technological progress of the past decades), rather than a unilinear approach, will make it possible to engage the findings of this type of research with those more traditionally focused on psychopathology per se. The discovery of the crucial moment and the key setting in which the cultural becomes biological and results in new normal, prepathological, or overtly pathological behaviors will add enormous consistency to the diagnostic and therapeutic tasks of mental health professionals.

Special Topics

Stigmatization and Racism

Stigmatization is an overwhelming cultural feature in the social scene in general, and in the health care field in particular. Beyond its historical origins or its symbolic implications, (reaffirmation of beliefs, however wrong or outdated, or invocation of distorted historical assumptions), stigmatization of individuals, groups, or specific conditions effectively stops any attempt at an objective assessment of such subjects. Stigmatization leads to isolation and to the continuous reinforcement of public neglect and social rigidity toward the stigmatized (Penn and Martin 1998; C.A. Pinderhughes 1979). Mental illness is one of the most stigmatized human conditions in contemporary life. Stigma creates a stereotyped approach to the examination of patients or, worse yet, contributes to prejudiced, uncritically accepted versions and explanation of behaviors. This conceptual dyad (stigma-stereotype) can result in overestimation or underestimation of a variety of conditions. In the case of minorities and immigrants, stigma carries the double jeopardy of being attached to both mental illness and ethnic prejudices. Research is needed to measure the impact of stigmatization and stereotyping on psychiatric diagnoses and, most importantly, to identify methodological and conceptual approaches to the minimization (or elimination) of their consequences (Neighbors et al. 1989). To assess their real variance in diagnostic practices would shed some light on their experiential impact on clinicians, other care providers, administrative and clerical personnel, patients, and their relatives (Weiss et al. 2001b). Public education enterprises could provide the foundation of these research initiatives.

Racism is the practice of racial discrimination, segregation, persecution, and domination based on a feeling of racial differences or antagonisms, particularly referred to supposed racial superiority, inferiority, or purity. It is related to the universal human phenomena of prejudice and stereotyping (C.A. Pinderhughes 1972, 1979). Racism most usually results from a multitude of biopsychosocial factors that interact with one another in complex ways. Clinical experience informs us that racism may be a manifestation of a delusional process, a consequence of anxiety, or a feature of an individual's personality dynamics (Adorno 1950; Allport 1958). However, racism may also be a learned behavior that has no relationship to individual psychopathology. The proponents of the model of racism as a social ill in which cultural patterns are institutionalized and internalized by socialization believe that the solution to racism lies in politics and social change, and not in the diagnostic and interpretive techniques of psychiatry (Fannon 1967; Thomas and Sillen 1972).

Racism, as the systematic exaltation of assumed intrapersonal differences based on physiognomic characteristics, establishes the basis of a declared or hidden dominance-submission system in which the oppressor monopolizes the perceptions of the victim (Carter 1994; Pierce 1988, 1992; Shanklin 1998). The latter, coming from different quarters (immigrants, refugees, indigenous people, native-born ethnic minorities, or "sojourners"), may respond in a variety of ways, which would then be deemed clinical or diagnosable by clinicians trained in and by the agencies of the dominant group—the so-called ethnocentric monoculturalism of Western medicine (Kovel 1970; D.W. Sue and Sue 1999). The implications of all these issues include consideration of racism as a symptom or as a diagnostic category.

If racism can be of a delusional nature or can have an anxiety-based etiology (an example would be a woman who was raped by a man of a different racial group, and who then develops hostile racial attitudes toward the rapist's group) or a personality disorder–based etiology, including it as a symptom in diagnostic criteria sets has some merit. Considering racism as a symptom emphasizes that its underlying etiology could be multifactorial.

However, unlike violence, DSM-IV-TR does not specially highlight racism as a symptom. It could be argued that this inattention has encouraged professional disregard for this extremely destructive behavior. One solution would be to encourage research that seeks to delineate the validity and reliability of racism as a symptom and to investigate the possibility of including it in some diagnostic criteria sets in future editions of DSM.

Probably the most common form of racism originates in the psychodynamics of narcissism (Bell 1978; Kohut 1972). In this context, it could be considered a variation of narcissistic personality disorder, which may or may not reach clinical significance in terms of functional impairment for the racist individual—especially in a cultural milieu that supports such beliefs. Bell (1980) outlines the possibility that there may be two types of socially misinformed racists: those with an underlying narcissistic personality disorder in which the racist attitudes and behavior are incorporated into the narcissistic pathology, and those who are simply socially misinformed at an early age, and who with adequate education may relinquish their ignorant beliefs.

Furthermore, there is often a relational component to racism that may warrant clinical attention. Individuals may be involved in an interracial relational disorder by virtue of their work environment. For example, a racist factory supervisor of an African American employee who is "pro-black" but not anti-white will sooner or later find himself embroiled in a conflictual relationship that will cause considerable distress as the supervisee challenges the supervisor's experience or may request administrative or legal actions against his perceived racism. Because overt discrimination is illegal, racism has become more covert and is frequently characterized by "microinsults" and "microaggressions," which victimize an individual in proportion to the space, time, energy, and mobility that is yielded to the oppressor (Pierce 1988). An example of a microinsult is an African American patient going to a dermatologist's office and being asked by the receptionist for a Medicaid card despite being the chief executive officer of a multi-million-dollar comprehensive mental health center, simply because the patient is black. The more one regains or commands control of these elements, the less one is victimized.

Brantly (1983) addresses the psychological effects of antiblack racism on black patients. However, because the nature of racism has changed, many African American men are confused about the subject, which then accounts for the possibility of an interracial relational disorder. For example, sometimes it can be difficult for African Americans to distinguish between the supportive efforts of individual whites and the destructive action of whites as a group (Bell 1996; Trierweiler et al. 2000). Defining racism as a relational disorder, however, may have significant disadvantages—for example, it carries the risk of blaming the victim or excusing the perpetrator. A thoughtful research agenda could elucidate these risks and could determine ways to balance the risks with the utility of such categories.

A research agenda on racism as a clinical condition could include validity, reliability, and prevalence studies of this potential symptom as well as the empirical usefulness of listing it as part of the presentation of other psychiatric disorders (Jackson et al. 1996; Neighbors 1997). Operating on the basis that a prejudice dynamic exists (Sullaway and Dunbar 1996), it may be worthwhile to identify a subset of narcissistic personality disorder that is essentially manifested by racist behavior. Finally, the conceptualization of racism as a relational disorder and the exploration of important ethical and legal issues raised by the various definitions of racism deserve intensive research.

Gender Issues

Although the term *sex* designates chromosomal or biological phenomena linked to having one or two X chromosomes, *gender* is used to refer to the psychosocial expression of living as a man or a woman. *Gender* is a proxy term for a complex of biological, behavioral, and psychological processes. Public health specialists and advocates for women's health have lobbied for the inclusion of women in clinical trials and all aspects of mental health research. The National Institutes of Health (NIH) issued guidelines in 1990 that required the inclusion of women and minorities in all NIH-sponsored clinical research. In 1994, analysis of clinical trial outcomes by sex of the subjects was added to the requirements. However, a recent study revealed that about one-fifth of the NIH-sponsored studies in medicine published through 1998 did not include women, and only a small percentage of these provided any sex-specific analyses (Vidaver et al. 2000). No improvements were noted across the years 1993 through 1998.

Recent research has revealed the intuitively obvious but previously neglected fact that women are not merely "small men" from a physiologic perspective. For example, medication dosages are developed primarily for men and are applied to the treatment of women. Recent advances in drug metabolism have demonstrated important differences in hepatic cytochrome P450 function between males and females (Pollock 1997) that are directly relevant to treatment. Estrogen may hold promise for treatment of mood disorders with postpartum onset (Ahokas et al. 2000; Epperson et al. 1999). Differences in the expression of disease between the two sexes hold great promise for knowledge growth in psychiatry. Every aspect of disease phenomenology in a population (for example, vulnerability to disorder, symptomatology, natural history, treatment responsivity, and functional capacity) is affected by gender. Differences between groups provide clues to hypothesis development for therapeutic and preventive interventions (Fullerton et al. 2001).

In psychiatric epidemiologic research, gender is the single strongest correlate of risk for many types of mental disorders. Women are two to three times more likely to have depressive and anxiety disorders and are eight to 10 times more likely to have eating disorders. Males are more likely to suffer from developmental disorders such as autism and attention-deficit/hyperactivity disorder and from substance use and conduct disorders. Why are these disorders partitioned in the population by gender? Similarly, cultural and economic factors exert effects on gender role performance. Do women from other cultures experience similar rates of eating disorders? Do cultural rituals around femininity play a role? Gender is a variable that is always present no matter how pure the cultural definition; it also allows cultural partitioning for hypothesis generation.

The approach of DSM-IV, which was to include a category of specific culture, age, and gender features, captured the extant information and ensured that attention was given to these issues for each diagnosis. Yet, current DSM-IV-TR categories of prevalence, course, familial patterns, comorbidity, laboratory findings, and differential diagnosis do not include any discussion of gender, although the effects are frequently profound. Researchers must continue to expand knowledge of psychiatric illness with respect to these variables.

The Institute of Medicine (1988) published a report that, in addition to emphasizing a broad genetic-environmental interaction model, urged the use of a powerful analytical tool—the gender-focused analysis—that promotes hypothesis development by establishing comparative risk for disease in women and men. For example, entry of women into the workforce has created a cadre of stay-at-home fathers, whose behavior is different from that of their fathers. Changing societal norms may have long-term health consequences. It is known that mothers of young children have increased risk for developing mood disorders in the first 2 years after giving birth (Kendell et al. 1987). Will fathers of young children who perform the primary caregiving role develop similar risk for mood disorder?

To serve the goal of informing DSM-V, every investigator must consider a framework for inclusion of gender and culture variables into research plans. It is likely that large sample sizes will be needed to achieve this goal, which is consistent with the NIH goal of promoting larger-scale studies of major public health significance (Lebowitz and Rudorfer 1998). At the initial stages of research planning, investigators must ask how knowledge about the study question can be maximized by considering gender and culture variables in the population to be included. Advancement of knowledge in the field will consist of investigating populations along several domains of study types (Alarcón et al. 1999) related to the research hypotheses. The five domains are interpretive/explanatory, pathogenic/pathoplastic, diagnostic/nosologic, therapeutic/protective, and management/services (Figure 6–4).

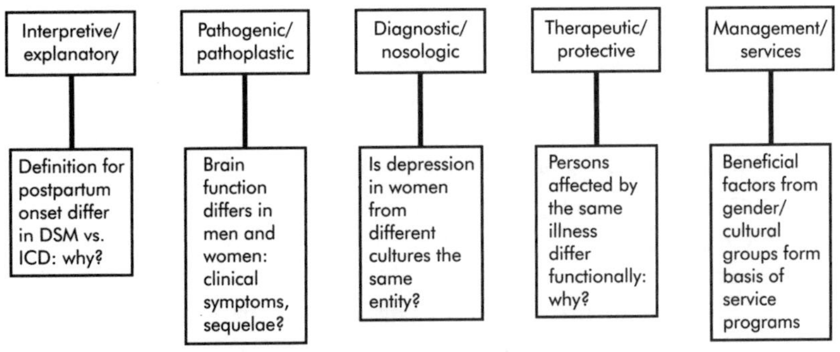

FIGURE 6–4. Domains of research on gender and culture: critical variables to dissect factors that contribute to disease risk or protection.

Interpretive/explanatory approaches allow clinicians to understand behaviors along the continuum of human experience. An example is that the course specifier "with postpartum onset" in DSM-IV-TR is defined only for four specific mood disorders, which must begin within 4 weeks of birth; however, the time criterion is 6 weeks in ICD-10, and diagnoses are not restricted. Understanding the observations that lead to varying classification definitions allows elaboration and challenge of core concepts. How did experts in different parts of the world come to develop nonidentical definitions? Did they draw different conclusions from the same phenomenological data, or did their observations of the episodes differ?

The pathogenic/pathoplastic domain focuses on mechanisms by which gender and culture are modulators of clinical symptoms. Neuroscientists evaluate brain differences in men compared with women with the same illnesses for clues to variability in disease expression. Researchers studying personality disorders, temperament disorders, or relational disorders might evaluate mental health outcomes in women who were abused as children in comparison with similarly abused men. Of the persons who do not exhibit serious psychopathology, what were (or are) the factors that decreased risk in these persons? Job stress, physiologic response to perceived stress, level of demands from and control over work life, quality of social support, income, child care responsibilities, and likelihood of sexual victimization are different between men and women.

The diagnostic/nosologic conceptual domain is more specifically used to explore the relationship between culture and psychiatric diagnosis, such as the many examples and lines of research described in this chapter—for example, whether instruments designed to assess depression in one population measure the same construct in a different culture (or in men compared with women in either group).

In the therapeutic/protective focus, cultural aspects related to resiliency that hold promise for therapeutic interventions are highlighted: that is, considering gender and culture variables that correlate with functional capacity in various types of psychopathology. For example, an exploration of the reasons that female patients with schizophrenia generally have more favorable interpersonal functioning (compared with male patients) could be considered.

Under management/services considerations, beneficial cultural factors or services in various communities might be identified (e.g., studying help-seeking patterns or investigating the relationship between structured after-school activities and rates of school and community violence, and whether such programs differentially affect females compared with males in the community) (Neighbors and Howard 1987).

Capturing variables that differentiate or partition populations related to disease expression is precisely the process that constitutes the rich opportunity for generating hypotheses, testing them, and gaining new knowledge in psychiatry. Research along these lines would lead to inquiries about the impact of cultural expectations and roles, age, and therapeutic and prognostic factors. Not to be forgotten is the viability of categorical and dimensional diagnostic approaches among women. As culture allows population partitioning for hypothesis generation, gender allows, in turn, a cultural partitioning for the generation of desirably converging hypotheses.

Violence and Trauma

The close relationship between stigmatization, racism, and socially prominent clinical areas such as violence (of political, domestic, or criminal nature) or trauma (chronic or acute, sustained or intermittent, subtle or blatant) also has diagnostic significance and noticeable cultural implications. From everyday statistics to well-conceived epidemiologic surveys, violence is a complex social, public health, and clinical reality in the United States (Gartner 1993; Protherow-Stith 1991). It is also a phenomenon that, except for a few features, does not seem to recognize ethnic boundaries. By the same token, the boundaries between nonclinical (i.e., criminal) and clinical (related to a mental disorder) violence are blurred at the center of a bell-shaped epidemiologic curve. In the case of children, adolescents, and other special populations acting as protagonists or witnesses, data are scarce and conflicting (Ember and Ember 1993).

Acculturation and Acculturative Processes

Acculturation, the process by which immigrants adapt (or try to adapt) to the rules and sociobehavioral characteristics of the host society, has unique, intense, and pervasive features, and its impact and outcome may reach, when unfavorable, true clinical dimensions. DSM-IV-TR includes "acculturation problem" as one of 13 conditions that may be a focus of clinical attention. When neglected or misunderstood by clinicians, acculturation may also generate bias in the assessment of certain personality measures; that is, it may make some features appear worse in the clinical narrative after a cursory workup (Montgomery and Orozco 1985; Williams and Berry 1991).

An ill-fated process of acculturation results in what is known as acculturative stress (Hovey and King 1996; Smart and Smart 1995), defined as a particular set of emotions and behaviors, including depression and anxiety, feelings of marginality and alienation, heightened psychosomatic symptoms, and identity confusion. Caught between the influence of traditional values and norms and their experiences in mainstream society, victims of this condition may be further weakened by low levels of family functioning and support. Acculturative stress stems from language barriers, "cultural shock" in facing a different social philosophy, changing socioeconomic status, and intergenerational conflict (Cortes and Rogler 1996). It occurs when environmental or internal demands tax the migrant's ability to cope and adapt. It obviously affects decision-making abilities, impairs occupational functioning, and contributes to role entrapment and status leveling, both of which limit the individual's future. It thrives on the lack of role models; puts pressure on inherently vulnerable social support systems; limits interpersonal transactions, including access to services; and magnifies other risk factors such as age, gender, educational status, nutritional patterns, or physical health.

Acculturation is therefore another of a long list of culturally based risk factors for stigmatization and alienation (Redfield et al. 1936). For acculturative stress to be considered a diagnostic construct would require both a precise phenomenological description and an assessment of its etiopathogenic impact. Future research should explore its connections with depression and suicidality; in turn, all these situations should be studied in relationship to different age and ethnic groups as well as other acculturating groups such as native peoples, refugees, and sojourners (Ahern and Athey 1991; Westermeyer 1989). Other factors—such as coping skills, self-esteem, adherence to traditional values and ethnic identification, prior knowledge of language and culture of the host society, motives for the move, and congruity between contact expectations and actual experiences—must be addressed by a functional analysis of behavior and by longitudinally designed studies examining the question of directionality. Finally, the steps and outcomes of the acculturative process require very well-defined instrumentation to cover important variables such as language, status evolution, discrimination, and social support (Guarnaccia 2000).

Religion and Spirituality Issues

Religion and spirituality are gaining legitimate importance as cultural variables operating in all the steps of the diagnostic and treatment processes. They have to do with the interpretive and explanatory function of culture in clinical psychiatry (Alarcón et al. 1999), but also with a possible influence on pathogenic and pathoplastic expressions of the clinical picture. Religion is to be examined in the history-taking and cultural formulation processes, and spirituality becomes a paramount component of self-identity, self-care, insight, self-reliance, and resiliency in the treatment arena (Lukoff et al. 1995; Murphy and Donovan 1988).

Research can also focus on the similarities and differences of religious and spiritual issues across ethnic and cultural groups. This can help in diagnostic characterizations as the clinician measures and compares information sources, age and gender differences, strength of beliefs and principles, and their relevance in the treatment and outcome of any condition. The transgenerational process of acquisition or transmission of religious and spiritual norms is an apt research item. Description of rules and rituals and their impact on diagnosis is also an appealing topic (Levin 1996).

Scope and Limits of Research on Culture and Diagnosis

The historical journey of culture and psychopathology has been stormy but also fascinating. From the first comparative observations made by European academicians at the end of the nineteenth century reporting (with an inevitable paternalistic flavor) on their visits to exotic lands, to the modern, solidly multidimensional perspective of cultural psychiatry, the relationship between humans and their environment, both in health and in illness, has lent itself to increasingly sophisticated research work. A spectrum of cultural variables ceased to be a peculiar anthropological collection and became rather a tangible set of powerful factors shaping the behavior of patients and clinicians in the context of a unique encounter. Psychiatric diagnosis has been and will continue to be enriched by an increasing cultural sensitivity, the demarcation of clinically significant or insignificant impairments, the impact of values, and the validation or refutation of boundaries. Diagnosis will result from the formulation of hypotheses and from the assessment of symptoms and their configuration into disorders reflecting the cumulative character of culture and cultural factors.

Mental illness is more than the insidious or acute disappearance of a previously healthy state, or the dramatic derailment of neurobiological structures or functions. It is a substantial distortion of lives and expectations as a result of multisystemic failures in molecular structures, organismic pathways, psychosocial settings, cultural precepts, and long-term projects of any given individual. This dynamic chain of events demands a thoroughly comprehensive evaluation, based on epistemological skills, multidisciplinary knowledge, and methodological sophistication of the highest order. It is clear that an accurate psychiatric diagnosis, with all the progress made so far, requires still an extraordinary series of research initiatives, particularly from the sociocultural domain.

Yet the whole cultural enterprise may be subverted by the effort to fit cultural issues within the straitjacket of a nosologic system. The nosologic perspective of DSM is disease centered, essentializing, individual-based, and driven by biomedical technologies and interests, especially the efficacy and availability of pharmacologic treatments. In contrast, a cultural perspective tends to be person centered, focused on context, oriented to social networks or communities, and concerned with psychosocial interventions in a pluralistic health care system.

Understanding the processes that lead to mental illness is only a first step. Individuals possess multiple cultural "templates" and may draw on them in different ways and in different situations (Anderson 1998). This requires, on the diagnostician's side, precise theoretical definitions, development of state-of-the-art research methods in both biological and social sciences, appropriate measurements (longitudinal, multilevel, experimental, comparative) in a broad set of social and cultural settings (beyond national boundaries), and safeguarding ethical standards dear to communities and the society at large (Susser and Susser 1996).

An Attempt at Prioritization

Investigations leading to a more comprehensive diagnosis lie initially in the *epidemiologic* realm. A cultural approach to instruments, actual surveys, and analysis of results will assist the clinician in achieving much clearer terminology, context, meaning, and explanation of the observed behaviors. This cultural epidemiology also examines risk and protective factors, quality-of-life issues, and microculture of families and social networks. The study of bias or errors in clinical judgment, of environmental stimuli, and social desirability complement this approach (Rogler 1996; Weiss 1997).

The field of *outcomes research* offers further support to a culturally strong psychiatric diagnostic system. A systematic examination of the cultural formulation, the glossary of cultural terms, and the cultural considerations included in the category subheadings of DSM-IV-TR would provide the clinician with crucially important information. Most or all existing clinical entities require research of their cultural components, from the study of factors contributing to or associated with their emergence, to the evaluation of the patient's intricate help-seeking efforts. These areas of investigation would also encompass family and other support systems, the impact of acculturation, and a more cogent and objective study of the intriguing culture-bound syndromes and idioms of distress. The many cultural nuances of the psychotherapeutic process and the variants related to the cultural makeup of special populations add strength to this objective.

Racism and stigmatization are topics that transcend the customary grounds of epidemiologic or outcomes research. The study of these conditions at the individual, structural, and institutional levels will increase the credibility of the diagnostic and nosologic effort. The same applies to the vast implications of *gender and psychopathology;* to social and cultural realities such as violence and trauma; and to sensitive yet culturally prominent variables such as sexual orientation, religion, and spirituality. In this area, for instance, Gartner (1993) advocates the exploration of mechanisms mediating macrosocial factors and punctual, individual outcomes. Similarly, cultural research on the large topic of *disparities* in mental health care and its many components (availability, accessibility, quality, and accountability) from patient to care agency and vice versa will have a significant effect on diagnosis. This process of cultural critique not only of psychiatry but also of the research process has been considered a conceptual antidote for such disparities.

The diagnostic assessment would not be complete, however, without an estimate of the broad common ground between *culture and neurobiology.* The old nature versus nurture debate, translated contemporaneously into the genetic-environmental interaction, requires research aimed not only at a definition of the magnitude of each parcel in the life of the mind, the brain, the chromosome, or the community, but mostly at the points of contact operating in each behavioral act or in the chain of events that result in the actions (behaviors) to be observed, diagnosed, cataloged, and treated. It is necessary to biologize culture by thinking through the ways in which culture is an aspect of the biological organization of human beings. By the same token, it is also necessary to culturalize biology by examining how biological models and metaphors are shaped by cultural values and assumptions. Ethnophysiology and ethnopsychopharmacology each have a role in the diagnostic task as confirming or modifying factors; within the next several decades the biocultural study of behavioral traits, specific emotions, and cognitive processes will add information that may very well change the whole nature and conduct of the diagnostic task in psychiatry. Another critical step in this whole process is the articulation of an efficient translation and dissemination system that would generate the development and testing of practical new strategies in diagnosis, service delivery, and treatment (U.S. Department of Health and Human Services 1999). How research on mental health diagnosis is understood by professionals and the public and is implemented by agencies and administrators are areas that should themselves be the subject of investigative efforts.

Conclusion

A diagnosis-oriented cultural psychopathology research agenda integrates ethnographic, observational, clinical, and epidemiologic approaches, each one providing useful information to crystallize into a comprehensive description of a clinical condition with different levels of impact. On the other hand, a systemic approach surpasses, despite some limitations, the mind-body dichotomy while accepting biological, psychological, social, religious, and spiritual components of the human experience. A crucial aspect of all these approaches consists of not ignoring the internal diversity of most communities in terms of ethnic and religious groups, rural versus urban settings, social class, and others—all sources of considerable variability in the clinical and epidemiologic data. In short, a culturally informed diagnosis uses multiple lenses as the researcher moves between lay and professional systems of meaning to make sense out of behavioral observations.

Teaching and training present and future professionals on the need to include cultural factors in the diagnostic process is a logical step in any attempt to develop comprehensive research programs in psychology, psychiatry, and related disciplines. Reasons for the slow development of these fields are not only methodological, curricular, or doctrinary. Reid (1994) goes so far as to say that the reasons are attitudinal, and Y.T. Lee (1994) asserts that the terms *culture* and *social group* appear to be "alien and strange to many researchers in the United States." Educational leaders must address current weaknesses in residency programs, graduate schools, and similar settings while attracting young scientists into research careers. Pellmar and Eisenberg (2000) recently examined the obstacles to interdisciplinary research and training, including attitudinal and communication barriers, the structures and promotion policies of academic institutions, and obstacles from funding organizations and peer review processes. Obviously, infrastructure needs for these efforts (different from those of a neurobiological nature) must be addressed. In sum, training of underrepresented minorities and the development of capabilities that integrate social and cultural dimensions in mental health and psychiatric diagnosis would be a crowning effort for a research agenda such as the one outlined in these pages.

References

Abroms GM: Psychiatric serialism. Compr Psychiatry 22:372–378, 1981

Adorno T: The Authoritarian Personality. New York, Harper, 1950

Aguilar-Gaxiola S: World mental health 2000 in the Americas: an initiative of the World Health Organization. Keynote lecture presented at the Congress of the World Federation for Mental Health, Santiago, Chile, September 9–11, 1999

Aguilar-Gaxiola S, Zelezny L, García B, et al: Linking mental health research to practice and policy to reduce mental health disparities in Hispanics. Paper presented at the National Institute of Mental Health Meeting on Disparities in Health Care for Latinos, Los Angeles, CA, May 21–23, 2000

Ahern FL, Athey JL (eds): Refugee Children: Theory, Research and Services. Baltimore, MD, Johns Hopkins University Press, 1991

Ahokas A, Aito M, Rimon R: Positive treatment effect of estradiol in postpartum psychosis: a pilot study. J Clin Psychiatry 61:166–169, 2000

Alarcón RD: A Latin American perspective on DSM-III. Am J Psychiatry 140:102–105, 1983

Alarcón RD: Identidad de la psiquiatría latinoamericana: voces y exploraciones en torno a una ciencia solidaria. México DF, Editorial Siglo XXI, 1990

Alarcón RD: Culture and psychiatric diagnosis. Impact on DSM-IV and ICD-10. Psychiatr Clin North Am 18:449–465, 1995

Alarcón RD: Conexiones biológico—culturales en psicopatología, in Psicopatologia Clínica: El Síntoma en las Neurociencias. Edited by Tellez-Vargas J, Taborda LC, Taborda CB. Bogotá, Fundación Cultural Javeriana, 2000, pp 487–509

Alarcón RD, Foulks EF: Personality disorders and culture: contemporary clinical views (part B). Cult Divers Ment Health 1:79–91, 1995

Alarcón RD, Ruiz P: Theory and practice of cultural psychiatry in the United States and abroad, in Review of Psychiatry, Vol 14. Edited by Oldham JM, Riba MB. Washington, DC, American Psychiatric Press, 1995, pp 599–626

Alarcón RD, Foulks EF, Vakkur M: Personality Disorders and Culture. Clinical and Conceptual Interactions. New York, Wiley, 1998

Alarcón RD, Westermeyer J, Foulks EF, et al: Clinical relevance of contemporary cultural psychiatry. J Nerv Ment Dis 187:465–471, 1999

Alegría M, Canino G, Rios R, et al: Inequalities in rates of specialty mental health use among Latinos, African Americans and Non-Latino Whites in the U.S. Paper presented at the National Institute of Mental Health Meeting on Disparities in Health Care for Latinos, Los Angeles, CA, May 21–23, 2000a

Alegría M, Kessler R, Bijl R: Comparing data on mental health service use between countries, in Unmet Need for Treatment. Edited by Andrews G, Henderson S. Cambridge, Cambridge University Press, 2000b, pp 97–118

Allport GW: The Nature of Prejudice. New York, Doubleday, 1958

Almeida R: Expansions of Feminist Theory Through Diversity. New York, Harworth Press, 1994

American Psychiatric Association: Diagnostic and Statistical Manual of Mental Disorders, 4th Edition. Washington, DC, American Psychiatric Association, 1994

American Psychiatric Association: Diagnostic and Statistical Manual of Mental Disorders, 4th Edition, Text Revision. Washington, DC, American Psychiatric Association, 2000

Anderson NB: Levels of analysis in health science: a framework for integrating sociobehavioral and biomedical research. Ann N Y Acad Sci 840:563–576, 1998

Andreasen NC: Creativity and mental illness: prevalence rates in writers and their first degree relatives. Am J Psychiatry 144:1288–1292, 1987

Aronowitz M: The social and emotional adjustment of immigrant children: a review of the literature. International Migration Review 18:237–257, 1984

Bell CC: Racism, narcissism, and integrity. J Natl Med Assoc 70:89–92, 1978

Bell CC: Racism: a symptom of the narcissistic personality disorder. J Natl Med Assoc 7:661–665, 1980

Bell CC: Treatment issues for African-American men. Psychiatric Annals 26:33–36, 1996

Benjamin LS: Psychosocial factors in the development of personality disorders, in Personality and Psychopathology. Edited by Cloninger CR. Washington, DC, American Psychiatric Press, 1999, pp 309–342

Berganza CE, Mezzich JE, Otero AA, et al: The Latin American Guide for psychiatric diagnosis: a cultural overview. Psychiatr Clin North Am 24:433–448, 2001

Bibeau G: Cultural psychiatry in a creolizing world: questions for a new research agenda. Transcultural Psychiatry 34:9–41, 1997

Bird HR, Canino G, Rubio-Stipec M: Essentials of the prevalence of childhood maladjustment in a community survey in Puerto Rico: the use of combined measures. Arch Gen Psychiatry 45:1120–1126, 1988

Blue HC, Griffith EEH: Sociocultural and therapeutic perspectives on violence. Psychiatr Clin North Am 18:571–587, 1995

Boehnlein JK, Alarcón RD: Aspectos culturales del trastorno de estrés post-traumático. Monografias de Psiquiatria 12:18–26, 2000

Boehnlein JK, Kinzie JD: DSM diagnosis of posttraumatic stress disorder and cultural sensitivity: a response. J Nerv Ment Dis 180:597–599, 1992

Brantly T: Racism and its impact on psychotherapy. Am J Psychiatry 140:1605–1608, 1983

Brislin R: Back-translation for cross-cultural research. J Cross Cult Psychol 1:185–216, 1970

Brody EB: Biomedical science and the changing culture of social practice. J Nerv Ment Dis 178:279–281, 1990

Brown DA, Eaton WV, Sussman L: Racial differences in prevalence of phobic disorders. J Nerv Ment Dis 178:434–441, 1990

Cabaj R, Stein T (eds): Textbook of Homosexuality and Mental Health. Washington, DC, American Psychiatric Press, 1996

Canino G, Lewis-Fernandez R, Bravo M: Methodological challenges in cross-cultural mental health research. Transcultural Psychiatry 34:163–184, 1997

Carr JE, Vitaliano PP: The theoretical implications on converging research on depression and the culture-bound syndromes, in Culture and Depression: Studies in the Anthropology and Cross-Cultural Psychiatry of Affect and Disorder. Edited by Kleinman A, Good B. Berkeley, CA, University of California Press, 1985, pp 244–266

Carter JH: Racism's impact on mental health. J Natl Med Assoc 86:543–547, 1994

Clark A: Being There: Putting Brain, Body and World Together Again. Cambridge, MA, MIT Press, 1995

Clark DM: Cognitive therapy for panic disorders, in National Institutes of Health Consensus Development Conference on Treatment of Panic Disorder. Bethesda, MD, National Institutes of Health, 1991, pp 20–24

Comas-Díaz L, Jacobsen FM: Ethnocultural transference and countertransference in the therapeutic dyad. Am J Orthopsychiatry 61:392–402, 1991

Compton WM, Helzer JE, Hwu HG, et al: New methods in cross-cultural psychiatry: psychiatric illness in Taiwan and the United States. Am J Psychiatry 148:1697–1704, 1991

Cortes DE, Rogler LH: Health status and acculturation among Puerto Ricans in New York City. Journal of Gender Culture and Health 1:267–276, 1996

Cowen PJ, Wood AJ: Biological markers of depression. Psychol Med 21:831–836, 1991

Cross TL, Bazron BJ, Dennis KW: Towards a Culturally Competent System of Care. Washington, DC, Technical Assistance Center at Georgetown University Child Development Center, 1989

de la Monte SM, Hutchins GM, Moore GW: Racial differences in the etiology of dementia and frequency of Alzheimer's lesions in the brain. J Natl Med Assoc 81:644–652, 1989

Desjarlais R, Eisenberg L, Good B, et al: World Mental Health. Problems and Priorities in Low-Income Countries. New York, Oxford University Press, 1995

Draguns JG: Culture and psychopathology: toward specifying the nature of the relationship, in Nebraska Symposium on Motivation 1989: Cross-Cultural Perspectives. Edited by Breman J. Lincoln, NE, University of Nebraska Press, 1990, pp 235–277

Duff RS, Hollingshead AB: Sickness and Society. New York, Harper & Row, 1968

Eaton WW, Dryman A, Weissman MM: Panic and phobia, in Psychiatric Disorders in America. Edited by Robins LN, Regier DA. New York, Free Press, 1991, pp 155–168

Eccles J: Expectancies, values, and academic behaviors, in Achievement and Achievement Motives: Psychological and Sociological Approaches. Edited by Spence JT. San Francisco, CA, Freeman, 1983, pp 75–146

Egeland J: Cultural factors and social stigma for manic-depression: the Amish Study. Am J Soc Psychiatry 4:279–286, 1986

Eisenberg L, Kleinman A: The Relevance of Social Science for Medicine. Rotterdam, Dordretch, 1981

Eisenbruch M: Toward a culturally sensitive DSM: cultural bereavement in Cambodian refugees and the traditional healer as taxonomist. J Nerv Ment Dis 180:8–10, 1992

Ember CR, Ember M: Issues in cross-cultural studies of interpersonal violence. Violence Vict 8:217–233, 1993

Epperson CN, Wisner KL, Yamamoto B: Gonadal steroid in the treatment of mood disorders. Psychosom Med 61:676–687, 1999

Escobar JI, Gomez I, Tuason VB: Depressive phenomenology in North and South American patients. Am J Psychiatry 140:47–51, 1983

Fabrega H: Culture and history in psychiatric diagnosis and practice. Psychiatr Clin North Am 24:391–405, 2001

Fabrega H, Ahn CW, Boster J, et al: DSM-III as a systemic culture pattern. Studying intracultural variation among psychiatrists. J Psychiatr Res 24:139–154, 1990

Fabrega H, Ulrich R, Pilkonis P, et al: On the homogeneity of personality disorder clusters. Compr Psychiatry 32:373–386, 1991

Fabrega H, Mulsant BM, Rifal H, et al: Ethnicity and psychopathology in an aging hospital-based population. J Nerv Ment Dis 182:136–144, 1994

Fannon F: The Wretched of the Earth. New York, Grove Press, 1967

Favazza AR, Oman M: Overview: foundations of cultural psychiatry, in Culture and Psychopathology. Edited by Mezzich JE, Berganza CE. New York, Columbia University Press, 1984, pp 17–31

Federal Interagency Forum on Aging-Related Statistics: Report on Older Americans 2000: Key Indicators of Wellbeing. Washington, DC, U.S. Government Printing Office, 2000

Flaherty JA, Gaviria FM, Pathak D, et al: Developing instruments for cross-cultural psychiatry research. J Nerv Ment Dis 176:257–263, 1988

Fullerton CS, Ursano RJ, Epstein RS, et al: Gender differences in posttraumatic stress disorder after motor vehicle accidents. Am J Psychiatry 158:1486–1491, 2001

Gartner R: Methodological issues in cross-cultural large-survey research on violence. Violence Vict 8:199–215, 1993

Geertz C: The Interpretation of Cultures. New York, Basic Books, 1973

George MS: Functional MRI of mood and emotion. Paper presented at the First Heidelberg Conference on Dynamic and Functional Radiological Imaging of the Brain, Heidelberg, Oct 31–Nov 2, 1996

Golding JM, Burnam MA, Benjamin B, et al: Risk factors for secondary depression among Mexican Americans and non-Hispanic whites. J Nerv Ment Dis 181:166–175, 1992

Good BJ, Delvecchio-Good MJ: Toward a meaning-centered analysis of popular illness categories: "fright illness" and "heart illness" in Iran, in Cultural Conceptions of Mental Health and Therapy. Edited by Marsella AJ, Wente GM. Dordrecht, Netherlands, Reidel, 1982, pp 41–166

Gordon RA: Anorexia and Bulimia: Anatomy of a Social Epidemic. Cambridge, MA, Blackwell, 1990

Gothe CJ, Molin C, Nilsson CG: The environmental somatization syndrome. Psychosomatics 36:1–11, 1995

Greenfield PM, Cocking RR (eds): Crosscultural Roots of Minority Child Development. Hillsdale, NJ, Erlbaum, 1996

Grier W, Cobbs P: Black Rage. New York, Basic Books, 1968

Grigsby J, Stevens D: Neurodynamics of Personality. New York, Guilford, 2000

Group for the Advancement of Psychiatry, Committee on Cultural Psychiatry: Cultural Assessment in Clinical Psychiatry. Washington, DC, American Psychiatric Publishing, 2001

Group for the Advancement of Psychiatry, Committee on the Family: The challenge of relational diagnoses: applying the biopsychosocial model in DSM-IV. Am J Psychiatry 146:1492–1494, 1989

Guarnaccia P: Memorandum for the Study of Acculturation II. Presented to the Hispanic Mental Health Care Disparities Meeting, Los Angeles, May 19, 2000

Guarnaccia PJ, Lopez SR: The mental health and adjustment of immigrant and refugee children. Child Adolesc Psychiatr Clin N Am 7:537–553, 1998

Guarnaccia PJ, Rogler LH: Research on culture-bound syndromes: new directions. Am J Psychiatry 156:1322–1327, 1999

Guarnaccia PJ, Parra P, Deschamps A, et al: "Si Dios quiere": Hispanic families' experiences of caring for a seriously mentally ill family member. Cult Med Psychiatry 16:187–215, 1992

Guarnaccia PJ, Canino G, Rubio-Stipec M, et al: The prevalence of ataques de nervios in the Puerto Rico disaster study: the role of culture in psychiatric epidemiology. J Nerv Ment Dis 181:157–165, 1993

Habermas T: The role of psychiatric and medical traditions in the discovery and description of anorexia nervosa in France, Germany and Italy, 1873–1918. J Nerv Ment Dis 179:360–365, 1991

Hannerz U: Cultural Complexity: Studies on the Social Organization of Meaning. New York, Columbia University Press, 1992

Harwood A (ed): Ethnicity and Medical Care. Cambridge, MA, Harvard University Press, 1981

Hathaway SR, McKinley JC: Minnesota Multiphasic Personality Inventory Manual (revised). New York, Psychological Corporation, 1967

Hatta SM: A Malay crosscultural worldview and forensic review of Amok. Aust N Z J Psychiatry 30:505–510, 1996

Heath AC, Madden PA, Cloninger CR, et al: Genetic and environmental structure of personality, in Personality and Psychopathology. Edited by Cloninger CR. Washington, DC, American Psychiatric Press, 1999, pp 343–368

Heggenhougen HK, Shore L: Cultural components of behavioral epidemiology: implications for primary health care. Soc Sci Med 22:1235–1245, 1986

Henningsen P, Kirmayer LJ: Mind beyond the net: implicators of cognitive neurosciences for cultural psychiatry. Transcultural Psychiatry 37:467–494, 2000

Herman JL: Trauma and Recovery: The Aftermath of Violence—From Domestic Abuse to Political Torture. New York, Basic Books, 1992

Hinton AL: Biocultural Approaches to Emotions. Cambridge, MA, Cambridge University Press, 1999

Hovey JD, King CA: Acculturative stress, depression, and suicidal ideation among immigrant and second-generation Latino adolescents. J Am Acad Child Adolesc Psychiatry 35:1183–1193, 1996

Howard University Symposium on Mental Health: Disparities in Mental Health Access for African Americans. Washington, DC, December 2000

Hu WH, Lee C, Yang Y, et al: Imipramine plasma levels and clinical response. Buletin of Chinese Society of Neurology and Psychiatry 9:40–49, 1983

Hutchins E: Cognition in the Wild. Cambridge, MA, MIT Press, 1995

Iancu I, Spivak B, Ratzoni G, et al: The sociocultural theory in the development of anorexia nervosa. Psychopathology 27:29–36, 1994

Insel TR: A neurobiological basis of social attachment. Am J Psychiatry 154:726–735, 1997

Institute of Medicine: Gender Differences in Susceptibility to Environmental Factors: A Priority Assessment. Washington, DC, Institute of Medicine, 1998

Jablensky A: Impact of the new diagnostic systems on psychiatric epidemiology, in International Review of Psychiatry. Edited by Costa e Silva JA, Nadelson CC. Washington, DC, American Psychiatric Press, 1993, pp 13–43

Jackson JS, Brown TN, Williams DR, et al: Racism and the physical and mental health status of African Americans: a thirteen year national panel study. Ethn Dis 61:132–147, 1996

Jadhav S, Weiss, MG, Littlewood R: Cultural experience of depression among white Britons in London. Anthropology and Medicine 8:47–69, 2001

Jenkins JH, Karno M: The meaning of expressed emotion: theoretical issues raised by cross-cultural research. Am J Psychiatry 149:9–21, 1992

Jenkins JH, Kleinman A, Good BJ: Cross-cultural studies of depression, in Advances in Mood Disorders. Edited by Becker J, Kleinman A. New York, Erlbaum, 1990, pp 67–99

Jilek WG, Jilek-Aall L: The metamorphosis of "culture-bound" syndromes. Soc Sci Med 21:205–210, 1985

Kandel ER: A new intellectual frame for psychiatry. Am J Psychiatry 155:457–469, 1998

Kandel ER: Biology and the future of psychoanalysis: a new intellectual framework for psychiatry revisited. Am J Psychiatry 156:505–524, 1999

Karno M, Jenkins JH: Cross-cultural issues in the course and treatment of schizophrenia. Psychiatr Clin North Am 16:339–350, 1993

Kaslow NJ, Celano M, Dreelin ED: A cultural perspective on family theory and therapy. Psychiatr Clin North Am 18:621–633, 1995

Kendell RE, Chalmers JC, Platz C: Epidemiology of puerperal psychosis. Br J Psychiatry 150:662–673, 1987

Kendler KS: A psychiatric dialogue on the mind-body problem. Am J Psychiatry 158:989–1000, 2001

Kendler KS, Neale MC, Kessler RC, et al: Major depression and generalized anxiety disorder: same genes, partly different environments. Arch Gen Psychiatry 49:716–722, 1992

Kendler KS, Sham PC, Maclean CJ: The determinants of parenting: an epidemiological, multi-informant, retrospective study. Psychol Med 27:549–563, 1997

Kessler C, Stang PE, Wittchsen H: Past-year use of outpatient services for psychiatric problems in the National Comorbidity Survey. Am J Psychiatry 156:115–123, 1999

Kinzie JD, Manson SM: The use of self-rating scales in cross-cultural psychiatry. Hosp Community Psychiatry 38:190–196, 1987

Kinzie JD, Leung P, Boehnlein J, et al: Tricyclic antidepressant plasma levels in Indochinese refuges: clinical implications. J Nerv Ment Dis 175:480–485, 1987

Kirmayer LJ: Cultural variations in the response to psychiatric disorders and emotional distress. Soc Sci Med 29:327–339, 1989

Kirmayer LJ: Landscapes of memory: trauma, narrative, and dissociation, in Tense Past: Cultural Essays on Memory and Trauma. Edited by Autze P, Lambek M. London, Routledge, 1996, pp 173–198

Kirmayer LJ, Minas IH: The future of cultural psychiatry: an international perspective. Can J Psychiatry 45:438–446, 2000

Kirmayer LJ, Young A: Culture and context in the evolutionary concept of mental disorder. J Abnorm Psychol 108:446–452, 1999

Kirmayer LJ, Young A, Hayton BC: The cultural context of anxiety disorders. Psychiatr Clin North Am 18:503–521, 1995

Kirmayer LJ, Brass GM, Tait C: The mental health of aboriginal peoples: transformation of identity and community. Can J Psychiatry 45:607–616, 2000

Kleinman A: Patients and Healers in the Context of Culture. Berkeley, CA, University of California Press, 1980

Kleinman A: The Illness Narratives: Suffering, Healing and the Human Condition. New York, Basic Books, 1988a

Kleinman A: Rethinking Psychiatry: From Cultural Category to Personal Experience. New York, Free Press, 1988b

Kleinman A, Eisenberg L, Good B: Culture, illness and care: clinical lessons from anthropological and cross-cultural research. Ann Intern Med 88:251–258, 1978

Kleinman A, Das V, Lock M (eds): Social Suffering. Berkeley, CA, University of California Press, 1997

Kohut H: Thoughts on narcissism and narcissistic rage, in The Psychoanalytic Study of the Child, Vol 27. New York, NY Times Book Co, 1972, pp 386–394

Kosten TR: Addiction as a brain disease. Am J Psychiatry 155:711–713, 1998

Kovel J: White Racism: A Psycho-history. New York, Vintage Books, 1970

Lawson WB: Racial and ethnic factors in psychiatric research. Hosp Community Psychiatry 37:50–54, 1986

Leathart JB, London SJ, Steward A, et al: CYP2D6 phenotype-genotype relationship in African-Americans and Caucasians in Los Angeles. Pharmacogenetics 8:529–541, 1998

Lebowitz BD, Rudorfer MV: Treatment research at the millennium: from efficacy to effectiveness. J Clin Psychopharmacol 18:1–13, 1998

Lee S: Reply to Drs. J. Yager and C. Davis: Transcultural Psychiatry Research Review 30:296–304, 1993

Lee S: From diversity to unity: the classification of mental disorders in 21st-century China. Psychiatr Clin North Am 24:421–432, 2001

Lee S, Wing YK, Wong KC: Knowledge and compliance towards lithium therapy among Chinese psychiatric patients in Hong Kong. Aust N Z J Psychiatry 26:444–449, 1992

Lee YT: Why does American psychology have cultural limitations? (letter) Am Psychol 49:524, 1994

Leff J, Vaughn C: Expressed Emotions in Families. New York, Guilford, 1985

Lefley HP: Culture and chronic mental illness. Hosp Community Psychiatry 41:177–186, 1990

Lefley HP: Expressed emotion: conceptual, clinical and social policy issues. Hospital and Community Psychiatry 43:591–598, 1992

Leo RJ, Narayan DA, Sherry C, et al: Geropsychiatric consultation for African American and Caucasian patients. Gen Hosp Psychiatry 19:216–222, 1997

Levin JS: How religion influences morbidity and health: reflections on natural history, salutogenesis, and host resistance. Soc Sci Med 43:849–864, 1996

Levine RE, Gaw A: Culture-bound syndromes. Psychiatr Clin North Am 18:523–536, 1995

Lewis-Fernandez R: Cultural formulation of psychiatric diagnosis. Cult Med Psychiatry 20:133–144, 1996

Lewis-Fernandez R, Kleinman A: Culture, personality and psychopathology. J Abnorm Psychol 103:67–71, 1993

Lewis-Fernandez R, Tun H, Reyes F, et al: Los "sindromes dependientes de la cultura": Un dilema nosológico recurrente en la psiquiatría cultural. Monografias de Psiquiatria 12:24–28, 2000

Lilienfeld SO, Waldman ID, Israel AC: A critical examination of the term and concept of comorbidity in psychopathology research. Clinical Psychology: Science and Practice 1:71–83, 1994

Lin K-M: Hwa-byung: a Korean culture-bound syndrome? Am J Psychiatry 140:105–107, 1983

Lin K-M: Asian American perspectives, in Culture and Psychiatric Diagnosis. A DSM-IV Perspective. Edited by Mezzich JE, Kleinman A, Fabrega H, et al. Washington, DC, American Psychiatric Press, 1996, pp 35–38

Lin KM, Kleinman A: Psychopathology and clinical course of schizophrenia: a cross-cultural perspective. Schizophr Bull 14:555–567, 1988

Lin KM, Smith MW: Psychopharmacotherapy in the context of culture and ethnicity, in Ethnicity and Psychopharmacology. Edited by Ruiz P. Washington, DC, American Psychiatric Press, 2000, pp 1–36

Lin K-M, Poland RE, Nakasaki G (eds): Psychopharmacology and Psychobiology of Ethnicity. Washington, DC, American Psychiatric Press, 1993

Lin K-M, Anderson D, Poland RE: Ethnicity and psychopharmacology: bridging the gap. Psychiatr Clin North Am 18:635–647, 1995

Littlewood R: From categories to contexts: a decade of the "new cross-cultural psychiatry." Br J Psychiatry 156:308–327, 1990

Littlewood R, Lipsedge M: The butterfly and the serpent: culture, psychopathology and biomedicine. Cult Med Psychiatry 11:289–336, 1987

Livesley WJ: Suggestions for a framework for an empirically based classification of personality disorders. Can J Psychiatry 43:137–147, 1998

Lopez S: The empirical basis of ethnocultural and linguistic bias in mental health evaluation of Hispanics. Am Psychol 43:1095–1097, 1988

Lopez SR: Patient variable biases in clinical judgement: conceptual overview and methodological considerations. Psychol Bull 106:184–203, 1989

Lopez SR: Latinos and the expression of psychopathology: a call for the direct assessment of cultural influences, in Current Research and Policy Perspectives. Edited by Telles C, Karno M. Los Angeles, CA, University of California Press, 1994, pp 109–116

Lopez SR: Teaching culturally informed psychological assessment, in Handbook of Cross-Cultural and Multicultural Personality Assessment. Edited by Dana RH. Mahwah, NJ, Erlbaum, 2000, pp 669–687

Lopez SR, Guarnaccia PJ: Cultural psychopathology. Uncovering the social world of mental illness. Annu Rev Psychol 51:578–598, 2000

Lopez SR, Hernandez P: How culture is considered in evaluations of psychopathology. J Nerv Ment Dis 176:598–606, 1986

Lopez S, Nunez JA: Cultural factors considered in selected diagnostic criteria and interview schedules. J Abnorm Psychol 96:270–272, 1987

Lopez SR, Taussig IM: Cognitive-intellectual functioning of Spanish-speaking impaired and non-impaired elderly: implications for culturally sensitive assessment. Psychol Assess 3:448–454, 1991

Lu FG, Lin RF, Mezzich JE: Issues in the assessment and diagnosis of culturally diverse individuals, in Review of Psychiatry, Vol 14. Edited by Oldham JM, Riba MB. Washington, DC, American Psychiatric Press, 1995, pp 477–510

Lukoff D, Lu FG, Turner R: Cultural considerations in the assessment and treatment of religious and spiritual problems. Psychiatr Clin North Am 18:467–485, 1995

Malgady RG: The question of cultural bias in assessment and diagnosis of ethnic minority clients: let's reject the null hypothesis. Prof Psychol Res Pr 27:73–77, 1996

Malgady RG, Rogler LH, Constantino G: Ethnocultural and linguistic bias in mental health evaluation of Hispanics. Am Psychol 42:228–234, 1987

Manson SM: Culture and major depression: current challenges in the diagnosis of mood disorders. Psychiatr Clin North Am 18:487–501, 1995

Manson SM: Cultural considerations in the diagnosis of DSM-IV mood disorders, in Sourcebook for DSM-IV, Vol 3. Edited by Widiger TA, Frances AJ, Pincus HA. Washington, DC, American Psychiatric Press, 1997, pp 909–924

Marsella AJ, Sartorius N, Jablensky A, et al: Cross-cultural studies of depressive disorders: an overview, in Culture and Depression: Study in the Anthropology and Cross-Cultural Psychiatry of Affect and Disorder. Edited by Kleinman A, Good BJ. Berkeley, CA, University of California Press, 1985, pp 299–324

Marsella AJ, Friedman MJ, Gerrity ET, et al (eds): Ethnocultural Aspects of Posttraumatic Stress Disorder. Issues, Research and Clinical Applications. Washington, DC, American Psychological Association, 1996

Matsuda KT, Cho MC, Lin KM, et al: Clozapine dosage, serum levels, efficacy, and side effect profiles: a comparison of Korean Americans and Caucasian patients. Psychopharmacol Bull 32:253–257, 1996

McKelvey RS, Webb JA: A comparative study of Vietnamese Amerasians, their non-Amerasian siblings, and unrelated like-aged Vietnamese immigrants. Am J Psychiatry 153:561–563, 1996

Mendlewicz J, Kerkhofs M: Sleep electroencephalography in depressive illness: a collaborative study by the World Health Organization. Br J Psychiatry 159:505–509, 1991

Mezzich JE: International diagnostic systems and Hispanic populations, in Research Agenda for Hispanic Mental Health (Supplement). Edited by Gaviria M, Arana J. Chicago, IL, University of Illinois Press, 1984, pp 1–28

Mezzich JE, Kleinman A, Fabrega H, et al (eds): Culture and Psychiatric Diagnosis: A DSM-IV Perspective. Washington, DC, American Psychiatric Press, 1996

Mezzich JE, Kirmayer LJ, Kleinman A, et al: The place of culture in DSM-IV. J Nerv Ment Dis 187:457–464, 1999

Mezzich JE, Berganza CE, Ruiperez MA: Culture in DSM-IV, ICD-10, and evolving diagnostic systems. Psychiatr Clin North Am 24:407–421, 2001

Millon T: Millon Multiaxial Clinical Inventory Manual. Minneapolis, MN, National Computer Systems, 1977

Molesky J: Understanding the American linguistic mosaic: a historical overview of language maintenance and language shift, in Language Diversity: Problem of Resource. Edited by McKay J, Wong SC. New York, Newburg House, 1988, pp 98–112

Montgomery GT, Orozco S: Mexican Americans' performance on the MMPI as a function of level of acculturation. J Clin Psychol 41:203–212, 1985

Murphy M, Donovan S: The Physical and Psychological Effects of Meditation: A Review of Contemporary Meditation Research With a Comprehensive Bibliography 1931–1988. Oakland, CA, Dharma Enterprises, 1988

Murray CJL, Lopez AD: The Global Burden of Disease. A Comprehensive Assessment of Mortality and Disability From Diseases, Injuries, and Risk Factors in 1990 and Projected to 2020. Cambridge, MA, Harvard University Press, 1999

Ndetei DM, Vadher A: A comparative cross-cultural study of the frequencies of hallucinations in schizophrenia. Acta Psychiatr Scand 70:545–459, 1984

Neff JA: Race differences in psychological distress: the effects of SES, urbanicity and measurement strategy. Am J Community Psychol 12:337–351, 1984

Neighbors HW: The (mis)diagnosis of mental disorder in African Americans. African American Research Perspectives 3:1–11, 1997

Neighbors HW, Howard CS: Sex differences in professional help seeking among adult black Americans. Am J Community Psychol 15:403–417, 1987

Neighbors HW, Jackson, JS, Campbell L, et al: The influence of racial factors on psychiatric diagnosis: a review and suggestions for research. Community Ment Health J 25:301–311, 1989

Nichter M: Idioms of distress: alternatives in the expression of psychosocial distress. Cult Med Psychiatry 5:379–408, 1981

Okasha A, Saad A, Kahlil AH, et al: Phenomenology of obsessive-compulsive disorder: a transcultural study. Compr Psychiatry 35:191–197, 1994

Olatawura M: Culture and child psychiatric disorders: a Nigerian perspective. Psychiatr Clin North Am 24:497–506, 2001

Oldham JM: Personality disorders: current perspectives. JAMA 272:1770–1776, 1994

Oyama S: Evolution's Eye: A Systems View of the Biology-Culture Divide. Durham, NC, Duke University Press, 2000

Paradis CM, Friedman S, Hatch MJ: Isolated sleep paralysis in African Americans with panic disorder. Cult Divers Ment Health 3:69–76, 1995

Parker G, Gladstone G, Chee KT: Depression in the planet's largest ethnic group: the Chinese. Am J Psychiatry 158:857–864, 2001

Patcher LM, Harwood RL: Culture and child behavior and psychosocial development. Developmental and Behavioral Pediatrics 17:191–198, 1996

Paulesu E, McCrory E, Fazio F, et al: A cultural effect on brain function. Nat Neurosci 3:91–96, 2000

Pellmar TC, Eisenberg L (eds): Bridging Disciplines in the Brain, Behavioral, and Clinical Sciences. Washington, DC, National Academy Press, 2000

Penn DL, Martin J: The stigma of severe mental illness: some potential solutions for a recalcitrant problem. Psychiatr Q 69:235–247, 1998

Pescosolido BA: Beyond rational choice: the social dynamics of how people seek help. American Journal of Sociology 97:1096–1138, 1992

Pierce CM: Stress in the workplace, in Black Families in Crisis. Edited by Conner-Edwards AF, Spurlock J. New York, Brunner/Mazer, 1988, pp 27–33

Pierce CM: Public Health and Human Rights: Racism, Torture and Terrorism. Paper presented at the annual meeting of the American Psychiatric Association, Washington, DC, May 1992

Pinderhughes CA: Managing paranoia in violent relationships, in Perspectives on Violence. Edited by Usdin G. New York, Brunner/Mazel, 1972, pp 131–138

Pinderhughes CA: Differential bonding: toward a psychophysiological theory of stereotyping. Am J Psychiatry 136:33–37, 1979

Pinderhughes E: Understanding Race, Ethnicity and Power. New York, Free Press, 1989

Pollock B: Gender differences in psychotropic drug metabolism. Psychopharmacol Bull 32:235–241, 1997

Prince R, Tcheng-Laroche F: Culture-bound syndromes and international disease classifications. Cult Med Psychiatry 11:3–19, 1987

Pritchard DA, Rosenblatt A: Racial bias in the MMPI: a methodological review. J Consult Clin Psychol 48:263–267, 1980

Protherow-Stith D: Deadly Consequences. New York, Harper-Collins, 1991

Raguram R, Weiss MG, Channabasavanna SM, et al: Stigma, depression, and somatization in South India. Am J Psychiatry 153:1043–1049, 1996

Raguram R, Weiss MG, Keval H, et al: Cultural dimensions of clinical depression in Bangalore, India. Anthropology and Medicine 8:31–46, 2001

Redfield R, Linton R, Herskovits M: Memorandum for the study of acculturation. American Anthropologist 38:147–151, 1936

Regier DA, Kaelber CT, Rae DS, et al: Limitations of diagnostic criteria and assessment instruments for mental disorders: implications for research and policy. Arch Gen Psychiatry 55:109–115, 1998

Reid PT: The real problem in the study of culture. Am Psychol 49:529–530, 1994

Riso LP, Klein DN, Anderson RL, et al: Concordance between patients and informants on the Personality Disorder Examination. Am J Psychiatry 51:568–573, 1994

Ritenbaugh C, Shisslak CL, Teufel N, et al: Eating disorders: a cross-cultural review, in Sourcebook for DSM-IV, Vol 3. Edited by Widiger TA, Frances AJ, Pincus HA. Washington, DC, American Psychiatric Press, 1997, pp 959–973

Roberts RE, Vernon SW: The Center for Epidemiological Studies–Depression Scale: its use in a community sample. Am J Psychiatry 140:41–46, 1983

Roberts RE, Roberts CR, Chen YR: Ethnocultural differences in prevalence of adolescent depression. Am J Community Psychol 25:95–110, 1997

Robins LN, Helzer JE, Croughan J, et al: National Institute of Mental Health Diagnosis Interview Schedule: Its History, Characteristics, and Validity. Arch Gen Psychiatry 38:381–389, 1981

Rogler LH: The role of culture in mental health diagnosis: the need for programmatic research. J Nerv Ment Dis 180:745–747, 1992

Rogler LH: Framing research on culture in psychiatric diagnosis: the case of the DSM-IV. Psychiatry 59:145–155, 1996

Rogler LH: Making sense of historical changes in the Diagnostic and Statistical Manual of Mental Disorders: five propositions. J Health Soc Behav 38:9–20, 1997

Rogler LH: Implementing cultural sensitivity in mental health research: convergence and new directions (part I). Psychline 3:3–12, 1999a

Rogler LH: Methodological sources of cultural insensitivity in mental health research. Am Psychol 54:424–433, 1999b

Rogler LH, Cortes DE: Help-seeking pathways: a unifying concept in mental health care. Am J Psychiatry 150:554–561, 1993

Rogler LH, Malgady RG, Rodriguez O: Hispanics and Mental Health: A Framework for Research. Malabar, FL, RE Kreiger, 1989

Root MP: Women of color and traumatic stress in "domestic captivity": gender and race as disempowering statuses, in Ethnocultural Aspects of Posttraumatic Stress Disorder: Issues, Research and Clinical Applications. Edited by Marsella AJ, Friedman MJ, Gerrity RM, et al. Washington, DC, American Psychological Association, 1996, pp 363–388

Rousseau R: A critique of DSM-IV's Cultural Formulation. Paper presented at the annual meeting of the Society for the Study of Psychiatry and Culture, Chantilly, France, Oct 18–21, 2000

Rubio-Stipec M, Bird H, Canino G, et al: The internal consistency and concurrent validity of a Spanish translation of the Child Behavior Checklist. J Abnorm Child Psychol 18:393–406, 1990

Rush AJ, Giles DE, Roffwarg HP, et al: Sleep EEG and DST findings in outpatients with unipolar major depression. Biol Psychiatry 17:327–340, 1982

Sartorius N, Jablensky A, Korten A, et al: Early manifestations and first contact incidence of schizophrenia in different cultures. Psychol Med 16:909–928, 1986

Sartorius N, Kaelber CT, Cooper JE, et al: Progress toward achieving a common language in psychiatry. Arch Gen Psychiatry 50:115–124, 1993

Satcher D: Eliminating disparities, promoting partnerships. Mayo Clin Proc 74:838–840, 1999

Schermerhorn RA: Comparative Ethnic Relations: A Framework for Theory and Research. Chicago, IL, University of Chicago Press, 1970

Schildkraut JJ, Otero A (eds): Depression and the Spiritual in Modern Art: Homage to Miró. New York, Wiley, 1996

Schissel B: Coping with adversity: testing the origins of resiliency in mental health. Int J Soc Psychiatry 39:34–46, 1993

Schumman JH: Research on the acculturation model for second language acquisition. Journal of Multilingual and Multicultural Development 7:379–392, 1986

Sclar DA, Robison LM, Skaer TL, et al: Ethnicity and the prescribing of antidepressant pharmacotherapy 1992–1995. Harv Rev Psychiatry 7:29–36, 1999

Shanklin E: The profession of the color blind: sociocultural anthropology and racism in the 21st century. American Anthropologist 10:669–679, 1998

Siever L, Davis K: A psychobiological perspective on the personality disorders. Am J Psychiatry 148:1647–1658, 1991

Silove D: The psychosocial effects of torture, mass human rights violations, and refugee trauma. J Nerv Ment Dis 187:200–207, 1999

Simons RC, Hughes CC (eds): The Culture-Bound Syndromes: Folk Illnesses of Psychiatric and Anthropological Interest. Dordrecht, Netherlands, Reidel, 1985

Smart JF, Smart DW: Acculturative stress. Couns Psychol 23:25–42, 1995

Smith M, Lin KM, Mendoza R: "Non-biological" issues affecting psychopharmacotherapy: cultural considerations, in Psychopharmacology and Psychobiology of Ethnicity. Edited by Lin KM, Poland R, Nakasaki G. Washington, DC, American Psychiatric Press, 1993, pp 37–59

Solís JM, Marks G, García M: Acculturation, access to care, and use of preventive services by Hispanics: findings from HHANES 1982–1984. Am J Public Health 80 (suppl):11–19, 1993

Sue DW, Sue D: Counseling the Culturally Different: Theory and Practice. New York, Wiley, 1999, pp 31–52

Sue S: In search of cultural competence in psychotherapy and counseling. Am Psychol 53:440–448, 1998

Sullaway M, Dunbar E: Clinical manifestations of prejudice in psychotherapy: toward a strategy of assessment and treatment. Clinical Psychology: Science and Practice 3:296–309, 1996

Susser M: Disease, illness, sickness: impairment, disability, and handicap. Psychol Med 20:471–473, 1990

Susser M, Susser E: Choosing a future for epidemiology, II: from black boxes to Chinese boxes and ecoepidemiology. Am J Public Health 86:674–677, 1996

Svrakic DM, Przybeck TR, Whitehead C, et al: Emotional traits and personality dimensions, in Personality and Psychopathology. Edited by Cloninger CR. Washington, DC, American Psychiatric Press, 1999, pp 245–267

Takeuchi DT, Chung RC-Y, Lin K-M, et al: Lifetime and 12-month prevalence rates of major depressive episodes and dysthymia among Chinese Americans in Los Angeles. Am J Psychiatry 155:1407–1414, 1998

Thomas A, Sillen S: Racism and Psychiatry. New York, Brunner/Mazel, 1972

Thompson J: Report to the House Appropriations Subcommittee on Interior and Related Agencies. American Psychiatric Association, Washington, DC, April 2000

Trierweiler SJ, Neighbors HW, Munday C, et al: Clinician attributions associated with the diagnosis of schizophrenia in African American and non–African American patients. J Consult Clin Psychol 68:171–175, 2000

U.S. Department of Health and Human Services: Mental Health: A Report of the Surgeon General. Rockville, MD, U.S. Department of Health and Human Services, Substance Abuse and Mental Health Services Administration, Center for Mental Health Services, National Institutes of Health, 1999

U.S. Department of Health and Human Services: Healthy People 2010 Initiative. Washington, DC, U.S. Department of Health and Human Services, 2000

Üstün TB, Sartorius N: Mental Illness in General Health Care: An International Study. Chichester, UK, Wiley, 1995

Üstün TB, Chatterji S, Bickenbach JE, et al (eds): Disability and Culture. Universalism and Diversity. London, Hogrefe & Huber, 2000

Vaillant G: Cultural factors in the etiology of alcoholism: a prospective study. Ann N Y Acad Sci 472:142–148, 1986

Vega WA: Latino Mental Health Research and Disparities in Services. Paper presented at the National Institute of Mental Health Meeting on Disparities in Health Care for Latinos. Los Angeles, CA, May 21–23, 2000

Vega WA, Kolody B: The meaning of social support and mediation of stress across cultures, in Stress and Hispanic Mental Health. Relating Research to Service Delivery. Edited by Vega WA, Miranda MR. Rockville, MD, National Institute of Mental Health, 1985, pp 95–112

Vega WA, Kolody B, Aguilar-Gaxiola S, et al: Lifetime prevalence of DSM-III-R psychiatric disorders among urban and rural Mexican Americans in California. Arch Gen Psychiatry 55:771–778, 1998

Vidaver RM, Lafleur B, Tong C, et al: Women subjects in NIH-funded clinical research literature: lack of progress in both representation and analysis by sex. J Womens Health Gend Based Med 9:495–504, 2000

Wakefield JC: The concept of mental disorder: on the boundary between biological facts and social values. Am Psychol 47:373–388, 1992

Wakefield JC: Evolutionary versus prototype analyses of the concept of disorder. J Abnorm Psychol 108:374–399, 1999

Walker RD, Howard MO, Anderson B, et al: Substance dependent American Indian veterans: a national evaluation. Public Health Rep 109:235–242, 1994

Weber WW: Pharmacogenetics. New York, Oxford University Press, 1997

Weiss MG: Eating disorders and disordered eating in different cultures. Psychiatr Clin North Am 18:537–553, 1995

Weiss MG: Explanatory Model Interview Catalogue (EMIC): framework for comparative study of illness. Transcultural Psychiatry 34:235–263, 1997

Weiss MG: Cultural epidemiology: an introduction and overview. Anthropology and Medicine 8:5–30, 2001

Weiss MG, Kleinman AK: Depression in cross-cultural perspective: developing a culturally informed model, in Psychology, Culture and Health. Edited by Dasen P, Sartorius N, Berry J. Beverly Hills, CA, Sage, 1988, pp 179–206

Weiss MG, Cohen A, Eisenberg L: Mental health, in Introduction to International Health. Edited by Merson M, Black B, Mills A. Gaithersburg, MD, Aspen, 2001a, pp 159–178

Weiss MG, Jadhav S, Raguram R, et al: Psychiatric stigma across cultures: local validation in Bangalore and London. Anthropology and Medicine 8:71–87, 2001b

Westermeyer J: Cultural factors in clinical assessment. J Consult Clin Psychol 55:471–478, 1987

Westermeyer J: Psychiatric Care of Migrants: A Clinical Guide. Washington, DC, American Psychiatric Press, 1989

Westermeyer J: Cultural aspects of substance abuse and alcoholism. Assessment and management. Psychiatr Clin North Am 18:589–605, 1995

Westermeyer J, Canino GJ: Culture and substance-related disorders, in Sourcebook for DSM-IV, Vol 3. Edited by Widiger TA, Frances AJ, Pincus HA. Washington, DC, American Psychiatric Press, 1997, pp 893–900

Westermeyer J, Janca A: Language, culture and psychopathology: conceptual and methodological issues. Transcultural Psychiatry 34:291–311, 1997

Widiger TA, Clark LA: Toward DSM-V and the classification of psychopathology. Psychol Bull 126:826–834, 2000

Widiger TA, Sankis L: Adult psychopathology: issues and controversies. Annu Rev Psychol 51:377–404, 2000

Wierzbick A: Human emotions: universal or culture-specific. American Anthropologist 88:584–594, 1986

Williams CL: Issues surrounding psychological testing of minority patients. Hosp Community Psychiatry 38:184–189, 1987

Williams CL, Berry JW: Primary prevention of acculturative stress among refugees: application of psychological theory and practice. Am Psychol 46:632–641, 1991

Wilson EO: Consilience. The Unity of Knowledge. New York, AA Knopf, 1998

Wittchen HU, Robins LN, Cottler LB, et al: Cross-cultural visibility, reliability and sources of variance of the Composite International Diagnostic Interview (CIDI). Br J Psychiatry 159:645–658, 1991

Witzig R: The medicalization of race: scientific legitimization of a flawed social construct. Ann Intern Med 125:675–679, 1996

Wohlfarth TD, vanden Brink W, Ormel J, et al: The relationship between social dysfunctioning and psychopathology. Br J Psychiatry 163:37–44, 1993

World Health Organization: The International Pilot Study of Schizophrenia, Vol 1. Geneva, World Health Organization, 1973

World Health Organization: Schizophrenia: An International Follow-up Study. Chichester, UK, Wiley, 1979

World Health Organization: The ICD-10 Classification of Mental and Behavioural Disorders: Clinical Descriptions and Diagnostic Guidelines. Geneva, World Health Organization, 1992

World Health Organization: International Classification of Functioning, Disability and Health. Geneva, World Health Organization, 2001

Yilmaz AT, Weiss MG: Clinical case study. Cultural formulation: depression and back pain in a young male Turkish immigrant in Basel, Switzerland. Cult Med Psychiatry 24:259–272, 2000

Young A: Harmony of Illusions. Princeton, NJ, Princeton University Press, 1995

Zheng YP, Lin K-M, Takeuchi D, et al: An epidemiological study of neurasthenia in Chinese-Americans in Los Angeles. Compr Psychiatry 38:249–259, 1997

APPENDIX 6–1

Preliminary List of Suggested Areas and Topics of Research in Culture and Psychiatric Diagnosis

1. Culture and Psychopathology Issues
   - Role of specific individual uses of culture in psychopathological processes
   - Role and implications of cultural variables in psychiatric diagnosis
   - Studies on the commission of category fallacies and the structure, characteristics, and distinctiveness of explanatory models of illness
   - Terminological distinctions across cultural or ethnic groups (distress, dysfunction, impairment, disability, and handicap)
   - Studies on comorbidities and cultural factors
   - Social desirability factor in diagnosis-making processes
   - Ethnocultural and linguistic biases in mental health evaluations
2. Methodological Issues

   General Topics

   - Research on adjustment of diagnostic thresholds, addition of subthreshold categories, and use of the dimensional approach
   - Combination of and/or comparisons between different diagnostic methods: cultural, ethnographic, epidemiologic, and experimental
   - Programmatic and longitudinal research on diagnostic process, predictive power of alternative categories, criteria, axes, and help-seeking pathways
   - Cultural aspects of case ascertainment and case definition
   - Study of psychiatric entities as relational disorders
   - Novel interviewing methods that tap knowledge structures and symptom experience
   - Intracultural variations among psychiatrists through use of protocols in different settings and professionals of different theoretical orientations

- Studies on ecological validators of psychiatric diagnoses

Assessment Instruments

- Emic complementation of existing scales, questionnaires, or survey instruments
- Incorporation of indigenous categories of experience into assessment schedules to ascertain normative uncertainty of the instruments
- Comparisons in the use of psychological tests among different cultural and ethnic groups
- Development of instruments focused on specific areas of functioning (e.g., quality of life, personal and cultural identity)
- Stepwise validations of selected instruments

Context, Meaning, and Interpretation

- Risks of overdiagnosing or underdiagnosing of psychiatric disorders because of distorted or subclinical use of idioms of distress, differences between illness behaviors, or help-seeking patterns
- Studies of child-rearing practices, sociopolitical contexts, community factors, migratory status, and associated stresses
- Studies on victims of torture or other human rights violations
- Problems of patients who do not meet any diagnostic criteria to typify their predicament

3. Epidemiology

General Topics

- Community-based surveys on age, gender, occupational, socioeconomic, and linguistically different populations
- Use of expanded pools of symptoms, alternative criteria, and alternative key or core symptoms (with use of anchor points in current nosology to allow for comparison and cumulative knowledge)
- Rethinking place of social-interactional problems and predicaments in nosology

Cultural Epidemiology

- Use of multivariate statistics to derive effects of specific sociocultural variables in epidemiologic surveys
- Development of interactional models of the role of cultural factors in psychiatric disorders
- Use of cultural epidemiology instruments focused on the study of locally valid representations of illness experience and its meaning, associated behaviors, narratives, and distribution

International Studies

- Differences in national nosologies and their roots in specific cultural histories
- Comparative studies using DSM and ICD nosologic categories
- Studies on the use of assessment guidelines and criteria for research on disabilities, distress, and handicaps in different countries and regions of the world
- Differences between urban and rural areas, human resources needs and skills, care strategies, technology transfer, and primary care interactions

4. Clinical and Health Services and Outcomes Research

Cultural Formulation

- Assessment of the usefulness and relevance of the cultural formulation (CF) in the diagnostic process
- Proposals and testing of content refinement, standardization, organization, and possibilities of quantitative structure
- Impact of different cultural variables on the CF
- Exploration of cultural explanations of illness and of cultural and personal identity
- Value of CF in assessing naturalistic clinical contexts, treatment effectiveness, and outcomes prediction
- Essential components of cultural competence vis-à-vis diagnosis and CF.

Specific Clinical Entities

- How clinicians deploy concepts of culture in everyday practice settings: diagnostic assessment processes and outcomes research to identify best practices
- Cultural components of the patient's illness experience of specific clinical entities (SCEs)
- Implications of labeling for clinical reasoning related to SCEs
- Frequency of symptoms of SCEs in different ethnic groups
- Assessment of clinical course and outcomes of large samples of patients belonging to different cultural and ethnic groups
- Cultural validity of expressed emotions (EE) protocols
- Perception of time, duration of symptoms, and psychotic-like and somatization features in most or all SCEs
- Clinical and cultural contributions to definitions of selfhood, indigenous categories of emotions, precipitating events, and ethnophysiological accounts of emotionality

- Characterization of stressors and memory distortions created by traumatic events in different populations
- Pathogenic/pathoplastic roles of shame, guilt, anger, and resentment in different populations
- Studies of posttraumatic stress disorder in survivors of massive collective traumas, refugees and other displaced groups, military populations of diverse ethnicities, and victims of natural and technological disasters or political persecution
- Relevance, efficacy, and impact of Western-based treatment modalities on diagnostic practices in non-Western populations
- Studies on groups and community tolerance of psychopathology
- Cultural prescriptions for and proscriptions against substance use and abuse
- Patterns of substance use throughout the life cycle; family response; and idiosyncratic aspects of definitions, sanctions, social tolerance, and religious/spiritual interactions
- Comparisons of categorical and dimensional approaches to diagnosis of personality disorders in different cultural and ethnic groups
- Assessment of homogeneity or heterogeneity of diagnostic criteria within and across the existing clusters and different cultural groups
- Measurements of cultural distance, cultural lenses, and cultural profile in different SCEs

Family and Support Systems

- Impact of child-rearing practices and family-based experiences on the expression, intensity, and severity of observable behaviors
- Comparisons between patient- and family-provided clinical data to identify possible differential factors
- Study of explanatory models of illness, behavior-labeling practices, and family attitudes vis-à-vis the helping professions

Culture-Bound Syndromes

- Ethnographic research examining culture-bound syndromes (CBSs) in social context to determine which of them can be mapped onto existing disorders, which require new categories, and/or which are causal explanations or idioms of distress that cut across other categories
- Clinical usefulness of diagnoses of local syndromes or CBSs
- Study of CBSs as final common pathways of culturally sanctioned behaviors or as a function of interactions of physiologic reactions, experiences that trigger specific personality manifestations, cognitive processes, and problem-solving skills

- Examination of CBSs as semantic networks
- Studies on defining clinical characteristics of CBSs, position in social and personal contexts, and sequence vis-à-vis the experience of traumatic events

Special Populations

- Demographic, clinical, health-related, and socioeconomic features of cultural issues in the diagnosis of psychiatric disorders among
  - Children
  - Adolescents
  - The elderly
  - Women
  - Gays and lesbians
  - Homeless persons
  - Ethnic and other minorities
- Access, availability, use, and accountability of mental health diagnostic and treatment services to special populations of different ethnic and cultural backgrounds
- Sensitivity of assessment instruments used in special populations

Care Disparities

- Impact of working with interpreters and culture brokers on the accuracy of diagnosis
- Causal mechanisms of care disparities at individual, interpersonal, and organization levels and their relevance for diagnostic tasks
- Studies on misdiagnosis, assessment measures, omitted factors in clinical evaluations, linguistic features, and coping styles
- Assessment of the role of primary care providers and their diagnostic skills, determinants of relapse, and profiles of successful case managers
- Translational research—from findings to policy and concrete operational changes in diagnostic and treatment processes

5. Culture and Neurobiology

General Topics

- Models of multilevel descriptions and explanations of normal and abnormal behaviors
- Inclusion of subjects with multiethnic and multicultural backgrounds and effects of ethnicity on biological markers and neurophysiologic correlates

Biocultural Linkages in Psychopathology

- Study of microsocial and macrosocial influences on psychopathology
    - Genetic-epidemiologic perspectives
    - Ethnophysiological approaches (i.e., neuropsychology)
    - Cognitive-interpretive views (i.e., changes in genetic expressiveness)
    - Psychopathology-creativity model

Ethnopsychopharmacology

- Ethnic variations in pharmacokinetics and pharmacodynamics of psychotropic agents
- Nonbiological processes in ethnopsychopharmacology (i.e., therapeutic alliance, compliance, placebo effect, side effects, and sociocultural factors affecting clinicians' prescription patterns)
- Research on potential reorganization of nosology to reflect differential therapeutics (not only psychopharmacology but also alternative and traditional healing methods)

Behavioral Traits and Emotional Processes

- Heritability and sociocultural components of different types of temperaments
- Animal and human models of resilience, fear, shyness, altruism, love, social attachment, and other culturally charged behaviors and emotions

6. Special Topics

Stigmatization and Racism

- Estimation of risks of overdiagnosis or underdiagnosis of clinical conditions as a result of stigma or stereotype-related influences
- Study of the impact of ethnocentric monoculturalism in diagnostic practices
- Identification of methods aimed at minimization (or elimination) of consequences of stigmatization in clinical and diagnostic procedures
- Assessment of racism and probable co-occurring or preceding behavioral features as diagnostic criteria of personality disorder(s)

Gender Issues

- Studies on clinical and diagnostic gender-based distinction of psychopathological conditions
- Viability of categorical versus dimensional diagnostic approaches among women

- Inclusion of gender issues in prevalence, course, familial patterns, comorbidity, laboratory findings, and differential diagnosis of psychiatric entities
- Development of hypotheses related to comparative risk for disease in women and men

Violence and Trauma

- Assessment of clinical and diagnostic implications of different types of violence and trauma
- Study of violence and trauma in special populations

Acculturation and Acculturative Processes

- In-depth clinical and diagnostic studies of the acculturation problem of DSM-IV-TR and its implications vis-à-vis established diagnostic entities
- Systematic longitudinal studies on acculturative stress as a potential clinical entity or behavioral syndrome (including phenomenology, connections with depression and suicidality, posttraumatic stress disorder, psychoses, etc.)
- Measurement instruments of acculturative stress

Religion and Spirituality Issues

- Religion and spirituality as pathogenic/pathoplastic and interpretive/explanatory factors in psychiatric diagnoses
- Transgenerational similarities and differences of religious and spiritual issues across ethnic and cultural groups

Index

Page numbers printed in **boldface** type refer to tables or figures.

Note: The authors have worked to ensure that all information in this book is accurate at the time of publication and consistent with general psychiatric and medical standards, and that information concerning drug dosages, schedules, and routes of administration is accurate as of the time of publication and consistent with standards set by the U.S. Food and Drug Administration and the general medical community. As medical research and practice continue to advance, however, therapeutic standards may change. Moreover, specific situations may require a specific therapeutic response not included in this book. For these reasons and because human and mechanical errors sometimes occur, we recommend that readers follow the advice of physicians directly involved in their care or the care of a member of their family.

The findings, opinions, and conclusions of this report do not necessarily represent the views of the officers, trustees, or all members of the American Psychiatric Association. The views expressed are those of the authors of the individual chapters.

Typeset in Adobe's Janson Text and Frutiger

Manufactured in the United States of America on acid-free paper
06 05 04 03 02 5 4 3 2 1
First Edition

American Psychiatric Association
1400 K Street, N.W., Washington, DC 20005
www.psych.org

Library of Congress Cataloging-in-Publication Data
A research agenda for DSM-V / edited by David J. Kupfer, Michael B. First, Darrel A. Regier.— 1st ed.
p. ; cm.
Includes bibliographical references and index.
ISBN 0-89042-292-3 (alk. paper)
1. Diagnostic and statistical manual of mental disorders. 2. Mental illness—Diagnosis.
3. Mental illness—Classification. I. Kupfer, David J., 1941- II. First, Michael B., 1956- III. Regier, Darrel A. IV. Dagnostic and statistical manual of mental disorders.
[DNLM: 1. Mental Disorders—diagnosis. 2. Research. WM 141 R432 2002]
RC455.2.C4 R463 2002
616.89'075—dc21

2002021556

British Library Cataloguing in Publication Data
A CIP record is available from the British Library.

A Research Agenda for DSM-V

Edited by

David J. Kupfer, M.D.
Michael B. First, M.D.
Darrel A. Regier, M.D., M.P.H.

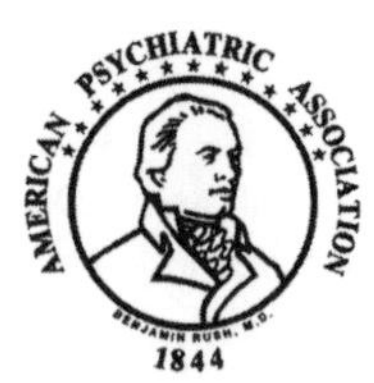

Published by the
American Psychiatric Association
Washington, D.C.